HANDBOOK OF
Musculoskeletal Tumors

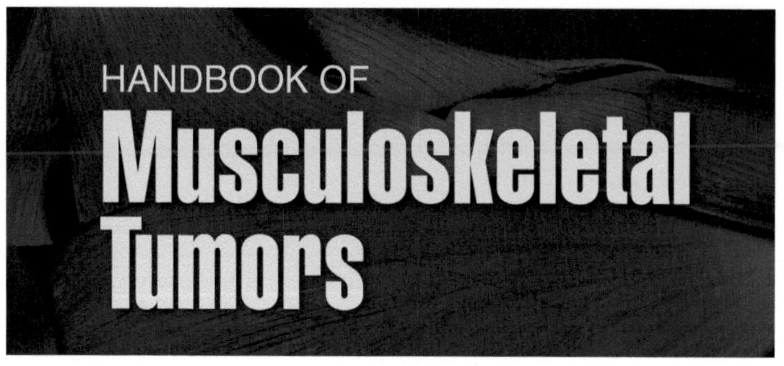

Editor

Matthew T. Wallace, MD, MBA

Assistant Professor of Oncology
Georgetown University Medical Center
Orthopaedic Oncologist
National Center for Bone and Soft Tissue Tumors
MedStar Cancer Institute
Baltimore, Maryland

Associate Editor

Frank J. Frassica, MD

Orthopaedic Oncologist
Renowned Orthopaedic Educator

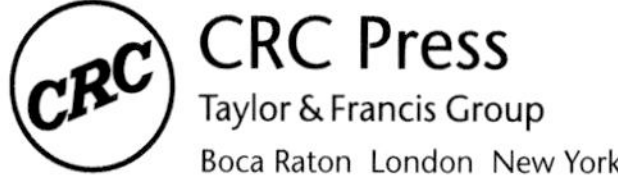

CRC Press is an imprint of the
Taylor & Francis Group, an **informa** business

Cover Artist: Katherine Christie

First published 2020 by SLACK Incorporated

Published 2024 by CRC Press
2385 NW Executive Center Drive, Suite 320, Boca Raton FL 33431

and by CRC Press
4 Park Square, Milton Park, Abingdon, Oxon, OX14 4RN

CRC Press is an imprint of Taylor & Francis Group, LLC

Library of Congress Cataloging-in-Publication Data:

LCCN: 2019057250

LC record available at https://lccn.loc.gov/

ISBN: 9781630916350 (pbk)
ISBN: 9781003524526 (ebk)

DOI: 10.1201/9781003524526

Dedication

To Tristan, Lily, and my dearest Audrey.

CONTENTS

Acknowledgments

A special thank you to Audrey Wallace for the original artwork and illustrations contained within this book.

On behalf of my team of colleagues and collaborators, I would first like to thank all of the patients and their families and caretakers who have privileged us by allowing us the honor of contributing to their care. We are made wiser and more humble with every experience. We cannot express enough gratitude to you for the relationships we build together, and for our shared adventures that continue to fuel the passion, curiosity, and exploration that makes our vocation so fulfilling.

I would like to extend a special thanks to my mentors in medicine who have guided me and provided so many opportunities to me. In chronological order this includes Dr. J. William Eley, Dr. Robert J. Neviaser, Dr. Panos Labropoulos, Dr. Robert Henshaw, Dr. Valerae Lewis, Dr. Patrick Lin, Dr. Bryan Moon, Dr. Justin Bird, Dr. Robert Satcher, Dr. Albert Aboulafia, and Dr. Frank Frassica, several of whom contributed patient cases to this book.

Lastly, I would like to thank my family, Beverly, James, Audrey, Amy, and Sydney of clan Wallace, for their unwavering love and support.

—Matthew T. Wallace, MD, MBA

I would like to thank my spouse Dr. Deborah Frassica, for advice and encouragement, and my mentor Dr. Frank Sim from the Mayo Clinic for a lifetime of encouragement and support.

—Frank J. Frassica, MD

We would like to thank Dr. Jeffrey S. Iding and Dr. Diana W. Molavi for their tremendous help with the histology section of the appendix.

—Matthew T. Wallace, MD, MBA & Frank J. Frassica, MD

About the Editors

Dr. Wallace is an orthopaedic oncologist with the National Center for Bone and Soft Tissue Tumors and Assistant Professor of Oncology at Georgetown University Medical Center. After undergraduate studies at the University of Virginia, he completed his medical degree at Emory University, Masters in business administration and orthopaedic surgery residency at George Washington University, and fellowship in musculoskeletal oncology at the University of Texas M.D. Anderson Cancer Center. Dr. Wallace's research efforts and publications are focused on bridging specialist oncology practices with generalists in the community to promote safer clinical practices. Dr. Wallace is a passionate educator of students and physicians and a highly popular lecturer at the regional and national levels.

Dr. Frassica is a world leader in teaching the concepts of oncology. He has published over 150 peer-reviewed publications and 5 books. He received the American Orthopaedic Association Distinguished Educator Award. He gives review courses both nationally and internationally.

Introduction

In the United States, more than 1.6 million new cancers and several-fold more benign neoplasms are seen in practitioner offices every year, which suggests with statistical certainty that every health care worker will encounter a number of tumors in his or her career. However, less than 1% of all surgical, medical, and radiological trainees will pursue any degree of specialization in musculoskeletal tumors. Specialists in bone and soft-tissue tumors are therefore rare, which limits easy patient and practitioner access to an expert opinion. Some practitioners may benefit from a specialist colleague working down the hall who can provide quick input or see patients on short notice, but for most, a specialist opinion may be located hours away, so the burden of work-up and short-term management of musculoskeletal tumors falls to the diligent generalists who serve their communities.

In the *Handbook of Musculoskeletal Tumors,* we aim to provide a high-yield, quick-reference resource to assist students, trainees, primary care and surgical practitioners, and midlevel practitioners who seek a guide to how to approach musculoskeletal tumors that will inevitably present in clinical practice. We will emphasize the general points of work-up and management, and provide helpful algorithms that will help the reader recognize suspicious lesions, order appropriate testing, and avoid errors that could compromise the life or limb of a patient.

Mismanagement of musculoskeletal tumors can have significant consequences for the patient, as well as professional consequences for practitioners and health care organizations. We therefore stress that the *Handbook of Musculoskeletal Tumors* is not designed to be a comprehensive manual of tumor management, nor a definitive treatise on musculoskeletal oncology. Many of the tumors we describe are rare and complex, and the nuances of their natural history and treatment must be assessed and definitively managed by a multidisciplinary team led by a trained musculoskeletal oncologist. For these unusual and often dangerous entities, the *Handbook* aims to serve as a practical guide to assist the practitioner in making an accurate diagnosis so as to facilitate a prompt referral and keep clinicians practicing safely.

Thank you for your time and interest. We hope the *Handbook of Musculoskeletal Tumors* will provide concise and helpful guidance in your clinical practice. Whether you are triaging a pathologic fracture in the emergency department, evaluating a new soft-tissue lump in the clinic, or just reviewing high-yield information for examination purposes, we hope this manual serves you and your patients so that everyone involved has a safe and mutually beneficial encounter.

—Matthew T. Wallace, MD, MBA

Section **I**

Evaluation of Musculoskeletal Tumors

1

Clinical Presentation of Bone Tumors

Overview

Making sense of a newly identified bone lesion can be daunting, but a well-thought-out patient and radiographic evaluation will often reveal specific patterns that aid in a quick and efficient diagnosis. We will discuss the presentation of bone tumors based on patient age at presentation, anatomic location, and associated symptoms (or lack thereof). We will present an algorithm for approaching incidentally discovered lesions, and introduce staging systems of bone tumors that dictate subsequent management.

Bone tumors can present in a myriad of different ways, and the discovery of a tumor can elicit alarm, fear, despair, and panic both for patient and practitioner. However, a well-thought-out, careful, and systematic evaluation can reveal patterns of presentation that will guide the practitioner to the correct diagnosis safely. This process begins with an extremely thorough history and physical examination process, followed by a careful interpretation of appropriate imaging studies, building a differential diagnosis, and ultimately deciding on a plan of care. It is important that the clinician confidently determine whether to observe, biopsy, or perform surgery on a skeletal lesion, and not simply "play the odds" or guess at a plan of action based on an assumption of what is most likely. Misdiagnosis or mismanagement both of benign and malignant lesions can have limb- or life-threatening consequences. For this reason, any practitioner who is not completely confident in his or her plan

Wallace, MT
Handbook of Musculoskeletal Tumors (pp 3-16).

Table 1-1

Commonly Encountered Tumors by Age

AGE GROUP	BENIGN	MALIGNANT
Young child, age 0-10 years	Eosinophilic granuloma (histiocytosis X) Osteomyelitis Nonossifying fibroma Unicameral bone cyst Aneurysmal bone cyst Osteoid osteoma Osteoblastoma Chondroblastoma	Metastatic neuroblastoma Lymphoma Leukemia (chloroma) Osteosarcoma Ewing sarcoma
Adolescent and young adult, age 11-39 years	Giant cell tumor Osteomyelitis Stress fracture Osteochondroma Fibrous dysplasia Enchondroma	Lymphoma Osteosarcoma Ewing sarcoma
Mature adult, age 40+ years	Enchondroma Juxta-articular cyst (geode) Bone infarct/avascular necrosis Osteomyelitis Paget's disease	Metastatic carcinoma Lymphoma Metastatic melanoma Multiple myeloma Chondrosarcoma

of care should refer that patient to a musculoskeletal oncology specialist, or otherwise seek a specialist's input.

An important step in building differentials is identifying likely classes of disease based on factors such as age, location, and symptomatology.

Age

Table 1-1 provides a grouping of commonly encountered bone tumors based on patient age. With notable exceptions, bone tumors frequently display a grouping or peak incidence around specific ages, so much so that common tumors are often thought of as either pediatric or adult diseases. For example, a destructive bone lesion in a child has a very different differential diagnosis from the exact same lesion in an adult older than 40 years.

Location

Many tumors display a curious predilection for specific anatomic regions, presenting within specific bones or in particular locations within the bone. Figure 1-1 depicts common long-bone lesions based on age and location. The metaphysis is a typical location for bone tumors, but specific lesions demonstrate a slight preference for diaphyseal and epiphyseal (or apophyseal) locations. Figure 1-2 demonstrates common spinal lesions based on location. With exceptions, lesions of the posterior elements are more likely to be benign compared with those of the vertebral body. Figure 1-3 lists tumors with a predilection for the flat bones of the pelvis and scapula.

Great Mimickers: Variable Appearance and Location

The following lesions have no anatomic preference and should be included on every differential:

- Osteomyelitis
- Eosinophilic granuloma (histiocytosis X)
- Metastatic bone disease
- Metabolic bone disease
- Lymphoma

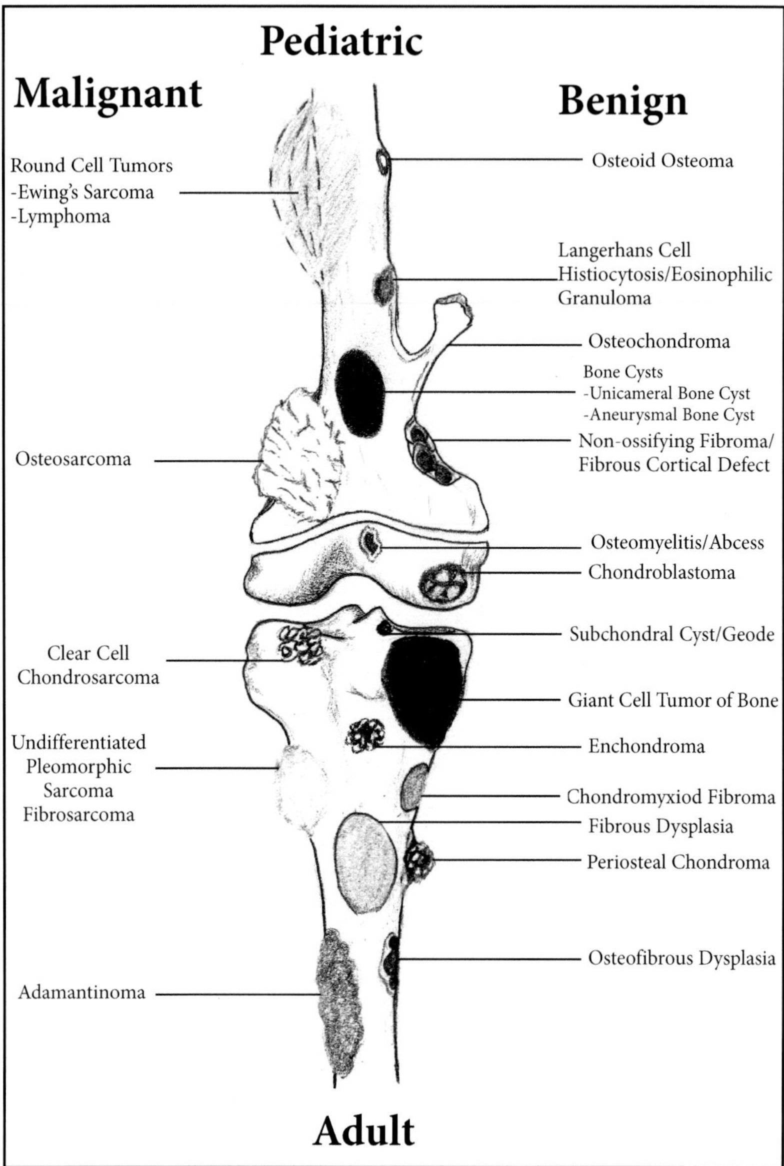

Figure 1-1. Locations of common pediatric and adult bone tumors.

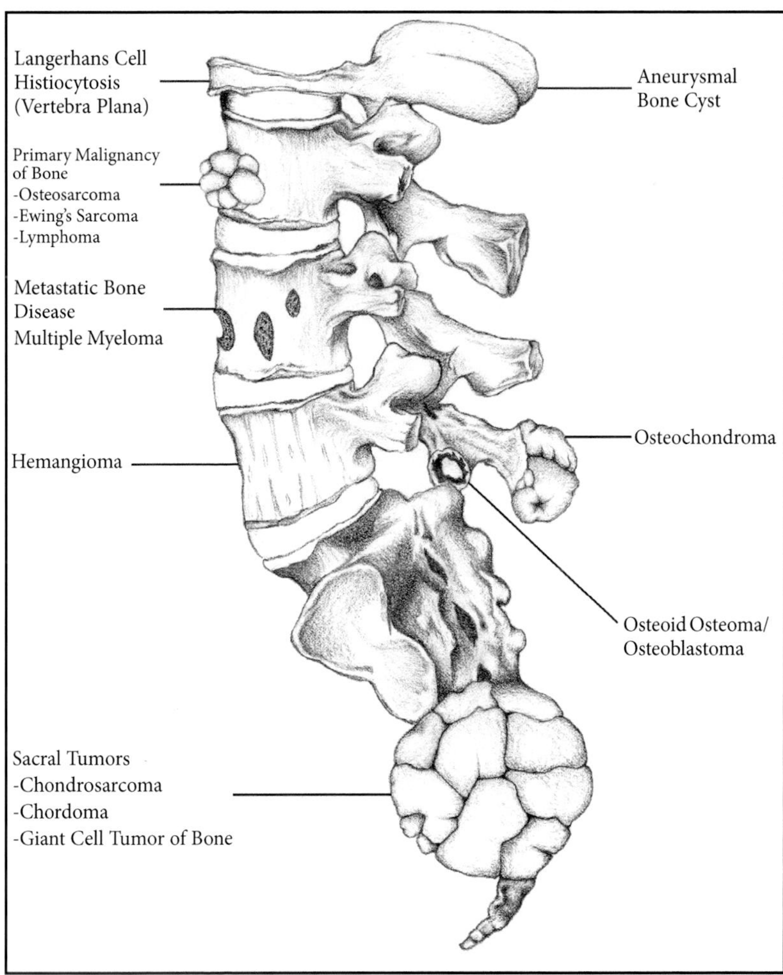

Figure 1-2. Common spine tumors by location.

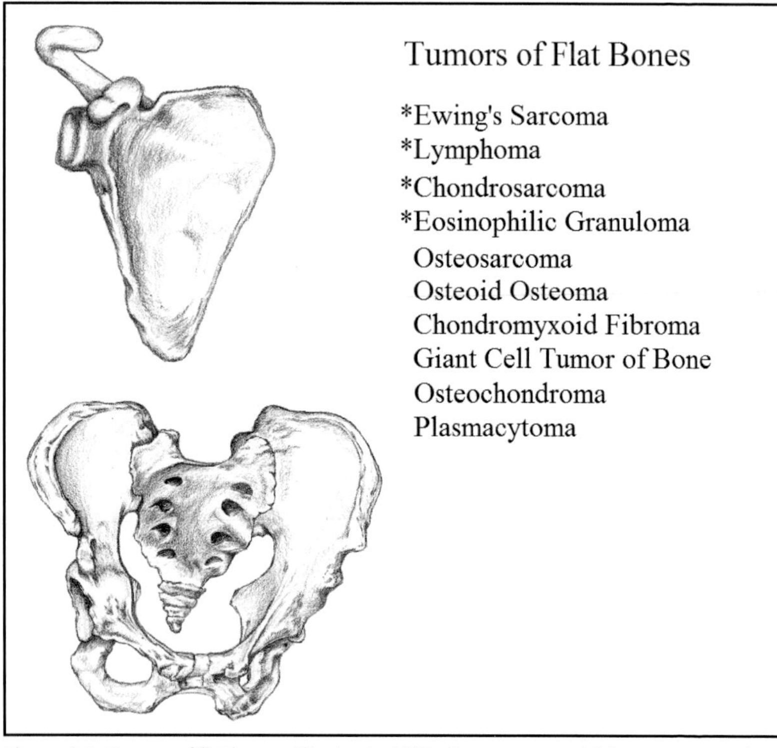

Figure 1-3. Tumors of flat bones. (Black asterisk) Indicates tumor with known propensity for flat bone involvement.

Common Pediatric and Adult Bone Tumors

Common lesions of the epiphysis/apophysis include the following:

- Chondroblastoma
- Clear cell chondrosarcoma
- Subchondral cyst/geode/intraosseous ganglion
- Giant cell tumor of bone (meta-epiphyseal)

Common lesions of the diaphysis include the following:

- Fibrous dysplasia
- Ewing sarcoma
- Lymphoma
- Osteoid osteoma
- Osteoblastoma

- Osteofibrous dysplasia (tibia/fibula)
- Adamantinoma (tibia/fibula)

Common lesions of the bony cortex include the following:

- Nonossifying fibroma
- Osteoid osteoma
- Osteochondroma
- Chondromyxoid fibroma
- Osteofibrous dysplasia (tibia/fibula)
- Adamantinoma (tibia/fibula)

Common Spine Tumors

Anterior (Vertebral Body)

Benign

- Eosinophilic granuloma (histiocytosis X)
- Hemangioma
- Fibrous dysplasia
- Giant cell tumor of bone

Malignant

- Metastatic bone disease
- Multiple myeloma/plasmacytoma
- Lymphoma
- Osteosarcoma
- Ewing sarcoma
- Chondrosarcoma
- Malignant fibrous histiocytoma
- Chordoma

Posterior Elements

Benign

- Aneurysmal bone cyst
- Osteochondroma
- Osteoid osteoma
- Osteoblastoma

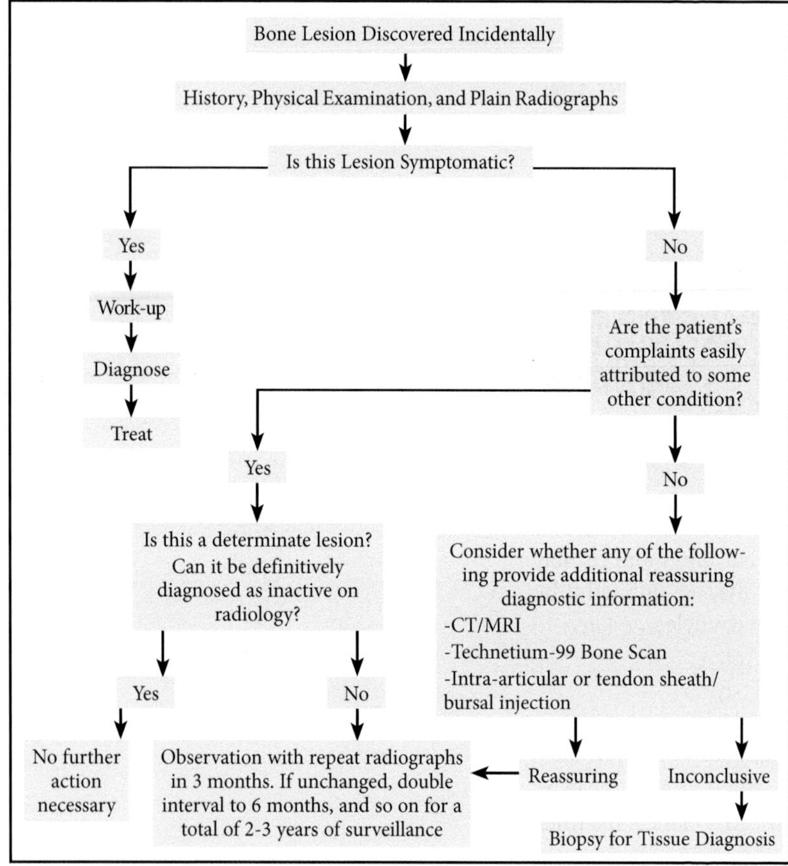

Figure 1-4. Algorithm for incidental bone lesions. CT, computed tomography; MRI, magnetic resonance imaging.

Malignant

- Metastatic bone disease
- Multiple myeloma/plasmacytoma

Symptomatology

Bone tumors may present as incidental findings during the work-up of an unrelated issue, as part of a staging work-up for a new diagnosis of malignancy identified elsewhere, or as a symptomatic primary bone lesion.

Figure 1-4 depicts an algorithm for the evaluation of incidentally discovered bone lesions. After a thorough history and physical, it is important to

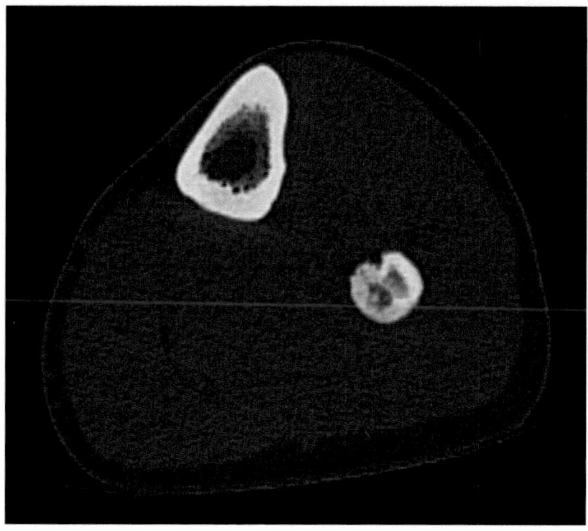

Figure 1-5. A 14-year-old boy presents with intense left lower leg pain relieved with nonsteroidal anti-inflammatory drugs. Axial CT demonstrates a well-defined cortical nidus with surrounding sclerosis and central ossification in the fibula, diagnostic of osteoid osteoma.

determine whether the lesion is symptomatic or if the patient's complaints (if any) are more reliably attributed to a different underlying cause, such as trauma, tendinopathy, bursitis, or degenerative joint disease. If the presentation is unclear, referral to an oncologic specialist is always appropriate.

Active and aggressive bone tumors are typically accompanied by pain and dysfunction, which may result from swelling, soft-tissue invasion, neurovascular compression, deformity, or pathologic fracture. Benign and malignant bone tumors both cause pain by a variety of mechanisms.

Bone tumors cause pain by the following mechanisms:

- Mechanical insufficiency/pathologic fracture
- Irritation or invasion of endosteal/periosteal nerve endings
- Mass effect: compression of adjacent structures or mechanical impingement during motion
- Increased intraosseous pressure due to rapid growth within the confined bony compartment
- Production of prostaglandins, parathyroid hormone-related protein, and other hormones

Painful lesions warrant a more complete imaging work-up, and more often than not, a tissue diagnosis. Certain determinate lesions can be treated without performing a biopsy. For example, the osteoid osteoma has a characteristic clinical presentation of pain, often at night, that is completely relieved with nonsteroidal anti-inflammatory drugs. A fine-cut computed tomography (CT) scan (Figure 1-5) that conclusively identifies the eccentric or cortically based nidus reassures the practitioner that an invasive biopsy or en bloc resection is unnecessary to establish the diagnosis, and thermal ablation can be performed with confidence. This must be performed by a team experienced with such lesions.

Determinate lesions that do not require biopsy include the following:

- Nonossifying fibroma
- Osteochondroma
- Osteoid osteoma
- Enchondroma
- Intraosseous lipoma
- Hemangioma of bone
- Bone infarct
- Enostosis (bone island)
- Unicameral bone cyst
- Degenerative cyst/geode
- Fibrous dysplasia

Systemic symptoms such as fevers, chills, malaise, weight loss, and laboratory abnormalities such as hypercalcemia or anemia suggest a more worrisome, likely malignant diagnosis. Exceptions to this include classic mimickers of malignancy such as infection, metabolic bone diseases, and histiocytosis.

Bone deformation is a more chronic process, typically suggestive of a benign or non-neoplastic etiology, or tumorigenic syndromes that contribute to skeletal dysplasia (Figure 1-6).

Lesions that cause deformity include the following:

- Fibrous dysplasia
- Osteofibrous dysplasia
- Osteoid osteoma (may cause physeal overgrowth, bowing, or scoliosis)
- Metabolic bone disease
- Paget's disease of bone
- Multiple hereditary exostosis (osteochondromatosis)
- Ollier's disease (enchondromatosis)
- Maffucci syndrome (enchondromatosis and hemangiomatosis)

Staging of Bone Tumors

Imaging of the primary bone is generally all that is required for staging of benign bone tumors. Aggressive lesions such as giant cell tumor of bone and chondroblastoma may present with pulmonary spread at the time of diagnosis, so staging of these lesions should include chest radiography or CT

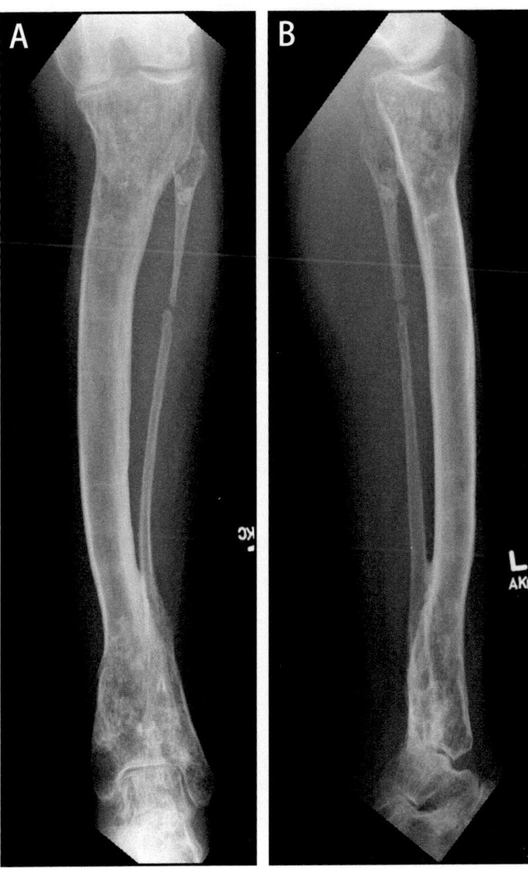

Figure 1-6. A 30-year-old woman presents with shortening and persistent deformity of the left lower extremity despite multiple corrective osteotomies and guided-growth procedures. (A) Anteroposterior and (B) lateral radiographs of the left tibia demonstrate persistent valgus and procurvatum of the tibia, and multiple underlying enchondromas consistent with Ollier's disease.

evaluation.[1] Benign bone tumors are staged with Arabic numerals according to the proposed Enneking staging system (Table 1-2).

Stage 1 lesions are well-defined lesions without significant growth potential. These are often identified incidentally, and do not generally require treatment. Examples of Stage 1 lesions include nonossifying fibromas and enchondromas.

Stage 2 lesions are lesions with activity and limited growth potential that generally respect anatomic confines, with some cortical thinning and bony expansion. Left untreated, these are prone to pathologic fracture. Examples of Stage 2 lesions include unicameral bone cysts, aneurysmal bone cysts, and chondroblastomas.

Stage 3 lesions are benign but locally destructive lesions with a tendency toward cortical bone loss, soft-tissue extension, and high rates of local

Table 1-2

Enneking System for Staging of Benign Bone Tumors

STAGE	TERM	NATURAL HISTORY
1	Latent	Inert; remains unchanged or may heal/resolve spontaneously
2	Active	Continued growth, limited by anatomic confines
3	Aggressive	Progressive growth and bony destruction, unchecked by anatomic confines
Adapted from Enneking WF.[2]		

Table 1-3

Musculoskeletal Tumor Society/Enneking System for Staging of Malignant Bone Tumors[3]

STAGE	GRADE	LOCATION
IA	Low (G1)	Intracompartmental (T1)
IB	Low (G1)	Extracompartmental (T2)
IIA	High (G2)	Intracompartmental (T1)
IIB	High (G2)	Extracompartmental (T2)
III	Any	Same bone (skip) or distant metastasis (M1)

recurrence. Giant cell tumor of bone is the most classic Stage 3 benign bone lesion.

Bone sarcomas are staged based on common patterns of metastatic spread, generally to the lung parenchyma, within the same bone, and to other bony sites. Staging work-up includes:

1. Magnetic resonance imaging of the entire involved bone
2. CT evaluation of the chest
3. Technetium-99 total body bone scan

Primary malignant bone tumors are staged with Roman numerals and subdivided based on histologic grade and the presence or absence of extraosseous extension and metastatic spread. The Musculoskeletal Tumor Society/Enneking Staging System (Table 1-3) considers skip metastases, or

TABLE 1-4

AMERICAN JOINT COMMITTEE ON CANCER SYSTEM FOR STAGING OF MALIGNANT BONE TUMORS[4]

STAGE	T	N	M	GRADE
IA	T1	N0	M0	G1, G2
IB	T2	N0	M0	G1, G2
IIA	T1	N0	M0	G3, G4
IIB	T2	N0	M0	G3, G4
III	T3	N0	M0	G3, G4
IVA	Any	N0	M1a	Any
IVB	Any	N0 or N1	M1b	Any

Abbreviations: T1, 8 cm or less in greatest dimension; T2, >8 cm; T3, discontinuous tumor (skip lesion); N0, no regional lymph node metastasis; N1, lymph node metastasis; M0, no distant metastasis; M1a, lung metastasis; M1b, other metastasis (including bone); G1, well-differentiated/low grade; G2, moderately differentiated/low to intermediate grade; G3, poorly differentiated/high grade; G4, undifferentiated.

discontinuous tumor, as prognostically identical to pulmonary and osseous metastatic disease, and thus considers these tumors Stage III. The American Joint Committee on Cancer prefers a conventional TNM staging system, detailed in Table 1-4.

TAKE-AWAYS

1. Evaluation of a new bone lesion starts with a comprehensive history and physical examination.
2. Age and location point to key patterns of bone tumor presentations that assist in building differentials and guiding future work-up.
3. Incidentally discovered lesions are most often benign, and most can be safely observed.
4. Painful or symptomatic lesions should always be pursued, diagnosed, and staged accordingly.

Commonly Tested Topics for Trainees

- Osteomyelitis and eosinophilic granuloma (histiocytosis) are commonly tested mimickers that can appear in ANY location of ANY bone, and must be included on every differential diagnosis.
- Chondroblastoma is the most common epiphyseal/apophyseal lesion in the child.
- Although extremely rare in clinical practice, adamantinoma is classically a destructive, cortically based, diaphyseal lesion of the tibia or fibula in the middle-aged patient.
- Nonossifying fibroma is an eccentric, cortically based lesion with determinate imaging findings that is most often diagnosed incidentally. It does not require biopsy or surgical intervention if asymptomatic.

References

1. Rosario M, Kim HS, Yun JY, Han I. Surveillance for lung metastasis from giant cell tumor of bone. *J Surg Oncol.* 2017;116(7):907-913. doi:10.1002/jso.24739.
2. Enneking WF. Staging tumors. In: Enneking WF, ed. *Musculoskeletal Tumor Surgery.* New York, NY: Churchill Livingston; 1983:87-88.
3. Enneking WF, Spanier SS, Goodman MA. A system for the surgical staging of musculoskeletal sarcoma. *Clin Orthop Relat Res.* 1980;153:106-120.
4. American Joint Committee on Cancer: Soft Tissue Sarcoma. In: Amin MB, Edge S, Greene F, et al, eds. *AJCC Cancer Staging Manual.* 8th ed. New York, NY: Springer; 2017.

2

Clinical Presentation of Soft-Tissue Tumors

Overview

Soft-tissue masses are a relatively common entity encountered by surgeons and primary care clinicians. Soft-tissue malignancies represent less than 1% of soft-tissue tumors, but their prompt recognition and appropriate management are important in keeping patient and clinician safe. We will discuss the clinical presentation of soft-tissue lumps and bumps, and identify findings that can be either reassuring or worrisome for malignancy. We will present an algorithm for approaching soft-tissue tumors, and discuss staging of soft-tissue malignancies that influence subsequent management.

Soft-tissue lumps and bumps are among the most common and sometimes most confounding lesions encountered by primary care practitioners and surgeons. Soft-tissue masses can ultimately be benign, malignant, infectious, reactive, or non-neoplastic. Unlike bone tumors, soft-tissue masses generally display fewer patterns of presentation that aid the clinician in diagnosis. Each year, approximately 13,000 new cases of soft-tissue sarcomas will be identified in the United States, and though the true incidence of benign soft-tissue masses cannot be determined, benign lesions are estimated to be at least 100-fold more common.[1] Despite their rarity, soft-tissue sarcomas that are misdiagnosed or mismanaged are associated with significant adverse outcomes. The clinical and radiographic presentation of benign and soft-tissue neoplasms may overlap considerably, and a careful evaluation is necessary to avoid compromising the life and limb of the patient.

Wallace, MT
Handbook of Musculoskeletal Tumors (pp 17-25).

History

Most patients with soft-tissue tumors will present with a palpable lump or growth, a tender nodule, or occasionally an incidentally discovered mass. The practitioner should spend ample time obtaining information regarding the circumstances of the discovery of the mass.

Chronicity

When was the mass discovered? For how long has the mass been present? A large mass that has only recently been discovered is more worrisome for malignancy, but some sarcomas, such as liposarcomas, synovial sarcomas, clear cell sarcomas, epithelioid sarcomas, and alveolar soft-part sarcomas may have an indolent presentation.

Size Changes

Has the mass grown since it was discovered? At what rate has it grown? A mass that fluctuates in size is generally non-neoplastic, suggestive of a cyst or vascular malformation. Progressively enlarging or rapidly growing masses must be thoroughly and aggressively evaluated.

Pain

Is the mass painful? Is it tender to touch? Is it exacerbated by anything in particular? Is there a history of trauma or injury? In contrast to malignant bone tumors, soft-tissue sarcomas are most often painless, and pain within a soft-tissue mass may be slightly reassuring.

Most Common Benign Painful Soft-Tissue Lumps and Bumps

- Abscess/Infection: warmth, erythema, and systemic symptoms often present
- Myositis ossificans
- Blue rubber bleb nevus
- Angiolipoma
- Neuroma
- Nerve sheath tumors (neurofibroma and schwannoma): pain generally elicited by palpation, with radiation along the course of the nerve (Tinel sign). The tumor is also mobile from side to side, but is tethered by the nerve proximally and distally

- Glomus tumor: pain and sensitivity to pressure and temperature in the subungual regions
- Eccrine spiradenoma
- Leiomyoma
- Ganglion cyst
- Inflammatory/Reactive granuloma

Important Caveat

Deep, painful, hemorrhagic lesions are deceptive. Sarcomas that undergo necrosis, internal bleeding, or cystic degeneration can present as rapidly enlarging and painful masses due to rapid changes in pressure on surrounding tissues (Figure 2-1). Before declaring a mass a benign "hematoma," the practitioner must be confident that the clinical history supports this diagnosis. There should be a clear history of trauma consistent with the location of the mass, symptoms should develop abruptly following the injury, and there must be a reasonable explanation for the degree of hemorrhage observed (significant injury, anticoagulant use, bleeding diathesis, etc). If unclear, consider biopsy. The risk of a potentially unnecessary biopsy or evacuation of a hematoma is minimal compared with the risk of delaying diagnosis of a high-grade or hemorrhagic soft-tissue sarcoma. The corollary recommendation is that all patients with a diagnosis of a hematoma must be followed carefully to ensure resolution of the mass over time.

Personal and Family History

Tumorigenic conditions such as neurofibromatosis, tumoral calcinosis, and lipomatosis should be investigated. Fibromatoses of the hands, feet, or penis should prompt evaluation of the other sites, and patients with extra-abdominal desmoids should be screened for familial adenomatous polyposis.

Physical Examination

Diagnosis of soft-tissue lumps and bumps by examination only is notoriously unreliable but can assist the clinician in identifying areas of further work-up and the most appropriate methods of imaging and biopsy.

Size

Masses larger than a golf ball or greater than 5 cm require a dedicated imaging work-up including magnetic resonance imaging (MRI). Small lesions may be difficult to assess on MRI, and other modalities should be considered.

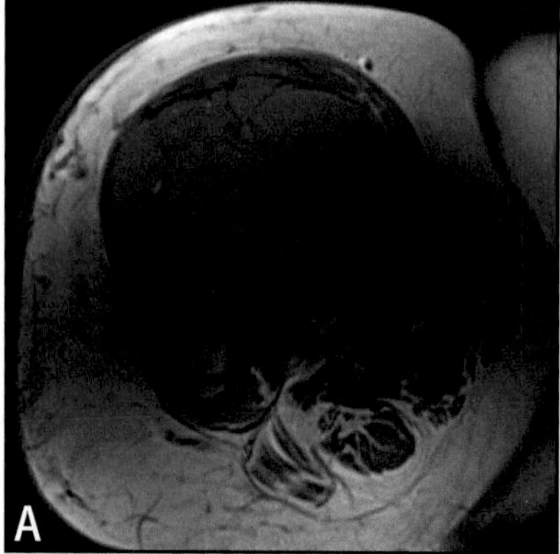

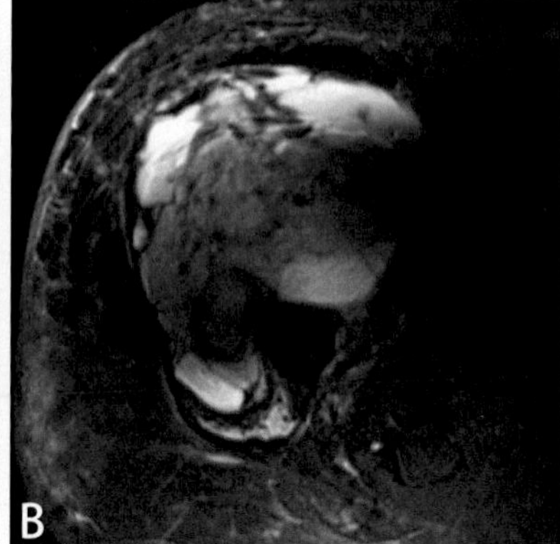

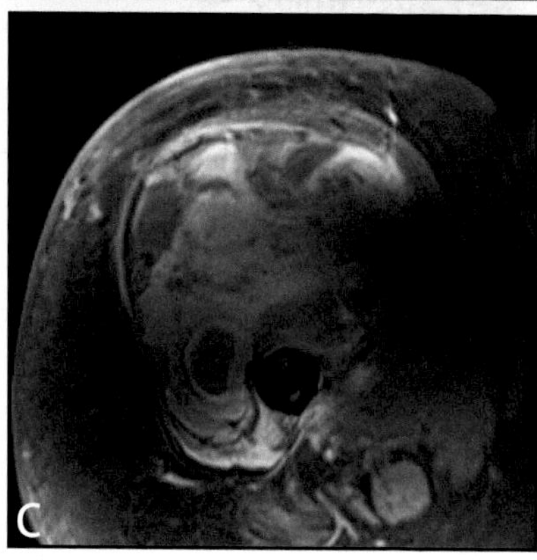

Figure 2-1. A 67-year-old woman presents with a rapidly enlarging and uncomfortable mass in the right thigh. Axial (A) T1, (B) T2, and (C) T1 postcontrast MRI demonstrate a soft-tissue mass with internal hemorrhagic and cystic components. Biopsy demonstrated pleomorphic liposarcoma.

Location and Mobility

Despite widely held belief, soft-tissue sarcomas can and frequently do occur in the subcutaneous space.[2,3] A subcutaneous mass that is large, firm, or immobile should be imaged. Small, soft, and mobile masses can be observed provided the examiner record clinical measurements at each evaluation. Masses that are deep to compartment fascia must be imaged.

Suggestive Findings

- Dense, rock-hard consistency: extra-abdominal desmoid tumor
- Compressible: cyst or vascular malformation
- Pulsations: pseudoaneurysm
- Warmth: nonspecific: infection, inflammation, or increased blood flow
- Regional lymphadenopathy: tender = inflammatory vs nontender = malignancy

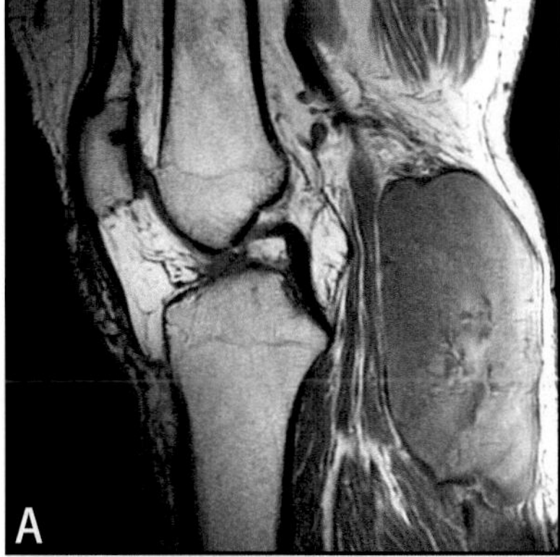

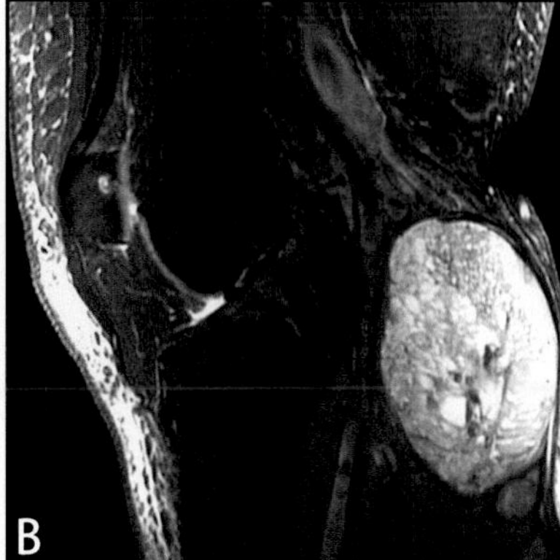

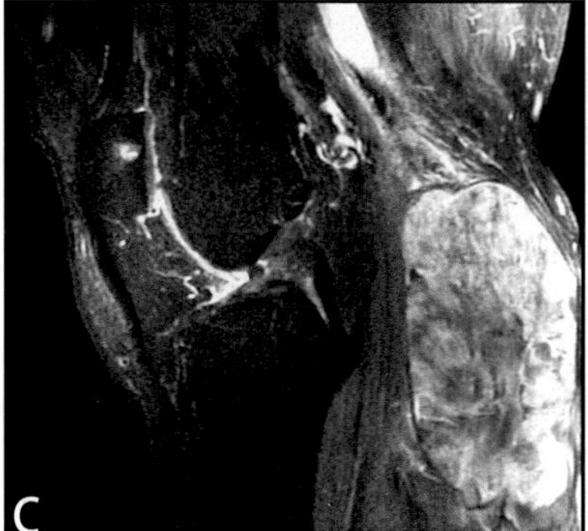

Figure 2-2. An 82-year-old man presents with painless swelling in the posterior left calf. Axial (A) T1, (B) T2, and (C) T1 post-contrast MRI demonstrate a large, deep, heterogeneous mass with significant internal enhancement with gadolinium. Biopsy confirmed a diagnosis of pleomorphic rhabdomyosarcoma.

- Neurological/Tinel signs: nerve sheath tumor
- Transillumination: ganglion cyst

Imaging

Large lesions, deep lesions, and lesions under consideration for biopsy or excision require an imaging work-up. MRI is the mainstay for evaluation of soft tissue, and must include axial T1- and T2-weighted sequences, and a T1 fat-suppressed sequence, preferably with contrast (Figure 2-2). Select masses, including benign lipomatous masses, hemangiomas, and ganglion cysts can be determinate on MRI, which can obviate the need for biopsy and further work-up.

Plain radiographs and computed tomography (CT) do not provide as much anatomic detail as MRI but are helpful in the evaluation of masses that may contain mineralization, gas, or bony invasion. Calcification patterns can

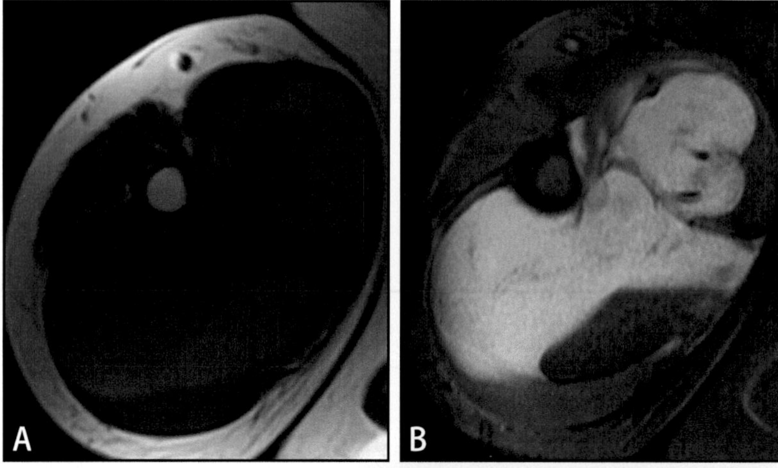

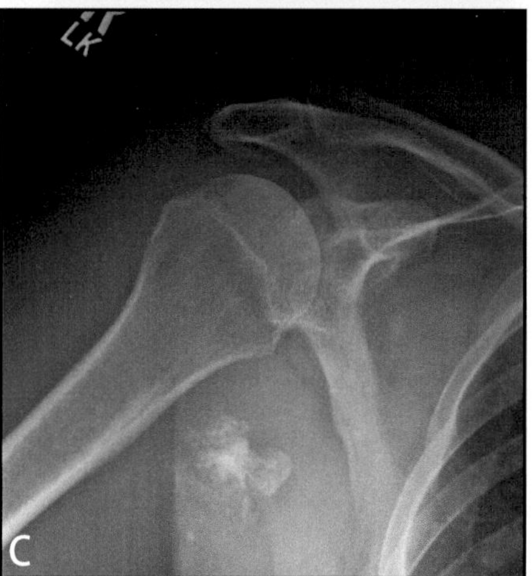

Figure 2-3. A 60-year-old man presents with painless swelling in the right upper arm. Axial (A) T1 and (B) T2 MRI demonstrate a large, deep, heterogeneous mass in the posterior compartment of the upper arm. (C) Plain radiographs of the shoulder demonstrate calcifications within the soft-tissue mass. Biopsy demonstrated biphasic synovial sarcoma.

be suggestive of particular diagnoses. Ultrasound can assist in the evaluation of vascular or fluid-containing soft-tissue masses.

Soft-Tissue Mineralization Patterns

- Phleboliths: soft-tissue hemangioma
- Indistinct, cloud-like ossification: extraskeletal osteosarcoma
- Ball-like ossification with a mature periphery: myositis ossificans
- Lobular dense calcification: tumoral calcinosis
- Lace-like or dystrophic calcification: synovial sarcoma (Figure 2-3)

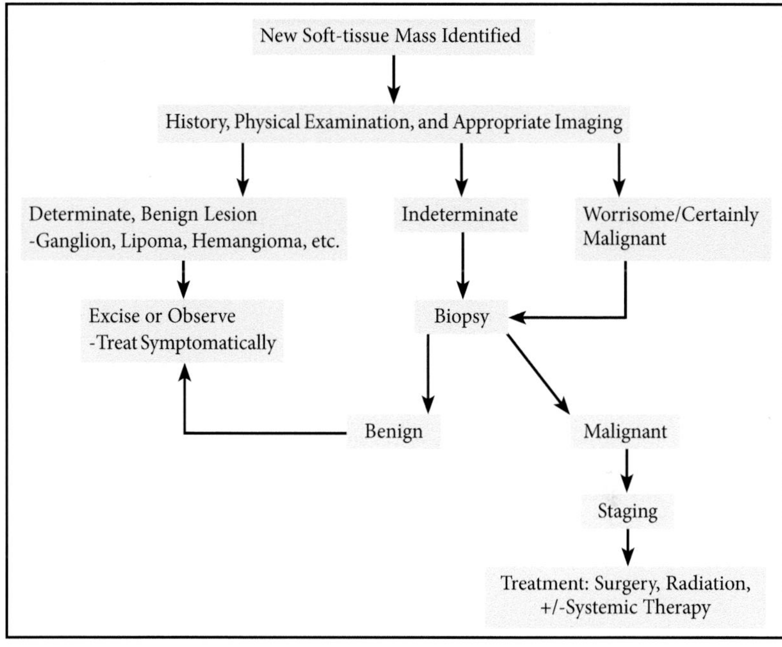

Figure 2-4. Algorithm for evaluation and work-up of soft-tissue tumors.

After careful history, physical examination, and imaging review, the practitioner must determine whether to observe, biopsy, or excise the soft-tissue mass. Figure 2-4 demonstrates a helpful algorithm for the work-up of soft-tissue tumors. It is always recommended that large tumors, deep tumors, and indeterminate lesions in need of biopsy be referred to a surgical specialist who is able to perform the definitive surgical resection. Biopsy complications are significantly higher when performed by inexperienced practitioners at referring institutions.[4]

Staging of Malignant Soft-Tissue Tumors

The broad category of primary soft-tissue malignancies is a heterogeneous group of entities with variable metastatic potential and patterns of spread. Sarcomas generally display a predilection for the lung parenchyma, which requires CT evaluation of the chest, but certain subtypes require additional studies for staging, detailed in Table 2-1. Staging is then performed based on the American Joint Committee on Cancer staging system, detailed in Table 2-2.

Table 2-1

Staging Studies Based on Soft-Tissue Sarcoma Subtype

DIAGNOSIS	PATTERNS OF METASTASIS	STAGING STUDIES
Undifferentiated pleomorphic sarcoma	Lung	CT chest
Liposarcomas (myxoid, round cell, dedifferentiated)	Lung, retroperitoneum	CT chest, abdomen, and pelvis
Myxoid liposarcoma, leiomyosarcoma	Lung, retroperi-toneum, bone	CT chest, abdomen, and pelvis Technetium-99 bone scan
Epithelioid sarcoma Synovial sarcoma Angiosarcoma Rhabdomyosarcoma Clear cell sarcoma	Lung, lymph nodes	CT chest PET Consider sentinel node biopsy
Alveolar soft-part sarcoma	Lung, brain	CT chest MRI brain

Abbreviations: CT, computed tomography; MRI, magnetic resonance imaging; PET, positron emission tomography.

Table 2-2

American Joint Commission on Cancer System for Staging of Malignant Soft-Tissue Tumors of the Trunk and Extremities

STAGE	GRADE	TUMOR	NODES/METASTASES
IA	G1	T1	N0, M0
IB	G1	T2, T3, T4	N0, M0
II	G2, G3	T1	N0, M0
IIIA	G2, G3	T2	N0, M0
IIIB	G2, G3	T3, T4	N0, M0
IV	Any	Any	N1 or M1

Abbreviations: G1, well-differentiated/low grade; G2, moderately differentiated/low-intermediate grade; G3, poorly differentiated/high grade; T1, 5 cm or less; T2, 5-10 cm; T3, 10-15 cm; T4, greater than 15 cm.

Take-Aways

1. Evaluation of a new soft-tissue mass starts with a comprehensive history and physical examination, with particular attention paid to size, firmness, location, pain, and mobility.
2. Imaging evaluation should include MRI for any large or deep mass, or any mass in need of biopsy or excision.
3. Benign and malignant soft-tissue tumors can present similarly and have similar radiographic appearances, so any indeterminate mass should be biopsied to establish a tissue diagnosis.

Commonly Tested Topics for Trainees

- The typical presentation of a soft-tissue sarcoma is a painless, growing mass, often larger than 5 cm, or larger than a golf ball.
- Painful masses are frequently benign, and a careful history and physical can differentiate those due to trauma, infection, or neoplasm.
- Soft-tissue hemangioma, myositis ossificans, and synovial sarcoma are commonly tested soft-tissue masses with notable mineralization patterns on plain radiographs.

References

1. Siegel RL, Miller KD, Jemal A. *Cancer Statistics. CA Cancer J Clin.* 2018;68(1):7-30. doi:10.3322/caac.21442.
2. Gibbs CP, Peabody TD, Mundt AJ, Montag AG, Simon MA. Oncological outcomes of operative treatment of subcutaneous soft-tissue sarcomas of the extremities. *J Bone Joint Surg Am.* 1997;79(6):888-897. doi:10.2106/00004623-199706000-00013.
3. Rhydholm A, Gustafson P, Rööser B, Willén H, Berg NO. Subcutaneous sarcoma: a population-based study of 129 patients. *J Bone Joint Surg Br.* 1991;73(4):662-667. doi:10.1302/0301-620X.73B4.2071656.
4. Mankin HJ, Mankin CJ, Simon MA. The hazards of biopsy, revisited. Members of the Musculoskeletal Tumor Society. *J Bone Joint Surg Am.* 1996;78(5):656-663. doi:10.2106/00004623-199605000-00004.
5. American Joint Committee on Cancer: Soft Tissue Sarcoma. In: Amin MB, Edge S, Greene F, et al, eds. *AJCC Cancer Staging Manual.* 8th ed. New York, NY: Springer; 2017.

3

Musculoskeletal Radiology and Imaging of Tumors

Overview

The accuracy and speed with which a clinician can diagnose musculoskeletal tumors relies heavily on the proper interpretation of imaging at presentation, followed by the thoughtful ordering of appropriate confirmatory imaging studies. We will discuss the essential fundamentals of imaging interpretation for musculoskeletal tumors, develop comfort with identifying indications for advanced imaging modalities, and recognize the limitations and pitfalls of these modalities. We will present an algorithm that will enable the practitioner to order appropriate studies so as to avoid misdiagnosis and limit unnecessary or expensive testing for patients.

After a thorough history and physical examination, the diagnosis of musculoskeletal tumors depends heavily on accurate imaging interpretation. The quality of image interpretation is determined by the experience, confidence, comfort level, and diligence of the interpreter. Similar to the orthopaedic traumatologist gaining expertise in the radiographic assessment of fracture patterns, so too can the tumor practitioner become adept at interpreting the appearance of lesions on a variety of imaging modalities. The treating clinician is often the only individual able to correlate the patient's presentation with the imaging findings. Therefore, it is essential that the treating clinician become confident in the imaging of tumors so as to arrive at a correct diagnosis quickly. It is also important to recognize when advanced imaging is appropriate or unnecessary. Given significant advances in imaging technology over

Wallace, MT
Handbook of Musculoskeletal Tumors (pp 27-48).

the past 30 years, it is tempting to pursue 3-dimensional (3D) or higher-resolution imaging to satisfy the clinician's curiosity or doubt, but this practice can be costly and unnecessary, and can occasionally impart risk to the patient. Ultimately, once a lesion is recognized, it is wise to defer the imaging work-up to the practitioner who will definitively manage the patient.

Radiographs

Plain radiographs are mandatory in the evaluation of any bone lesion and, as mentioned in Chapter 2, can be extremely helpful in the assessment of soft-tissue masses as well. Radiographs are cost-efficient, time tested, and frequently diagnostic.[1] They can accurately direct further work-up, assist in localization for biopsy, and often suggest the clinical behavior of lesions, which can be predictive of the ultimate diagnosis. Furthermore, radiography is often the imaging modality of choice used during treatment in the operating room and for the surveillance of lesions during long-term follow-up, so it is important to have a baseline study at the time of initial presentation (Figure 3-1).

For an accurate interpretation of x-rays, it is helpful to have a process that systematically evaluates every component of the images provided and obtains every important piece of information from the study.

1. Confirm the correct patient name and the date of the study. DO NOT get misled by interpreting images that may be out of date or not the correct patient
2. Check the patient's date of birth. Age is all-important in building differentials
3. Describe the location of the lesion
    a. What bone? Is this a long bone, flat bone, spinal segment, etc?
    b. In what region of the bone is the lesion? Diaphysis, metaphysis, epiphysis/apophysis?
    c. Is the lesion central, eccentric, cortically-based, or surface-based/periosteal?
4. What is the lesion doing to the surrounding bone?
    a. Is the lesion causing bony lysis or destruction?
    b. Is the cortex disrupted or is it intact?
    c. Is the bone expanded or deformed?
    d. Is the bone fractured?

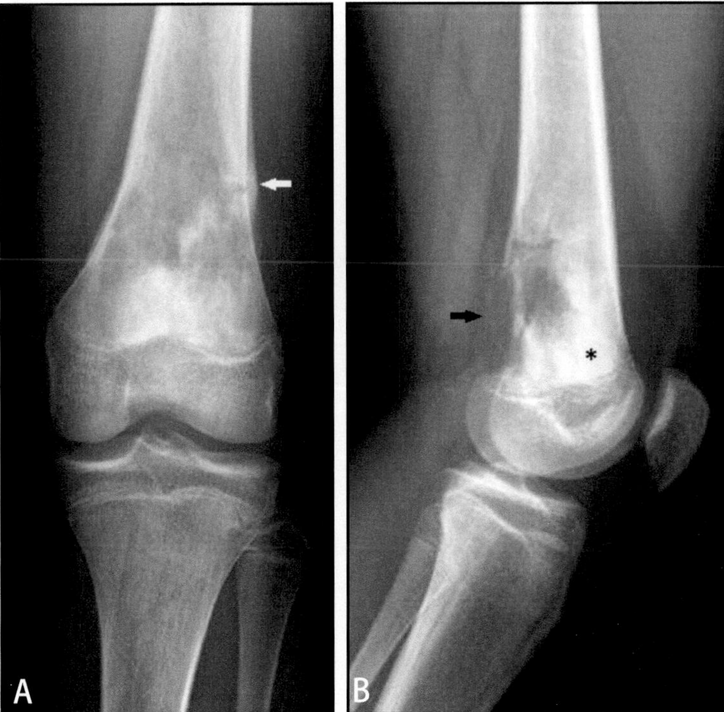

Figure 3-1. (A) Anteroposterior and (B) lateral x-rays of a 15-year-old boy with increasing left knee pain demonstrate an ill-defined destructive lesion in a skeletally immature patient, with indistinct margins, periosteal reaction (white arrow), cortical destruction (black arrow), and internal areas of osteoid matrix isodense to cortical bone (black asterisk). Biopsy confirmed a diagnosis of high-grade osteosarcoma.

5. Are there secondary changes in the bone?
   a. Is there reactive sclerosis around the lesion?
   b. Are there any patterns of periosteal reaction?
6. What do the margins look like around the lesion (Figure 3-2)?
   a. Well-defined: the extent of the lesion can be clearly identified from surrounding bone
   b. Ill-defined: the lesion becomes fuzzy or indistinct as it travels into surrounding bone
   c. Mixed/Changing: a combination of well-defined and ill-defined zones
   d. Permeative: a moth-eaten appearance of diffuse destruction
   e. Scalloped: endosteal (for intramedullary lesions) or periosteal (for surface-based lesions) round areas of cortical effacement

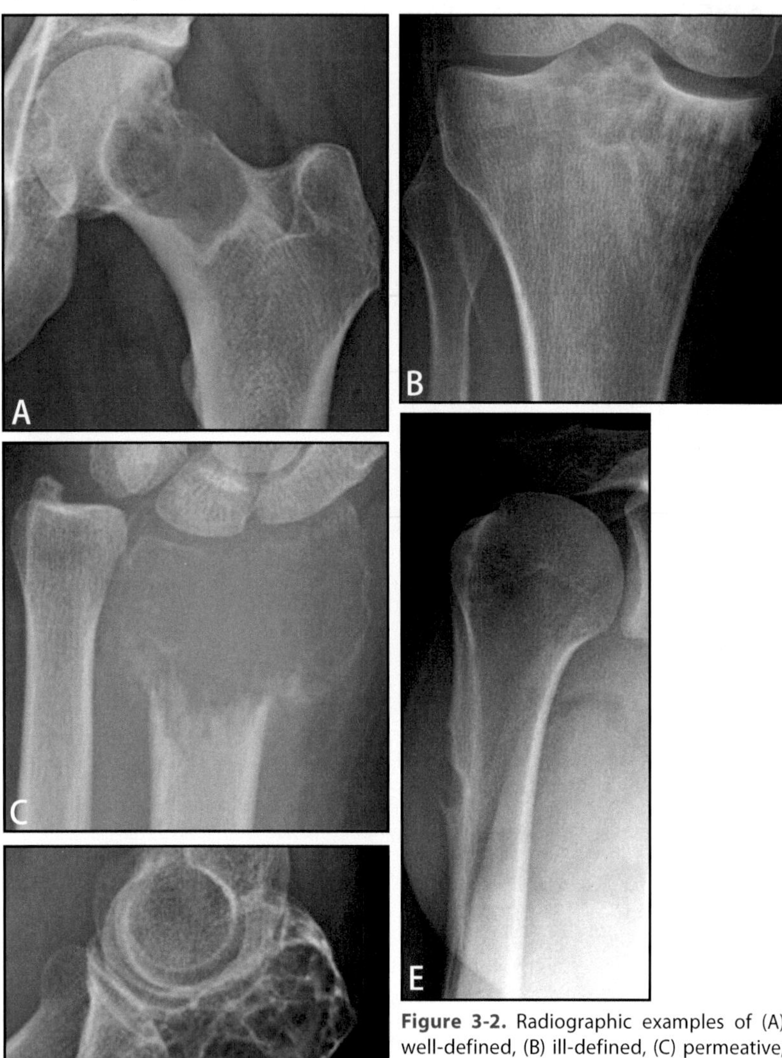

Figure 3-2. Radiographic examples of (A) well-defined, (B) ill-defined, (C) permeative, (D) scalloped, and (E) saucerized margins.

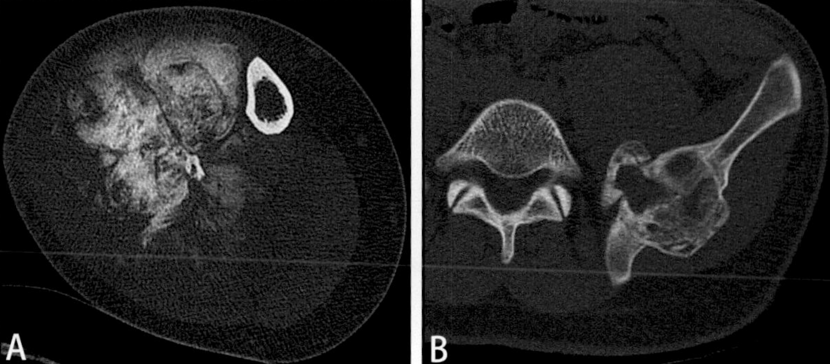

Figure 3-3. Axial CT demonstrating patterns of (A) malignant and (B) benign osteoid-producing tumors. Malignant osteoid tends to be more irregular and ill-defined, with greater density toward the center of the lesion and less mineralization at the periphery. Benign processes tend to form well-defined bone with trabecular markings, with a geographic, well-mineralized peripheral margin.

7. Is matrix present? Is there any pattern of internal radiodensity to suggest a dominant tissue type?
   a. Osteoid: bone. Fluffy, cloudlike, radiodense material with the same density as cortical bone. Malignant osteoid is often more dense centrally, becoming less dense at the periphery of the lesion. Benign bone-forming processes often demonstrate trabecular markings (Figure 3-3)
   b. Chondroid: cartilage. Lobules of sparsely mineralized tumor separated by rimming calcifications, which may be more or less radiodense than surrounding bone. This produces a pattern of rings, arcs, and stipples that are often described as "popcorn," or "packed beads" (Figure 3-4)
   c. Ground-Glass: fibrous lesions that produce a disorganized matrix of loose trabecular fragments will demonstrate a lesion with the same radiodensity as surrounding trabecular bone, but without any apparent trabecular markings, often appearing as if the trabeculae have been "smudged." This produces a pattern similar to opaque glass (Figure 3-5)
8. Evaluate the soft tissues. Has the lesion extended out of the bone into the soft tissues? Are tissue planes disrupted? Any calcifications? Is gas present?

The Lodwick classification is a system for describing margins of bone lesions and serves as a method to indicate the growth and aggressiveness of bony lesions. Features of cortical destruction, endosteal erosion, or

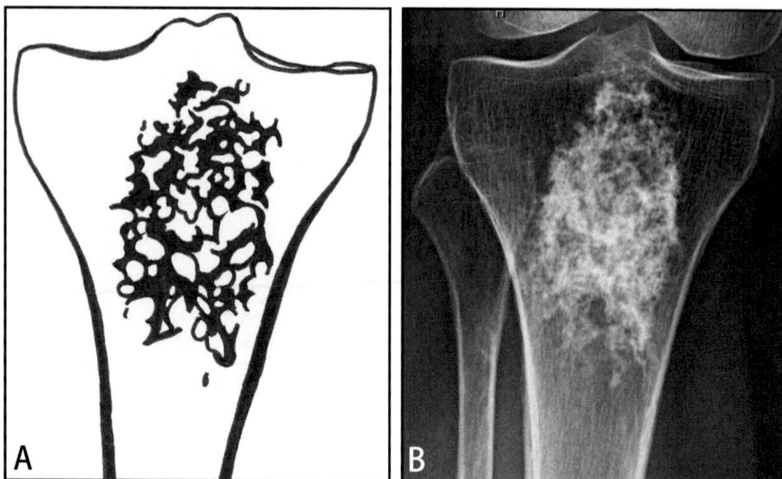

Figure 3-4. The mineralization patterns of (A) chondroid tissue form a series of radiodense arcs and rings in between the radiolucent lobules of cartilage. This is often informally called "packed beads," "tapioca pearls," or "popcorn." (B) This lobular growth pattern of chondroid tissue can be seen between the calcifications at the radiolucent zones on plain radiographs.

Figure 3-5. (A) Anteroposterior and (B) lateral radiographs of a 24-year-old woman with right lower leg pain demonstrate mild bowing through an irregular but well-defined lesion of the distal tibial diaphysis. The lesion is characterized by internal matrix isodense to cancellous bone, but without traditional trabecular markings, giving it a "ground-glass" appearance consistent with fibrous dysplasia.

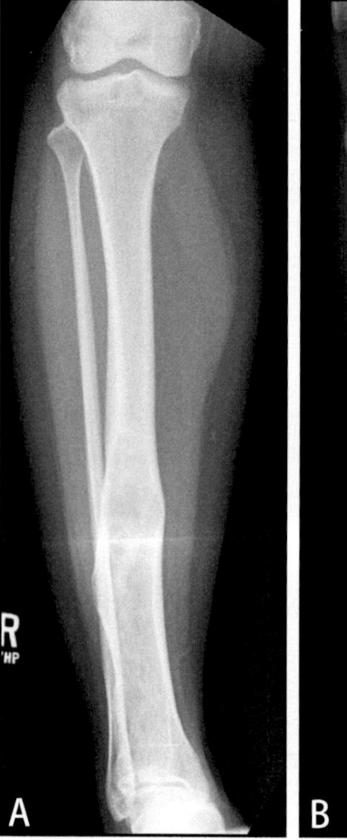

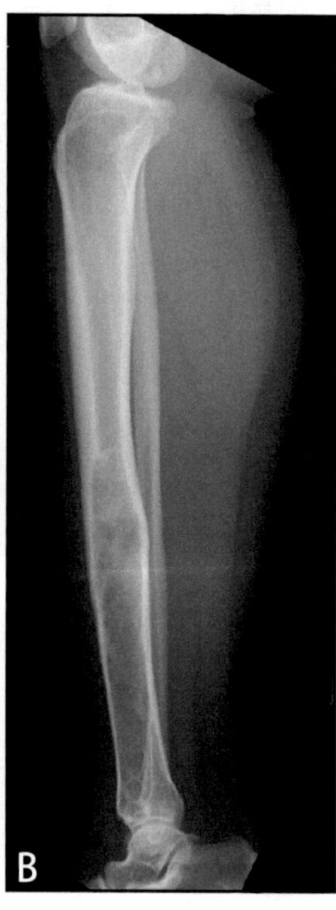

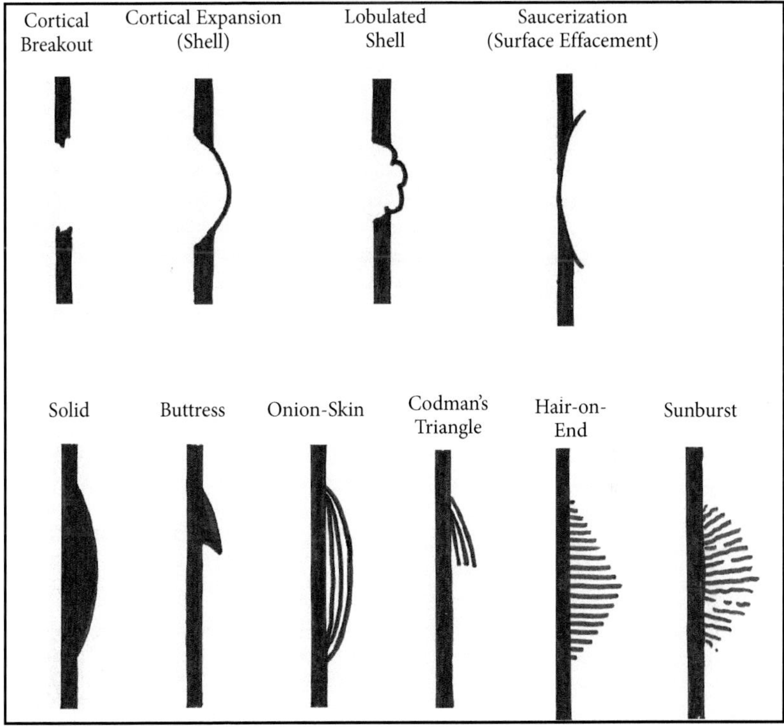

Figure 3-6. Patterns of (top row) cortical changes and (bottom row) periosteal reactions. Cortical effacement and expansion may indicate a slower-growing, more indolent process. Periosteal bone formation outside of the cortex suggests a more aggressive process that has penetrated the cortex and elevated the periosteum.

permeative margins are suggestive of aggressive growth, and cannot differentiate between benign and malignant processes, but well-defined, geographic lesions with a sclerotic rim are almost always benign[2] (Figures 3-6 and 3-7).

What should be apparent above is the considerable information that can be gleaned from an accurately interpreted radiograph. After correlation to the patient's age and clinical symptoms, the clinician should now have a clearer idea of the relative activity or aggressiveness of the lesion, and the most likely diagnoses. With exceptions, well-defined lesions that do not violate the cortex tend to be benign diagnoses, whereas ill-defined, destructive lesions with associated periosteal changes and soft-tissue extension are more commonly aggressive malignancies. Once the benign vs malignant assessment is judged, any further work-up at this point, if indicated, can proceed with the intent of confirming the suspected diagnosis, rather than exploring broader classes of disease without a clear direction. Advanced imaging modalities should be thought of in this context as confirmatory tests.

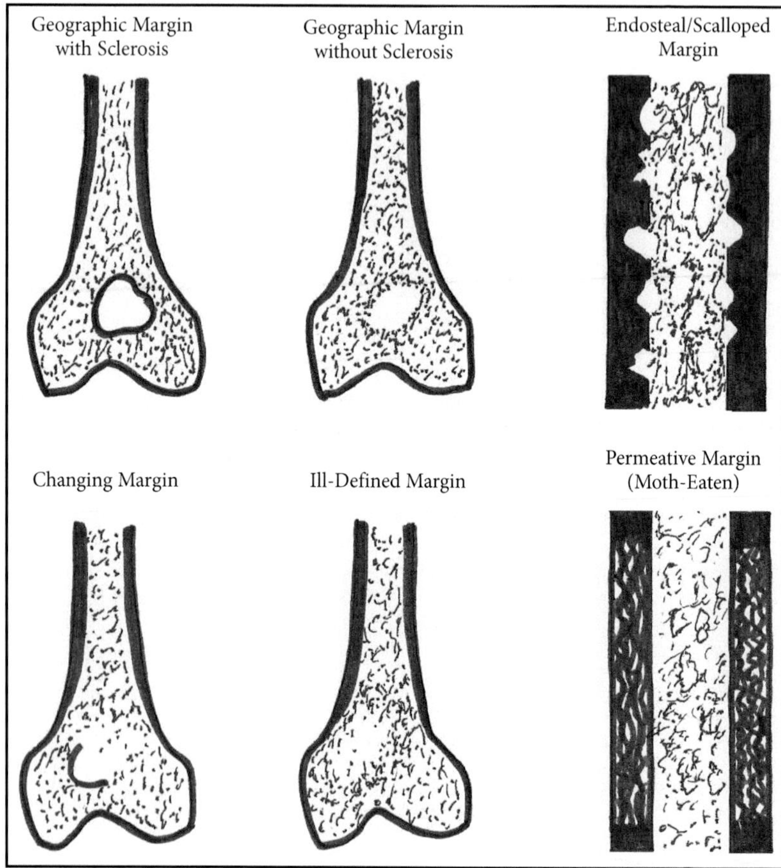

Figure 3-7. Intramedullary margins are described as well-defined (geographic), ill-defined, or changing/transitional. Surrounding sclerosis, when present, is more reassuring for a benign or indolent process. Scalloped margins indicate cortical effacement at the endosteal surface of the cortex. Permeative or moth-eaten patterns of destruction suggest aggressive tunneling through the cortex.

Computed Tomography

The computed tomography (CT) scan can be considered a high-resolution x-ray, capable of providing 3D imaging based on the relative densities of tissues. CT provides the finest detail of bone and other mineralized tissue, which is most helpful in musculoskeletal imaging when plain radiographs are unable to provide a comprehensive representation of the lesion in question. The corollary to this means that the CT is not necessary when plain radiographs are diagnostic.

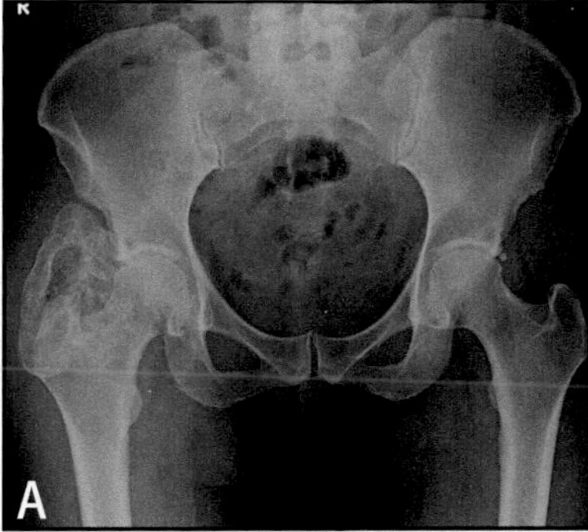

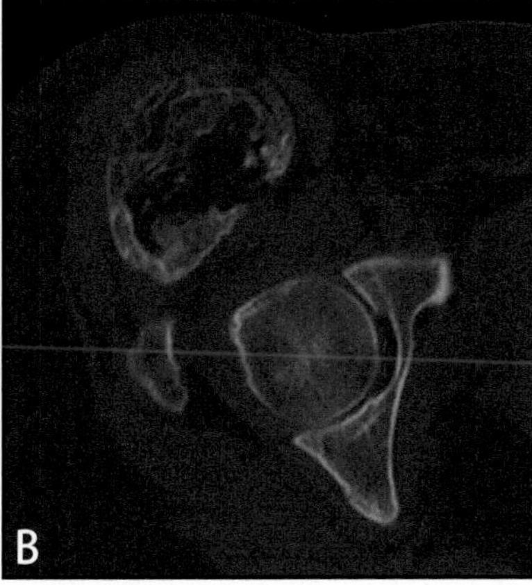

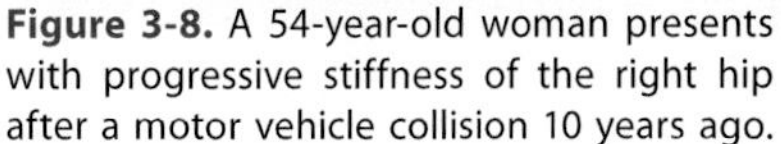

Figure 3-8. A 54-year-old woman presents with progressive stiffness of the right hip after a motor vehicle collision 10 years ago. (A) Anteroposterior radiograph and (B) axial CT demonstrate a soft-tissue mass composed of normal-appearing bone, with a mature periphery and fatty conversion within the center. This appearance is diagnostic of myositis ossificans.

Advantages of Computed Tomography

- Fast study: useful for claustrophobic patients
- More cost-efficient than magnetic resonance imaging (MRI) or nuclear medicine
- Can be combined with angiography to determine location of major blood vessels
- Quick thoracic and abdominopelvic staging of suspected malignancy

Disadvantages of Computed Tomography

- Ionizing radiation
- Less soft-tissue detail than MRI

Clinical Indications for Computed Tomography of Musculoskeletal Lesions

- Evaluating tumors in complex anatomic locations such as the spine, scapula, and pelvis, where overlapping structures can make plain radiographic evaluation challenging
- Evaluation of soft-tissue structures and mineralized soft-tissue lesions (Figure 3-8)
- Detailed evaluation of bony destruction and margins (Figure 3-9)

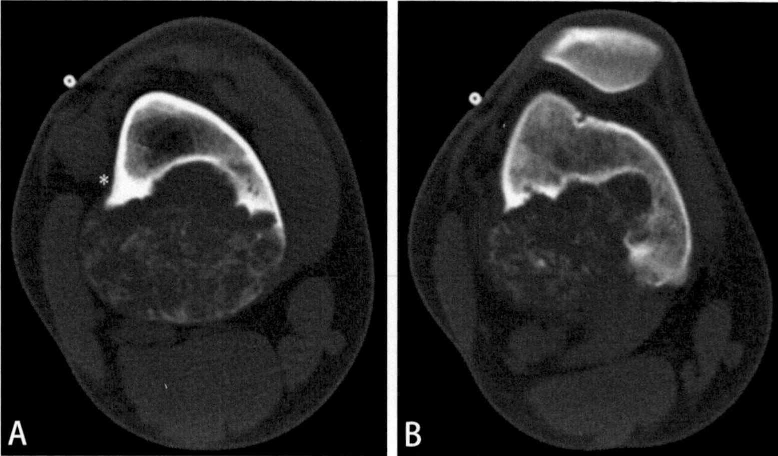

Figure 3-9. A 17-year-old boy presents with painless but diminished range of motion of the right knee. Axial CT demonstrates a lesion of the posterior distal femur with mineralization consistent with chondroid matrix. The periosteal buttress formation (white asterisk), well-defined geographic margin, and sclerotic boundary between the lesion and normal bony trabecular markings, confirming this lesion as a benign, surface-based periosteal chondroma with saucerization/effacement of the bone, and excludes the more serious diagnosis of chondroblastic osteosarcoma.

- Evaluation of lesional matrix
- Confirmation of suspected osteoid osteoma
- Preoperative planning/templating of resection
- Staging of malignant bone and soft-tissue tumors

CT is a density-based study, so lesions can be described as "radiolucent," "radiodense," or "radio-opaque" based on the attenuation of the x-ray beam through tissue. This is measured in Hounsfield units and can often be indicative of the type of tissue present within the lesion (Table 3-1).

Magnetic Resonance Imaging

The MRI can be a powerful diagnostic tool when ordered and interpreted appropriately, but can just as easily be a source of misdiagnosis or false confidence when the limitations of the study are not properly recognized. MR studies can provide outstanding detail of soft-tissue structures, delineate the relationship between tumors and neurovascular structures, specify a tissue type, and identify satellite lesions that may be indistinct on other imaging modalities. When combined with gadolinium contrast, MRI can help

Table 3-1

Hounsfield Measurements of Different Materials on Computed Tomography

MATERIAL	HU (APPROXIMATE OR WEIGHTED AVERAGE)
Air	−1,000
Fat (well-differentiated)	−105
Bodily fluids	0 to 30
Hemorrhage/Hematoma	40 to 100
Skeletal muscle	40
Soft-Tissue/Unmineralized tumor	100 to 300
Cancellous bone	350
Cortical bone	1,800
Foreign body (glass/rocks)	2,500
Metal	15,000+
Adapted from Feeman TG.[3]	

differentiate between posttreatment changes and recurrent/residual tumor for cancer restaging.

Advantages of Magnetic Resonance Imaging

- No ionizing radiation (preferable in children)
- Excellent soft-tissue imaging: strongly preferred for soft-tissue tumors
- Can be combined with angiography to determine location of major blood vessels
- Can be combined with contrast imaging to differentiate cystic lesions or fluid collections from solid tumor
- Accurate local staging of bone and soft-tissue malignancies
- Accurate, determinate diagnosis of lipomatous lesions, hemangiomata, and synovial proliferative tumors
- Most sensitive local restaging of soft-tissue sarcoma

Disadvantages of Magnetic Resonance Imaging

- Magnet-sensitive implants preclude many patients from undergoing MRI
- More expensive than other imaging modalities
- Slow and time-consuming study for patient
- Contained tubes may exacerbate claustrophobia
- Metallic artifact more difficult to suppress than CT, obscures structures and limits study

Clinical Indications for Magnetic Resonance Imaging of Musculoskeletal Lesions

- Evaluating tumors of or involving soft tissue
- Evaluation of intra-articular tumors
- Evaluation of cystic or fluid-containing lesions
- Preoperative planning of biopsy and resection
- Initial staging of malignant bone and soft-tissue tumors
- Postoperative staging of malignant bone or soft-tissue tumors

Interpreting Magnetic Resonance Imaging

MR uses magnetic fields to generate and receive radiofrequency energy, most often from hydrogen atoms that are particularly abundant in water and fat. By measuring the MR signal while adjusting the repetition time (TR) and echo time (TE), different materials can be weighted differently on a sequence. There are many methods for which MRI can be adjusted for different imaging purposes, but the main musculoskeletal sequences with which to become familiar are the traditional spin-echo sequences T1, T2, and proton density (Table 3-2). The T1 sequence is often called the "anatomy sequence" because the natural fat planes between muscles, compartments, and neurovascular structures make distinguishing anatomic boundaries easier. The T2 sequence is often called the "pathology sequence" because fluid from trauma, infection, or tumors is brighter and brought into better resolution.

Helpful Tip

A quick and easy way to determine whether the sequence is more fat sensitive (T1) or fluid sensitive (T2) is to glance at the TR value. A TR value between 400 and 900 is typically more T1 weighted. A TR value in the thousands is typically more T2 weighted.

Table 3-2

Appearance of Different Tissues on Magnetic Resonance Imaging Sequences

TISSUE TYPE	T1 SEQUENCE (ANATOMY STUDY) SHORT TR AND TE	T2 SEQUENCE (PATHOLOGY STUDY) LONG TR AND TE	T1 WITH FAT-SUPPRESSION SHORT TR AND TE
Fat (well-differentiated)	High	Low	Low
Fluid • Edema • Myxoid tissue	Low	High	Low
Tumor	Intermediate to low	High	With contrast: high Without contrast: intermediate to low
Hemorrhage	Acute: low Subacute: high Chronic: low	Acute: high	Low
Air	Low	Low	Low
Skeletal muscle	Intermediate	Intermediate	Intermediate
Paramagnetic contrast	High	Low	High
Fibrous tissue (ligament, tendon)	Very low	Very low	Very low
Bone/Mineralized tissue	Very low	Very low	Very low

Abbreviations: TE, echo time; TR, repetition time. (Adapted from Stark DD.[4])

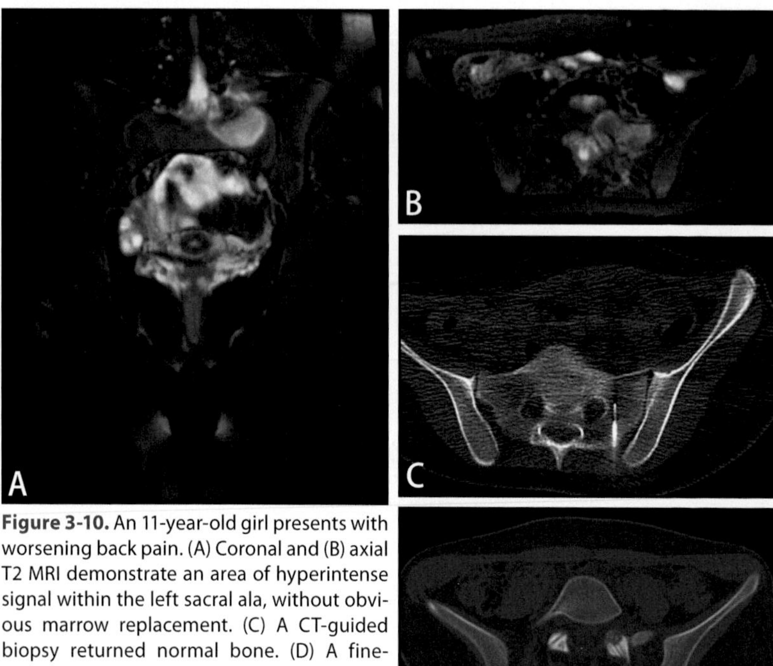

Figure 3-10. An 11-year-old girl presents with worsening back pain. (A) Coronal and (B) axial T2 MRI demonstrate an area of hyperintense signal within the left sacral ala, without obvious marrow replacement. (C) A CT-guided biopsy returned normal bone. (D) A fine-cut CT demonstrates a small, well-defined lucency with central ossification (nidus) in the superior articulating process of S1, confirmatory for osteoid osteoma.

Pitfalls of Imaging Musculoskeletal Tumors With Magnetic Resonance Imaging

- Lower size resolution than CT: MRI slices the area of interest into "cuts" averaging 5 mm to 7 mm or more. Lesions within this margin of measurement error (around 1 cm in size or less) can be missed entirely on MR (Figure 3-10)
- Fluid-containing lesions: Masses that are predominantly cystic, those with abundant high fluid signal, or those containing mostly blood products may be dismissed by an interpreter as benign cysts or hematomas if the imaging is not interpreted within the context of the clinical presentation of the patient. As discussed in Chapter 2, an MRI that does not demonstrate solid internal enhancement on postgadolinium imaging may provide false confidence of a benign diagnosis for an otherwise worrisome clinical entity (Figure 3-11)

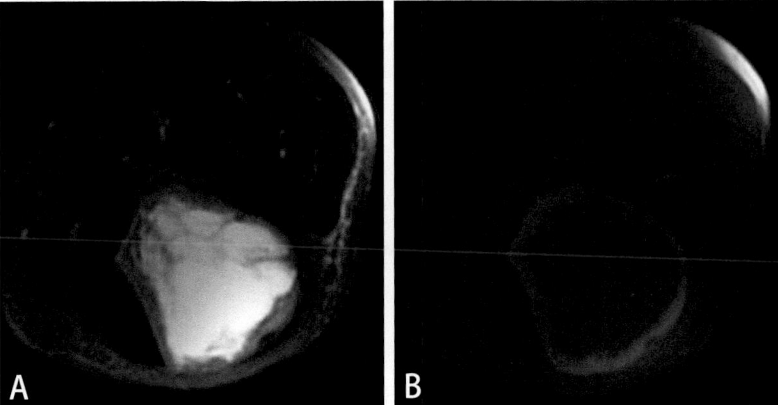

Figure 3-11. A 63-year-old man presents with a painful swelling in posterior aspect of the left thigh. (A) Axial T2 MRI demonstrates a large, complex fluid-filled mass within the biceps femoris muscle belly. (B) Fat-suppressed T1 MRI after administration of gadolinium contrast demonstrates a pattern of rim enhancement that can be mistaken for a benign cystic lesion without appropriate clinical correlation. The contrast pattern in this situation indicates that the most active tissue with the highest diagnostic yield for biopsy is at the periphery of the cystic cavity. Core-needle sampling confirmed the diagnosis of high-grade undifferentiated pleomorphic sarcoma with cystic degeneration.

- Bone lesions: It is tempting to obtain MRI for bony lesions because MR is often perceived as the "best" imaging study. This is far from accurate, and overdependence on MRI can be a source of misdiagnosis and lead to errors in management. Cortical destruction and periosteal changes may be subtle on MRI, and low-grade or heavily mineralized malignancies may be unimpressive on MR sequences. On the other side of the spectrum, occult trauma, overuse injuries, infections, and many benign bone lesions generate a substantial amount of intraosseous perilesional edema, which can appear alarming at first interpretation and generate panic, additional unnecessary testing, and anxiety-provoking referrals to oncologic specialists. Marrow edema can be distinguished from marrow-replacing lesions by the persistence of dark, speckled, trabecular markings within the area of interest (Figure 3-12). Not only should every imaging study be correlated to the patient's clinical symptoms, but it is essential practice that bony lesions be evaluated radiographically

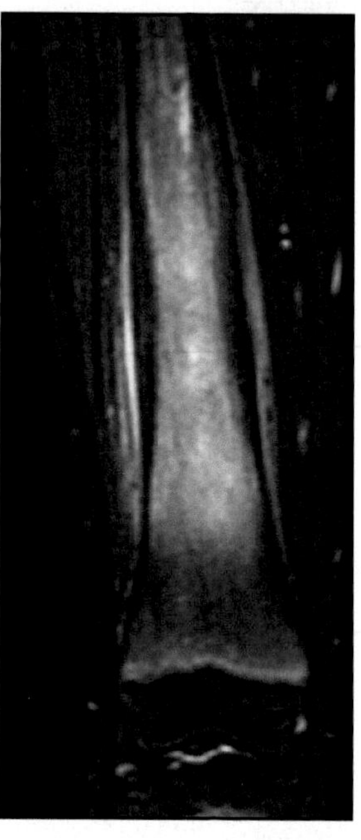

Figure 3-12. A 14-year-old girl presents with activity-related pain in the right thigh that is worse with sports participation. A MRI demonstrates a broad area of T2-hyperintense signal within the diaphysis of the distal femur, and she is promptly referred to an oncologic specialist. The MRI demonstrates symmetric cortical hyperostosis without periosteal reaction or soft-tissue extension. The fluid signal within the femur contains speckled, normal, trabecular markings and no evidence of marrow replacement. These findings are consistent with a stress fracture of the femur.

Important Lesson

Never interpret an MRI of a bone lesion without an x-ray or CT correlate.

When to Order Contrast

A common clinical scenario is that the patient returns after obtaining an MRI, only to find out that an indeterminate lesion was identified, and that the imaging interpreter has recommended additional sequences with administered contrast. When is it necessary to obtain a contrast-enhanced study? Strong indications for contrast include the following:

- Predominantly cystic or fluid-filled lesions
- Vascular lesions (Figure 3-13)
- Lesions identified in regions of trauma (fracture, muscle strain, post-surgery, etc)

However, as the treating clinician, one does not need to adhere to the dogma of always imaging lesions with contrast when the straightforward approach to ordering any additional testing is to determine whether such information is necessary to guide management and decision making. If the indication and location of a biopsy or resection is already determined, then contrast-enhanced sequences do not add value to the treating practitioner. If contrast can assist in identifying particular regions of a lesion that may be of

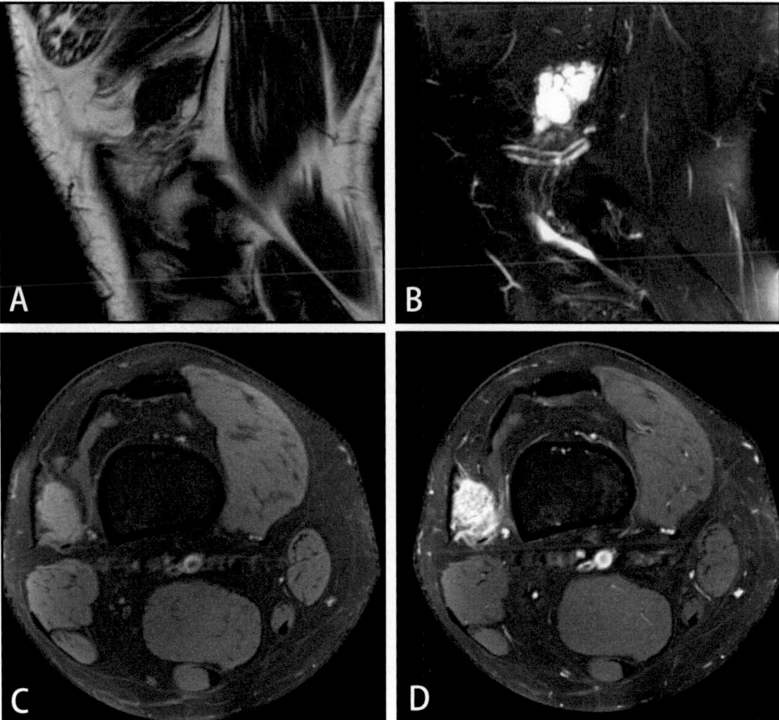

Figure 3-13. Sagittal (A) T1 and (B) T2 MRI demonstrate a lobular soft-tissue mass lateral to the right knee. Small streaks of fat between lobules are suggestive of hemangioma. Axial T1 fat-suppression sequences (C) before and (D) after administration of gadolinium contrast demonstrate significant internal enhancement consistent with a vascular malformation.

greater diagnostic yield for biopsy, if additional staging information can be obtained that will guide treatment, or if contrast enhancement can provide a definitive diagnosis that may obviate the need for biopsy, as in hemangioma, then it is appropriate to order contrast sequences. When in doubt, it is always acceptable to refer the patient to a musculoskeletal tumor specialist and allow the specialist to obtain any additional required studies.

Ultrasonography

Ultrasonic waves emitted from a probe echo off tissues of varying structure and density, which are then recorded and displayed as an image in real time. Though not often able to provide definitive imaging of musculoskeletal lesions, ultrasonography can be useful as an initial screening evaluation to determine the most appropriate subsequent testing, as a localizing tool for biopsy or excision, and occasionally as a restaging modality for superficial soft-tissue malignancies.[5]

Advantages of Ultrasonography

- No ionizing radiation, no side effects, no discomfort
- Can provide detail of cartilaginous skeletal structures in young children
- Inexpensive, easy to obtain
- Fast study, convenient for patient
- Useful for delineating solid from fluid-filled structures
- Renders "live" images, helpful for demonstrating blood flow or guiding biopsy/localizing needle placement

Disadvantages of Ultrasonography

- Unable to penetrate bone and other dense tissues: not helpful for bone lesions
- Depth-limited: may not image lesions deep to fascia or lesions in obese patients
- Operator dependent
- Orientation difficulty: no scout image from which to determine orientation of structures

Nuclear Scintigraphy

Technetium-99 bone scans (Tc-99) as well as positron emission tomography (PET) are "functional" studies that evaluate specific metabolic pathways through the uptake of a radiolabeled tracer. This uptake can be measured to determine the activity of the lesion or area in question. Nuclear medicine studies are helpful in the staging and surveillance of malignancy, for the assessment of treatment response within a lesion, and to assist in assessing the likelihood of malignancy when other imaging is equivocal.

Bone Scintigraphy

Tc-99m ("m" for medronic acid) is a phosphate derivative that is interchangeable with bone phosphate when taken up by activated osteoblasts. This tracer then localizes to areas of the skeleton under active turnover. Bone scans are therefore sensitive for sites of malignancy, and are useful as a

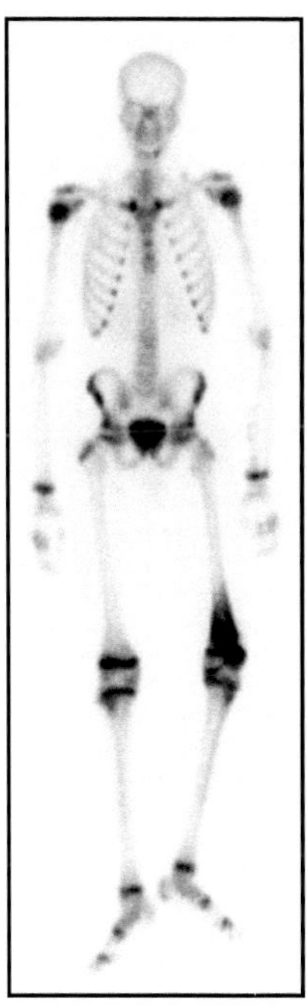

Figure 3-14. A 15-year-old boy with biopsy-proven osteosarcoma of the left distal femur undergoes technetium-99 total-body bone scintigraphy for staging. The primary tumor demonstrates significant activity, and no sites of synchronous skeletal metastases are demonstrated. There is normal uptake observed in the physeal plates. When uptake values are not provided, the area of the skeleton closest to the receiver, typically the anterior superior iliac spine or posterior superior iliac spine, can be used as an internal control to compare with the region of interest.

cost-efficient survey of the skeleton in the setting of metastatic bone disease. This comes at the expense of study sensitivity because the bone scan will also demonstrate activity within acute or healed fractures, infections, open growth plates, and degenerative joint disease (Figure 3-14). Therefore, when used to evaluate indeterminate or equivocal bone lesions, Tc-99m is reassuring only when activity is absent.

Potential Pitfall

Bone scintigraphy may be negative when the underlying process prevents osteoblast activation, typically when the lesion is so predominantly lytic that healing and remodeling of the lesion is not possible. Myeloma and aggressive malignancies such as metastatic lung and renal carcinoma may be deceptively "cold" on bone scan.

Positron Emission Tomography

Radiolabeled 18F-fluorodeoxyglucose (FDG) localizes to areas of active glucose consumption. The emitted radiation is reported as a standardized uptake value (SUV), which can be used to compare the lesion or area of

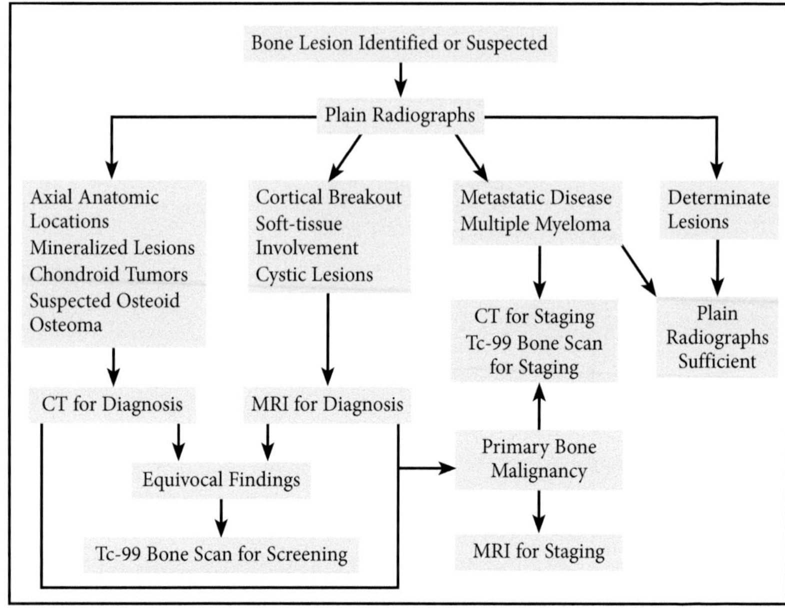

Figure 3-15. Algorithm for appropriate imaging of bone tumors. CT, computed tomography; MRI, magnetic resonance imaging; Tc-99m, technetium-99.

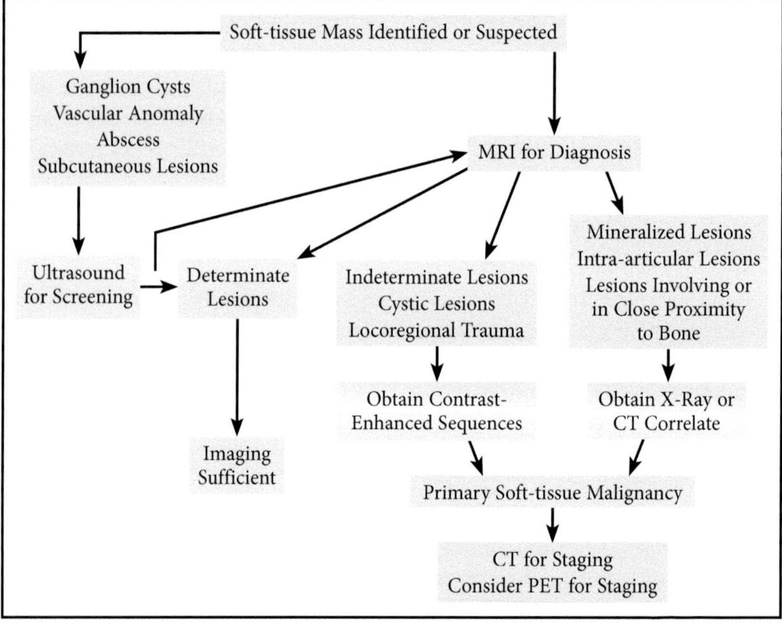

Figure 3-16. Algorithm for appropriate imaging of soft-tissue tumors. CT, computed tomography; PET, positron emission tomography.

interest with normal surrounding tissues. Cutoff values do vary widely, but an SUV below 3 is more reassuring of a benign process, and an SUV greater than 6 is more suspicious for malignancy. This has been used to differentiate benign tumors from malignant transformations in some patients with tumorigenic disorders such as neurofibromatosis, but the clinical utility of PET for solitary lesions is limited; PET studies are notoriously expensive, and their availability is often limited to patients with a proven diagnosis of malignancy.[6] Most PET studies are obtained for the staging of a newly diagnosed malignancy, for the assessment of treatment response during therapy, and for surveillance of high-risk diseases after treatment.

It is important that imaging studies be ordered for specific diagnostic and treatment purposes, and that ordering providers are aware of the advantages and limitations of specific imaging modalities. Figures 3-15 and 3-16 depict algorithms for ordering imaging studies for bone and soft-tissue tumors, respectively.

Take-Aways

1. Plain radiographs provide a wealth of diagnostic information at modest expense and should be considered a first-line tool for the evaluation of any new lesion.
2. CT is a high-resolution x-ray, helpful for complex anatomy and mineralized lesions. It is the study of choice for diagnosis of osteoid osteoma and cartilage tumors.
3. MRI is the modality of choice for soft-tissue structures but must be correlated with an x-ray–based study for bony lesions. It is the study of choice for imaging of the bone marrow.
4. Nuclear scintigraphy is most frequently used in staging and surveillance of malignancy but can be useful in the evaluation of indeterminate lesions.

Commonly Tested Topics for Trainees

- Well-defined lesions without extensive bony destruction or periosteal reaction are more likely to be benign entities.
- Fine-cut CT is the study of choice to identify a suspected osteoid osteoma.
- Myeloma is often cold on bone scintigraphy.

References

1. Sanders TG, Parsons TW III. Radiographic imaging of musculoskeletal neoplasia. *Cancer Control.* 2001;8(3):221-231. doi:10.1177/107327480100800302.
2. Lodwick GS, Wilson AJ, Farrell C, Virtama P, Dittrich F. Determining growth rates of focal lesions of bone from radiographs. *Radiology.* 1980;134(3):577-583. doi:10.1148/radiology.134.3.6928321.
3. Feeman TG. *The Mathematics of Medical Imaging: A Beginner's Guide.* 2nd ed. Cham, Switzerland: Springer; 2015.
4. Stark DD, Bradley WG, eds. *Magnetic Resonance Imaging.* 3rd ed. St Louis, MO: Elsevier; 1999:43-69.
5. Dangoor A, Seddon B, Gerrand C, Grimer R, Whelan J, Judson I. UK guidelines for the management of soft tissue sarcomas. *Clin Sarcoma Res.* 2016;6:20. doi:10.1186/s13569-016-0060-4.
6. Bredella MA, Torriani M, Hornicek F, et al. Value of PET in the assessment of patients with neurofibromatosis type 1. *AJR Am J Roentgenol.* 2007;189(4):928-935. doi:10.2214/AJR.07.2060.

4

Biopsy

Overview

The accurate diagnosis of a musculoskeletal lesion is made when the clinical, imaging, and histopathologic findings are concordant. We will discuss the ways in which tissue can be obtained for diagnosis and how to avoid mistakes in obtaining tissue. We will discuss the benefits and pitfalls for various methods of biopsy.

For the majority of tumors that cannot be definitively identified on clinical examination or imaging, a capably performed biopsy to establish a diagnosis is essential. Obtaining tissue for diagnosis can seem straightforward, but without appropriate planning for tissue handling and subsequent surgical treatment, avoidable errors in diagnosis and management are common. More than 90% of patients with primary musculoskeletal malignancies can be managed with effective limb salvage treatments, and the biopsy should be thought of as the first stage of limb salvage. However, an ill-advised or improperly executed biopsy can compromise bone, skin, and soft tissues, which can alter appropriate treatment, lead to more morbid surgical procedures, or necessitate an otherwise avoidable amputation.[1] The adverse effect on functional and oncologic outcomes is substantially higher when the biopsy is not performed by or directed by the practitioner providing definitive treatment to the patient, so it should not be considered a courtesy to perform a biopsy prior to referral to a treating institution.[2] Therefore it is strongly encouraged that any musculoskeletal lesion in need of a biopsy be referred

Wallace, MT
Handbook of Musculoskeletal Tumors (pp 49-57).

to a practitioner with the skill and comfort in the definitive treatment of the lesion in consideration, before tissue sampling is performed.

Prebiopsy Planning

Once a lesion has been evaluated and imaged and a biopsy is determined to be necessary, the appropriate method and approach to the lesion must be thoughtfully planned. Prebiopsy imaging must be sufficient to localize the tumor, identify its relationship to critical structures, and identify the approach that maximizes diagnostic yield while minimizing contamination and reducing adverse effects on treatment and patient outcome. This is best accomplished with an imaging modality that provides resolution in the axial plane. Such imaging can further identify areas that may provide more reliably diagnostic tissue; cystic, necrotic, and hemorrhagic zones within a mass are less likely to contain diagnostic tissue compared with solid, nodular, contrast-enhancing zones. A bone tumor with soft-tissue extension is best biopsied at the extraosseous component.

Principles of Biopsy

- A biopsy site must be chosen with the possibilities for definitive treatment in mind, typically in line with the incision one would use for a radical surgical resection (Table 4-1).
- The biopsy approach must minimize contamination of uninvolved compartments and structures that would not otherwise require resection. Biopsy approaches that expose nerves, vessels, intermuscular intervals, or joints are to be avoided.
- Incisions for biopsies should be oriented longitudinally so that subsequent en bloc resection of the biopsy tract can be performed and primary wound closure is possible. Transverse incisions often require skin grafting, tissue rearrangement, or flap coverage.
- For bone biopsies, it is essential to minimize the risk of postbiopsy fracture, and the risk of fracture must be discussed with the patient. Sample any soft-tissue component preferentially. For intramedullary sampling, the biopsy hole must be round or oval, and may be plugged with methyl methacrylate cement at the discretion of the surgeon. Weight-bearing restrictions for a few weeks postbiopsy may be appropriate. For high-risk lesions, particularly in the pediatric population, protective casting may be warranted.
- Meticulous hemostasis must be obtained. Postbiopsy bleeding can contaminate adjacent structures and compromise limb salvage. For

Table 4-1

Common Biopsy Approaches to Long-Bone Tumors

LOCATION	APPROACH	CONTAMINATED COMPARTMENT
Clavicle	Anterior, superior	Trapezius
Proximal humerus	Direct anterior	Anterior third deltoid
Humeral shaft/distal humerus	Anterolateral	Lateral biceps
Ulna	Direct ulnar	None/Extensor carpi ulnaris
Radius	Dorsoradial	Extensor carpi radialis brevis
Pelvis	Superior (ilioinguinal line)	Tensor fasciae
Proximal femur/femoral shaft	Direct lateral	Vastus lateralis
Distal femur	Anteromedial, anterolateral, or direct lateral	Vastus medialis or vastus lateralis
Tibia	Direct anterior, anteromedial	None (skin)
Fibula	Direct lateral	Peroneus longus/brevis

percutaneous sampling techniques, direct pressure must be held at the biopsy site twice as long as the clinician feels is appropriate (recommend at least 5 minutes). Other methods include:

- Preoperative embolization for high-risk or vascular tumors
- Local hemostatic matrix such as thrombin
- Open cautery or beam coagulation of bleeding surfaces
- Drain placement: the egress should be distal, in-line with the incision, and close to the end of the incision for later excision
- Methyl methacrylate plug or bone wax for bony openings

Needle Techniques

Percutaneous needle sampling is the most frequently employed method of obtaining tissue for diagnosis, with several advantages over open surgical biopsy. When combined with image guidance, percutaneous sampling can provide accurate diagnostic information in more than 90% of cases.[3]

Advantages of Percutaneous Biopsy

- Less invasive = less bleeding, less contamination
- Lower risk of postbiopsy infection or wound complication
- Decreased cost (local anesthetic, in-office procedure)
- Does not delay neoadjuvant treatment (radiation, chemotherapy) after diagnosis
- Able to sample different regions of heterogeneous lesions through same site
- More reliable localization for deeper lesions or lesions within complex anatomic locations

Disadvantages of Percutaneous Biopsy

- Smaller tissue quantity = lower diagnostic yield compared with open biopsy
- Risk of inadvertent injury to vital structures and uncontrolled bleeding

Fine-Needle Aspiration

Fine-needle aspiration (FNA) is a percutaneous sampling technique that uses small-gauge needles to sample cells within a lesion, which are then smeared and interpreted by a cytopathologist. This is the least invasive method of biopsy, quick and easy to perform, and commonly employed for tumors of endothelial or hematological origins and for confirmation of metastasis. There are several downsides to this technique, chief among them the paucity of material that can be obtained, which is often inadequate for immunohistochemical staining or cytogenetic evaluation. Furthermore, the lack of tissue architecture provided by FNA places increased reliance on the capabilities of the interpreting cytopathologist. For most primary musculoskeletal lesions, greater tissue sampling is required. FNA is therefore most valuable for confirming an infection, ganglion cyst, or suspected metastasis or recurrence of a known high-grade malignancy. FNA is not often helpful for low-grade tumors.

Core-Needle Sampling

Core-needle biopsy has the advantages of the availability and ease of FNA, but provides greater tissue sampling by obtaining a plug of solid tissue with a large-gauge needle. The preserved tissue architecture is generally adequate for specialized stains and studies (Figure 4-1).

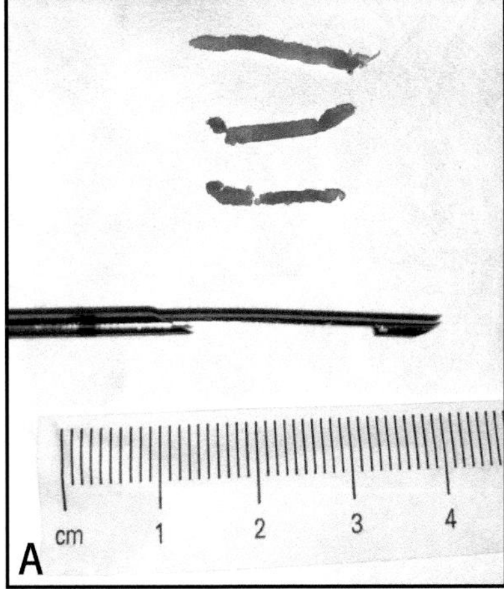

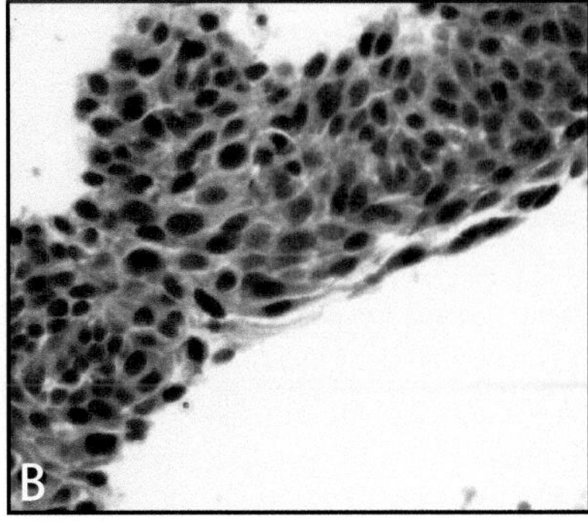

Figure 4-1. A 14G biopsy needle has a penetrating beveled end and a 20 mm open chamber for the specimen, which is captured by a beveled cutting sleeve. Cores can be up to (A) 2 mm in thickness and (B) better preserve tissue architecture compared with fine-needle aspiration.

Important: if the patient is referred to a percutaneous interventionalist for image-guided tissue sampling, the biopsy approach and subsequent tissue handling must be directed by the treating clinician and must adhere to the principles above. This requires close collaboration and communication between the individual performing the biopsy, the pathologist, and the patient care team to prevent diagnostic or treatment errors.

Surgical Biopsy

The gold standard for diagnostic yield of musculoskeletal lesions remains open surgical biopsy, even though it is not preferred over percutaneous sampling techniques. Surgical biopsy requires great care and adherence to the above principles to ensure that more aggressive tissue sampling does not compromise the functional or oncologic outcome of the patient.

Indications for Surgical Biopsy

- Percutaneous sampling nondiagnostic
- Lesions too small for accurate needle sampling
- Lesions involving or in proximity to critical neurovascular structures
- Patient unable to tolerate biopsy while conscious
- A secondary procedure is planned simultaneously (stabilization of bone or central venous catheter/port placement) after the diagnosis is made with some certainty and tissue is needed for confirmation

Incisional Biopsy

An intralesional surgical biopsy is performed via direct exposure of the tumor and removal of a portion of the mass. This provides significantly more tissue for diagnosis at the expense of increased local tissue contamination and a necessary delay in neoadjuvant therapies until the biopsy wound heals. This should be planned and performed by experienced clinicians, and it is recommended that an intraoperative "frozen section" pathology consultation be obtained prior to wound closure to confirm the adequacy of the biopsy via the presence of representative lesional tissue.[4]

Excisional Biopsy

Complete sampling of the lesion by primary excision is a "shoot first, ask questions later" approach that should be reserved for very specific cases. A marginal excision risks undertreatment of the lesion should the lesion prove to be malignant, and a wide or radical excision risks a more extensive or morbid procedure than is necessary if the lesion is benign. For malignant tumors that require adjuvant treatments, the absence of measurable disease renders the clinician unable to assess the efficacy of any therapy.

Relative Indications for Primary Excisional Biopsy

- Known, determinate benign lesions
- Well-differentiated lipomatous tumors (Figure 4-2). There is considerable sampling error with percutaneous biopsy of well-differentiated fatty lesions. Complete sampling is often required to differentiate benign lipomas from atypical lipomatous tumors[5]
- Small subcutaneous lesions
- Tumors for which obtaining a wide surgical margin can be performed without significant additional morbidity (Figure 4-3)

Specimen Handling

After tissue is obtained, it must be handled and processed appropriately so that specialized testing can be performed in addition to traditional hematoxylin and eosin staining. Direct communication with the pathologist before and after tissue sampling is helpful to ensure that biopsy material is not processed in a way that prevents required testing. For example, flow cytometry, cytogenetics, and other diagnostics may require tissue to be processed fresh or in specific solution. A touch preparation or separation of soft tissue from calcified lesions may be recommended before a

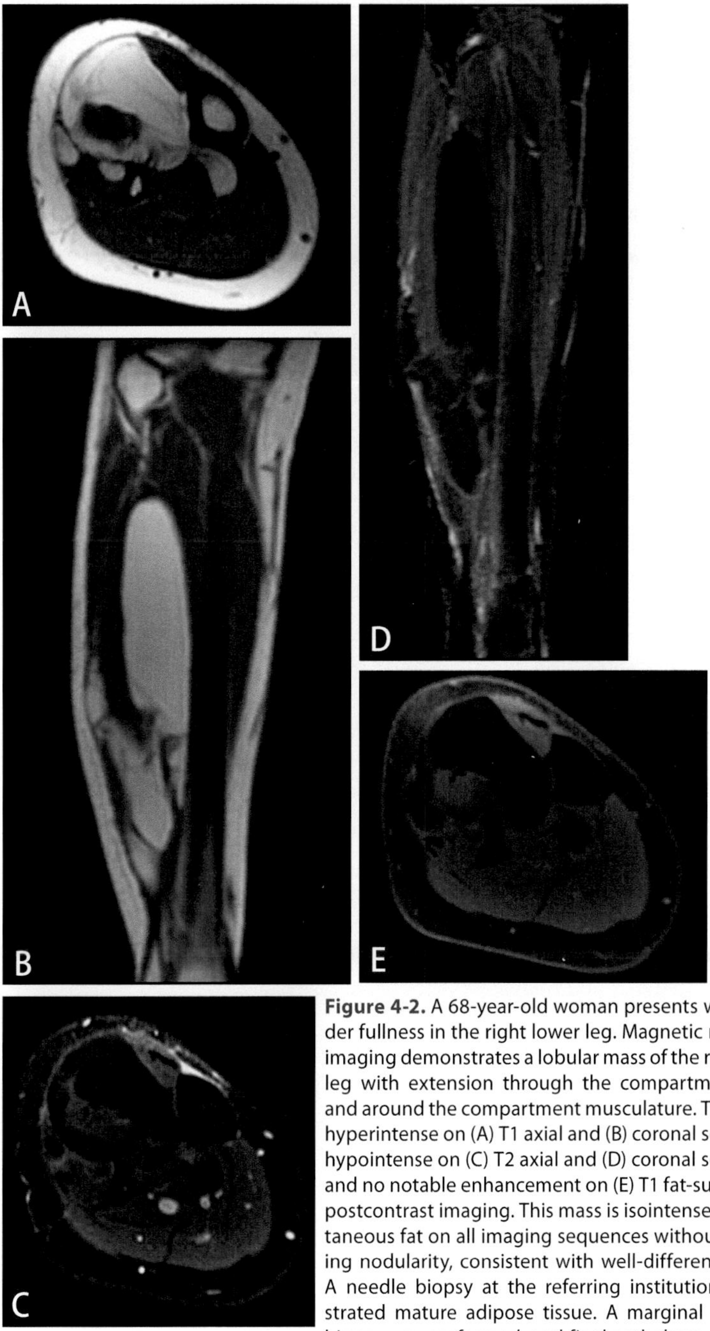

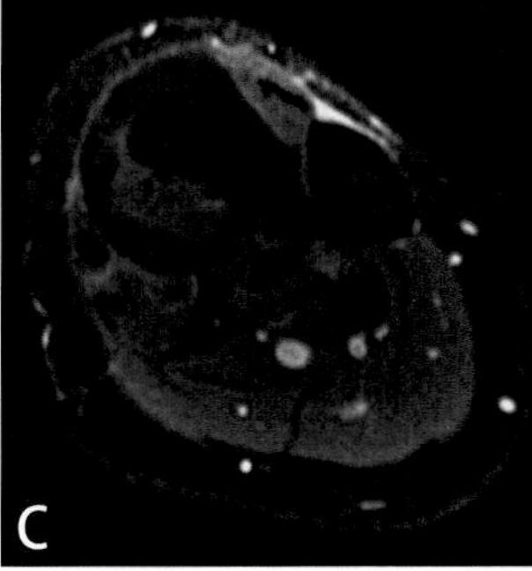

Figure 4-2. A 68-year-old woman presents with a tender fullness in the right lower leg. Magnetic resonance imaging demonstrates a lobular mass of the right lower leg with extension through the compartment fascia and around the compartment musculature. The mass is hyperintense on (A) T1 axial and (B) coronal sequences, hypointense on (C) T2 axial and (D) coronal sequences, and no notable enhancement on (E) T1 fat-suppression postcontrast imaging. This mass is isointense to subcutaneous fat on all imaging sequences without enhancing nodularity, consistent with well-differentiated fat. A needle biopsy at the referring institution demonstrated mature adipose tissue. A marginal excisional biopsy was performed, and final pathology confirmed diagnosis of atypical lipomatous tumor.

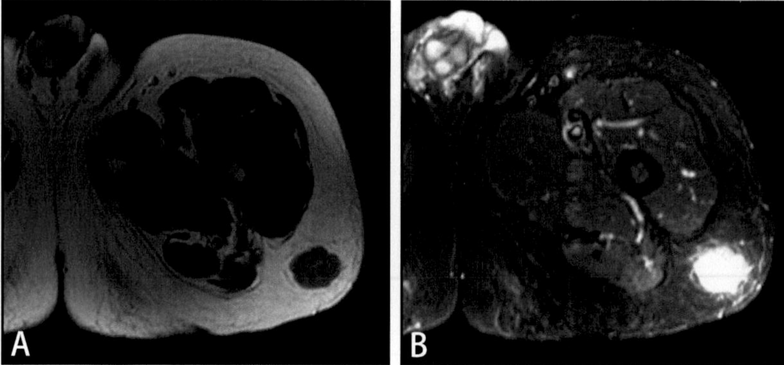

Figure 4-3. A 61-year-old man presents with a painless, enlarging mass over the lateral left hip. Magnetic resonance imaging demonstrates a subcutaneous mass with (A) intermediate signal on T1 and (B) increased signal on T2. A percutaneous core-needle sampling was performed, demonstrating a spindle cell tumor with atypical features and uncertain malignant potential. A wide excisional biopsy was performed because of the ability to obtain a wide margin without significant morbidity. Final pathology confirmed a diagnosis of benign fibrous histiocytoma.

demineralizing soak, which can render tissue unfit for genetic or molecular testing. A frozen section consultation at the time of biopsy will facilitate this discussion and can provide preliminary diagnostic information to guide appropriate specimen handling. If unsure, tissue can always be submitted fresh for evaluation, provided that the processing will be performed imminently; fresh tissue will desiccate over a few hours and become worthless.[6]

It is also good practice to send tissue for microbiological culture if infection cannot be definitively excluded at the time of biopsy. In addition to commonly encountered pyogenic abscesses, atypical infections such as fungus, acid-fast bacilli, and parasites can present with clinical signs and imaging features mimicking neoplasm. An old adage is to “biopsy what you culture, and culture what you biopsy.”

Take-Aways

1. Biopsies must be planned and performed or directed by the clinician providing definitive treatment for the patient.
2. Percutaneous sampling is the preferred method of obtaining tissue for diagnosis, and core-needle biopsy is recommended for primary musculoskeletal tumors.

3. It never hurts to know the diagnosis before treatment. Excisional biopsies should be reserved for selected cases for which the risk to the patient is minimal.
4. A descriptive pathologic diagnosis in which the tissue and cells are described without a named diagnosis is insufficient for proceeding with treatment. These cases should be referred for an additional opinion or work-up to establish a firm diagnosis.[7]

Commonly Tested Topics for Trainees

- Biopsy incisions must be longitudinal and aligned with the approach of definitive resection.
- Postbiopsy hemorrhage or fracture can lead to extensive local contamination and require an otherwise avoidable amputation.
- Although open biopsy is associated with a higher diagnostic yield, percutaneous needle sampling techniques are preferred because of their lower cost and minimal invasiveness.

References

1. Mankin HJ, Lange TA, Spanier SS. The hazards of biopsy in patients with malignant primary bone and soft-tissue tumors. *J Bone Joint Surg Am.* 1982;64(8):1121-1127.
2. Mankin HJ, Mankin CJ, Simon MA. The hazards of biopsy, revisited. Members of the Musculoskeletal Tumor Society. *J Bone Joint Surg Am.* 1996;78(5):656-663. doi:10.2106/00004623-199605000-00004.
3. Welker JA, Henshaw RM, Jelinek J, Shmookler BM, Malawer MM. The percutaneous needle biopsy is safe and recommended in the diagnosis of musculoskeletal masses. *Cancer.* 2000;89(12):2677-2686. doi:10.1002/1097-0142(20001215)89:12<2677::aid-cncr22>3.0.co;2-l.
4. Ashford RU, Scolyer RA, McCarthy SW, Bonar SF, Karim RZ, Stalley PD. The role of intra-operative pathological evaluation in the management of musculoskeletal tumors. *Recent Results Cancer Res.* 2009;179:11-24.
5. Rougraff BT, Durbin M, Lawerence J, Buckwalter K. Histologic correlation with magnetic resonance imaging for benign and malignant lipomatous masses. *Sarcoma.* 1997;1(3-4):175-179. doi:10.1080/13577149778272.
6. McCarthy EF, Frassica FJ. Management of orthopaedic pathology specimens from the operating room to the microscope. In: McCarthy EF, Frassica FJ. *Pathology of Bone and Joint Disorders.* 1st ed. Philadelphia, PA: WB Saunders; 1998:365-371.
7. Sim FH, Frassica FJ, Frassica DA. Soft-tissue tumors: diagnosis, evaluation, and management. *J Am Acad Orthop Surg.* 1994;2(4):202-211. doi:10.5435/00124635-199407000-00003.

5

Tumor-Mimicking Lesions—Tumor Simulators

Overview

Tumor-mimicking lesions, also known as pseudotumors, are lesions that simulate a palpable or radiologic mass that may be confused with a primary tumor. We will discuss the broad classes of tumor mimicking disorders, how they present clinically, and how best to identify them so as to avoid misdiagnosis and mismanagement.

Many common non-neoplastic conditions will present as a mass or a radiographic finding with features concerning for a tumor. The indeterminate and overlapping radiographic appearances of neoplastic and non-neoplastic conditions often prompt extensive work-ups, referrals to an oncologic specialist, and significant anxiety for the patient and family. Although many tumor mimickers may not be straightforward to assess and the typical algorithms for indeterminate lesions should be used, failure to recognize a pseudotumor can occur because of several correctable tendencies among clinicians.

- Inadequate history-taking and/or physical examination: specific events around the time of tumor presentation should be carefully considered. Associated medical comorbidities should not be overlooked
- Inadequacy of imaging: as discussed in Chapter 3, misdiagnosis based on magnetic resonance imaging (MRI) without a plain radiograph to correlate is common, particularly for bone and joint lesions

Wallace, MT
Handbook of Musculoskeletal Tumors (pp 59-74).

- Emphasis on imaging over clinical presentation: a diagnosis made presumptively without clinical correlation can blind the practitioner to the correct diagnosis if it is never considered in the differential

The key to identifying tumor mimickers is always to start with a thorough history-taking and physical examination, with particular attention paid to the presenting symptomatology, associated medical conditions, medication use, and a detailed review of systems. Investigation can then proceed with an appropriate work-up that keeps specific categories of common mimickers in mind based on the clinical presentation of the patient. This can help the practitioner avoid falling into a "rabbit hole" of random testing, unnecessary imaging studies, and escalating diagnostic procedures. When recognized properly, the treatment of pseudotumors is often significantly different from neoplastic lesions. Surgical treatment, if required, is often drastically different from oncologic resection, many conditions are reversible with medical management, and still other lesions will not require any treatment at all.

Injury—Trauma and Degenerative Conditions

Acute trauma, hemorrhage, and the subsequent healing and reactive reparative processes can produce painful, mass-like lesions. A history of recent or remote trauma, anteceding pain prior to the presentation of the mass, or pain that is reproducible with activity, weight-bearing, or specific motor-unit testing is suspicious for a posttraumatic or reactive lesion.

Myositis Ossificans

Heterotopic bone or calcium formation within the soft tissues can follow direct trauma, surgical trauma, burns, or central nervous system injury, and in the case of calcific myonecrosis, an untreated disruption in tissue perfusion such as compartment syndrome or infarct. At early presentation, these lesions are often unmineralized, with an indeterminate and concerning appearance on MRI. When mature, these lesions are typically well defined with a mature mineralized periphery. When accurately recognized, these lesions require little more than reassurance in asymptomatic patients. If pain or mechanical symptoms are present that do not respond to conservative management, marginal excision can be considered. This should be followed with either an extended course of prostaglandin-inhibiting chemoprophylaxis (often indomethacin) or prophylactic radiotherapy (typically 500-800 cGy), as surgical trauma through the initial zone of injury can reactivate the initial reparative process.[1]

Stress Injuries

Overuse injuries can induce hyperostosis and periostitis of the bone, thickening and prominence of tendons, or widening, fragmentation, or calcification of the apophysis or tendon insertion in the skeletally immature patient. On MRI, there is often diffuse, poorly localized, substantial edema that can raise alarm for an infiltrative neoplasm. These are most easily recognized by a history consistent with overuse, as well as the lack of overt marrow replacement on imaging. These are best managed with cessation of the offending activity followed by rehabilitation to optimize mechanics. Stress fractures of a lower extremity may require restricted weight-bearing or prophylactic stabilization (Figure 5-1).

Muscle and Tendon Ruptures

The rapid appearance of a painful, ball-like mass in the soft tissue with or without anteceding trauma should be suspicious for an acute musculotendinous injury. Cramping pain that is worse with testing of the involved muscle unit is frequently present (Figure 5-2). Imaging appearances can vary widely because the imaging features of hemorrhage change with chronicity. Feathery edema in multiple compartments is suspicious for posttraumatic swelling. For hematomas, a clinical history of injury and/or bleeding diathesis should be present, otherwise a biopsy to rule out hemorrhagic soft-tissue malignancy is recommended. The risk of evacuating a hematoma for diagnostic purposes is far outweighed by the risk of a missed malignancy.

Ganglion Cyst/Geode

Soft-tissue and intraosseous cysts can form when degenerative, traumatic, or developmental changes within the joint allow an egress of fluid into the juxta-articular structures. These are common around the wrist and ankle, and should be considered for epiphyseal lesions associated with degenerative joint disease. Transillumination on physical examination, or aspiration of jelly-like clear material are diagnostic.

Infection

Infection is such a ubiquitous and effective mimicker of tumors that it should always be considered in the differential until actively excluded. Osteomyelitis can have sclerotic, lytic, or mixed appearances, may have geographic, ill-defined, or even permeative margins, and may demonstrate soft-tissue extension, periosteal reaction, or bone deformation. Marrow edema is

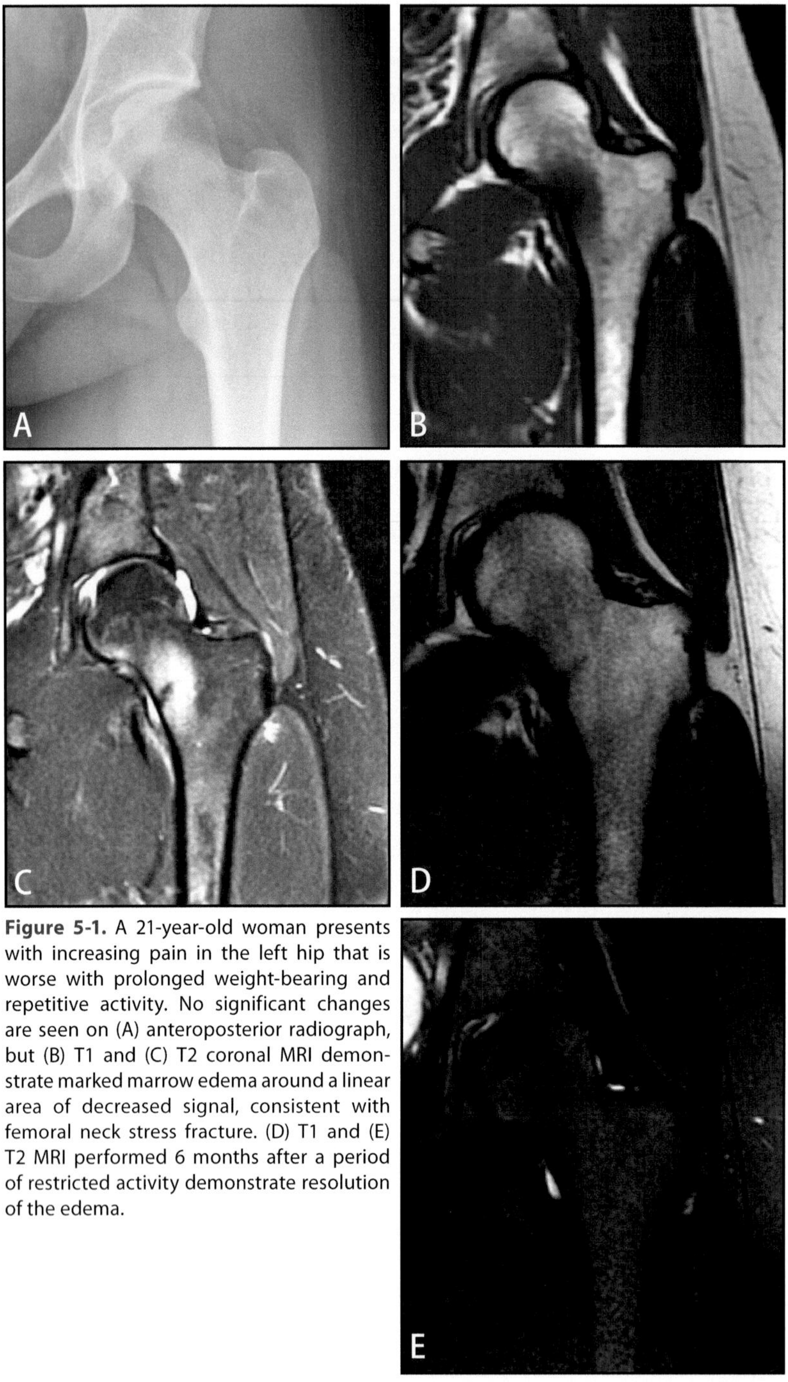

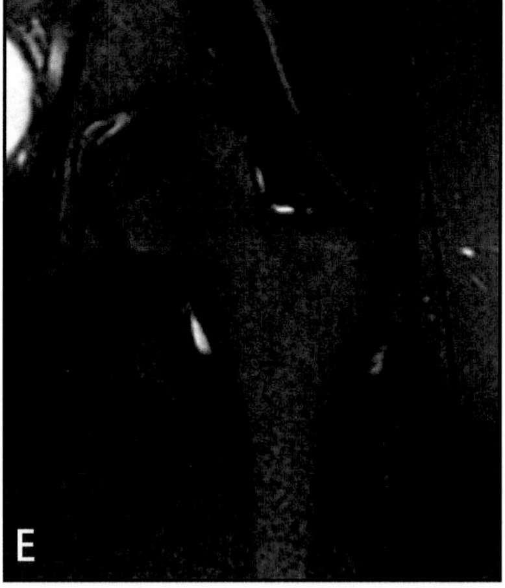

Figure 5-1. A 21-year-old woman presents with increasing pain in the left hip that is worse with prolonged weight-bearing and repetitive activity. No significant changes are seen on (A) anteroposterior radiograph, but (B) T1 and (C) T2 coronal MRI demonstrate marked marrow edema around a linear area of decreased signal, consistent with femoral neck stress fracture. (D) T1 and (E) T2 MRI performed 6 months after a period of restricted activity demonstrate resolution of the edema.

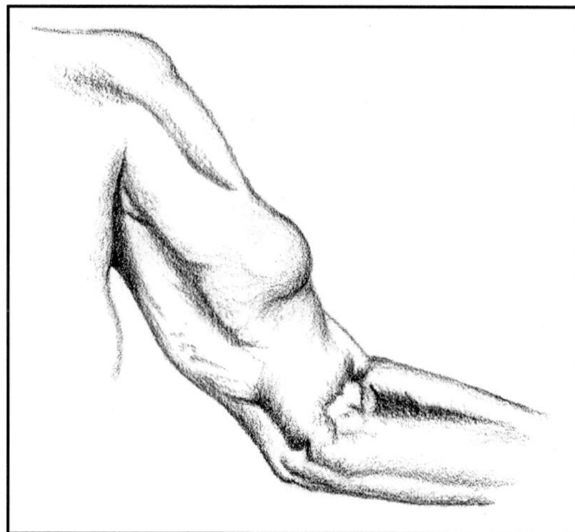

Figure 5-2. A popeye deformity is caused by an acute rupture of either the proximal or distal biceps tendon, with distal or proximal retraction of the muscle belly respectively, creating a large soft-tissue prominence.

often pronounced, without frank replacement or postcontrast enhancement. Appropriate management of osteomyelitis requires sequestrectomy, debridement of necrotic or devitalized tissue, and antimicrobial treatment based on the identification of the offending organism.

Pyogenic, or pus-producing infections are most commonly of bacterial origin and typically will present with deep bone pain, fever, localized tenderness, and elevated leukocyte count and inflammatory markers. A history of open wounds, penetrating trauma, recent dental procedures, or recent infections associated with bacteremia are suggestive of an infectious etiology.

Indolent, smoldering infections without substantial purulence is suggestive of lower-virulence organisms, and atypical organisms including fungus and acid-fast bacilli should be considered. Poor nutrition, immunosuppression, or travel to endemic zones should be investigated and identified.

A chronically draining or smoldering infection can drive dysplastic changes in surrounding tissues leading to malignant transformation. A change in pain or drainage should be investigated for underlying malignant transformation such as Marjolin squamous cell carcinoma.[2]

Vascular Disorders

The interruption of blood flow within the bone can produce dramatic imaging changes that may be mistaken for a primary or metastatic bone lesion. A history of trauma, alcohol abuse, long-term corticosteroid use, or other thrombogenic condition is often present. Juxta-articular

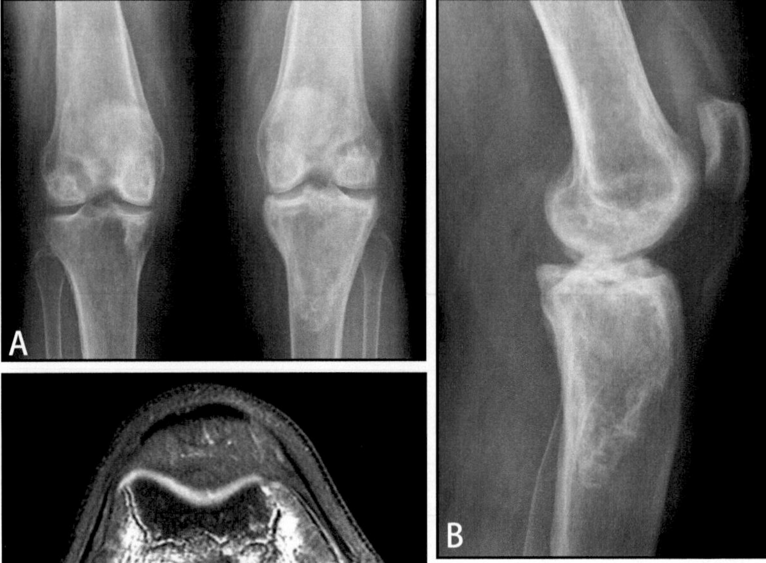

Figure 5-3. A 47-year-old woman with a history of substance abuse presents with progressive bilateral knee discomfort. (A) Anteroposterior and (B) lateral radiographs demonstrate multiple areas of irregular sclerosis. (C) T2 axial MRI shows multiple wedge-shaped lesions extending to subchondral bone, with paralleled lines of dark sclerotic bone and bright edema. This "double-line" sign is typical of osteonecrosis.

osteonecrosis characteristically produces wedge-shaped infarcts that extend to the subchondral bone, with softening and collapse of the joint in later stages. Metaphyseal infarcts are classically central, with a serpiginous appearance of parallel bands (Figure 5-3).

Transient osteoporosis is a painful condition associated with marked, diffuse hyperintensity of the bone marrow on MRI with normal radiographic and computed tomography findings at initial presentation, and subtle osteopenia in later stages (Figure 5-4). It is hypothesized that this is due to an interruption in intraosseous blood flow, with painful congestion within the marrow, due to an elevated risk of subsequent osteonecrosis. Another theory posits that transient osteoporosis is indicative of an occult subchondral fracture. Transient osteoporosis is most common in middle-aged men and

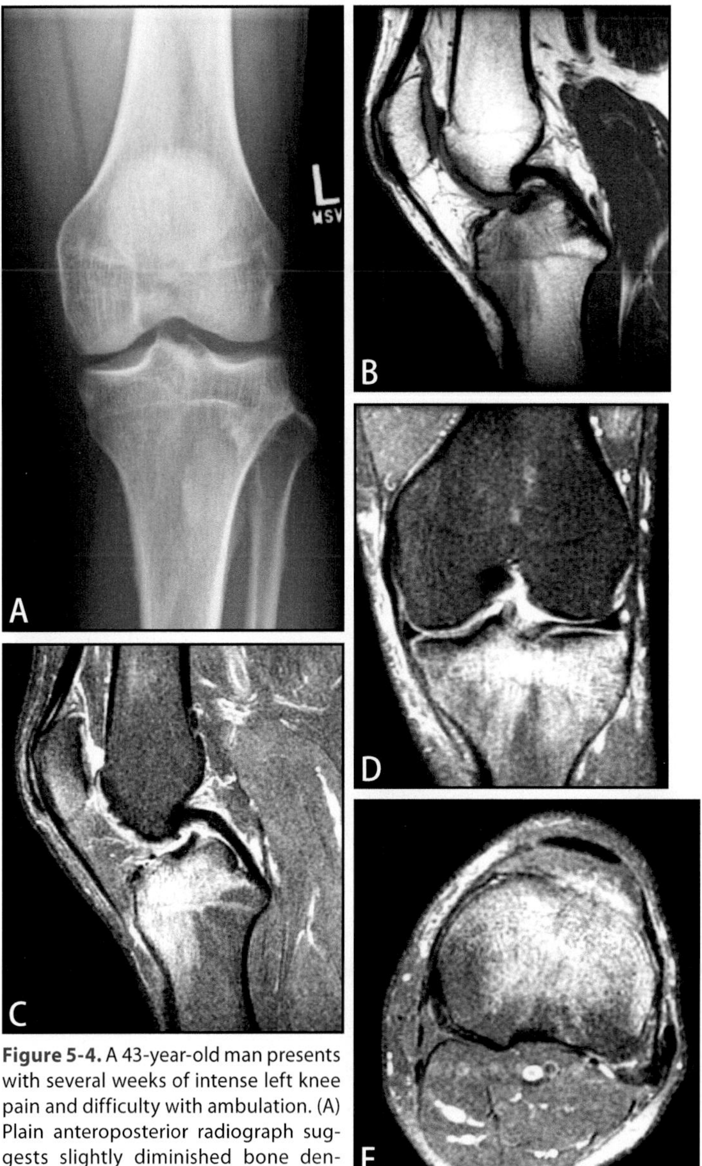

Figure 5-4. A 43-year-old man presents with several weeks of intense left knee pain and difficulty with ambulation. (A) Plain anteroposterior radiograph suggests slightly diminished bone density in the lateral proximal tibia without frank bony lysis. Sagittal (B) T1 and (C) T2, (D) coronal, and (E) axial MRI sequences demonstrate significant and diffuse marrow edema within the proximal tibia.

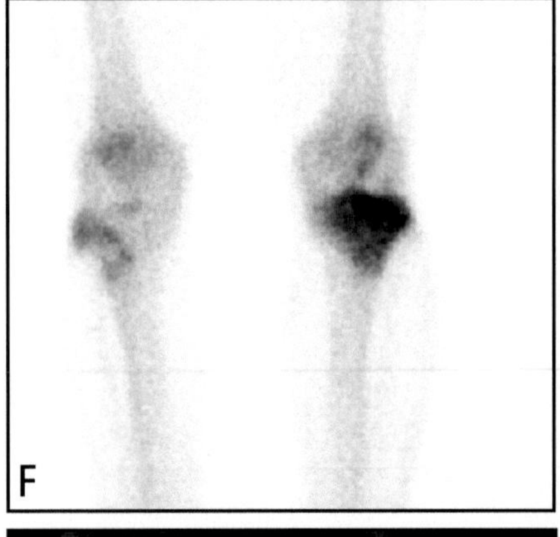

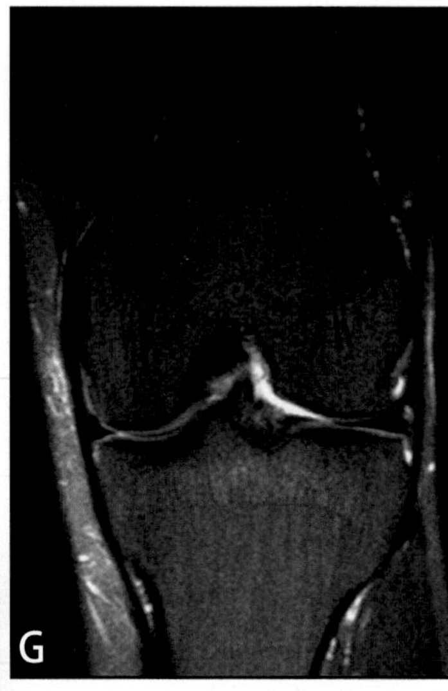

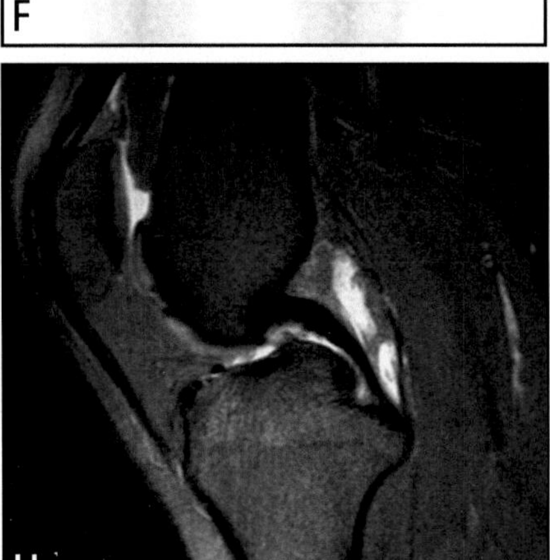

Figure 5-4 continued. A 43-year-old man presents with several weeks of intense left knee pain and difficulty with ambulation. (F) Bone scintigraphy shows diffuse intense uptake within the proximal tibia. These findings are characteristic of transient osteoporosis. After 8 months of observation, repeat (G) coronal and (H) sagittal MRI confirm resolution of the lesion without conversion to osteonecrosis.

postpartum women. Spontaneous resolution is expected with supportive management, but symptoms can last 6 months or longer.[3]

Metabolic Disorders

Endocrine disorders that affect calcium metabolism and bone turnover can generate solid masses and changes within bone that often mimic metastatic bone disease. Systemic complaints consistent with hypercalcemia, medical comorbidities such as renal insufficiency, and diffuse polyostotic changes should lead the clinician to investigate metabolic derangements during work-up.

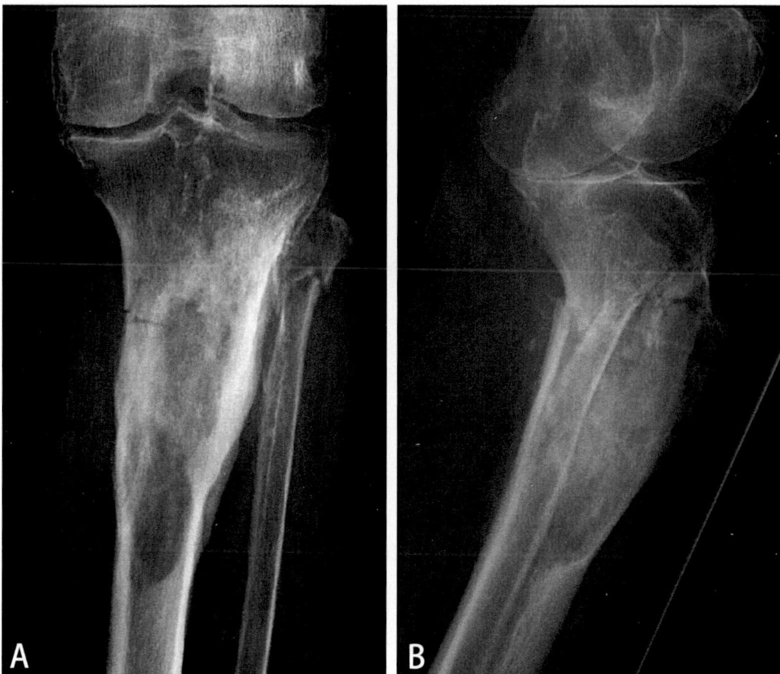

Figure 5-5. An 84-year-old man with dialysis-dependent renal insufficiency presents with pain and inability to bear weight on the left lower extremity. (A) Anteroposterior and (B) lateral radiographs demonstrate a pathologic fracture through an expansile, destructive lucent lesion of the proximal tibial metaphysis. Biopsy confirmed a diagnosis of brown tumor of secondary hyperparathyroidism.

Hyperparathyroidism

Increased production of parathyroid hormone or parathyroid hormone–related protein causes an increase in serum calcium levels by driving bone resorption (Table 5-1). This can produce polyostotic patterns of osteopenia, subperiosteal osteolysis, or multifocal lytic lesions suspicious for metastatic disease or myeloma. These hemosiderin-rich collections of osteoclastic giant cells are termed "brown tumors" (Figure 5-5). Management consists of correction of the underlying condition.

Tumoral Calcinosis

Gene mutations and endocrinopathies that disrupt the homeostasis of phosphate can lead to the deposition of calcium phosphates in juxta-articular soft tissues. These mass-like collections of fluid-calcium can cause pain,

Table 5-1

Pathways of Hyperparathyroidism

PATHWAY	CAUSE	PATHOGENESIS	MANAGEMENT
Primary hyperpara-thyroidism	Parathyroid-adenoma Parathyroid-hyperplasia Parathyroid-carcinoma	Isolated MEN 1 or MEN 2a Irradiation for acne	Parathyroid-ectomy
Secondary hyperpara-thyroidism	Renal osteodystrophy	Impaired calcitriol production Hyperphosphatemia	Correction of renal failure
	Nutritional osteomalacia	Decreased oral intake Malabsorption syndromes	Vitamin D supplementation
	Drug-Induced osteomalacia	Inhibition of bone mineralization or remodeling (bisphosphonates) Decrease parathyroid sensitivity to Ca (lithium) Inhibition of vitamin D absorption or metabolism (anticonvulsants, glucocorticoids, cholestyramine)	Discontinuation of drug Vitamin D supplementation
	Hereditary vitamin D–dependent rickets (type 1)	AR deficiency in 1 α-hydroxylase or 25-hydroxylase	High-dose activated vitamin D
Tertiary hyperpara-thyroidism	Autonomous PTH production unresponsive to Ca	Renal transplantation	Parathyroid-ectomy

Abbreviations: Ca, calcium; MEN, multiple endocrine neoplasia type 1; PTH, parathyroid hormone.

mechanical impingement, and loss of muscle function. Treatment consists of correction of serum phosphate levels and reversing correctable etiologies (most commonly dialysis-dependent renal insufficiency).

Paget's Disease of Bone

Paget's disease is a disorder of bone remodeling, resulting in alternating resorption and deposition of bone. This can result in expansion, deformity, and insufficiency as the overall density of the bone is diminished. Paget's disease may be monostotic and polyostotic, generally diagnosed in the later decades of life. The diagnosis is often confirmed radiographically by cortical thickening, coarsened trabeculae, and bony expansion with or without deformity (Figure 5-6). Elevated serum alkaline phosphatase is present in 95% of patients, and intense technetium-99 uptake is typical. Treatment for symptomatic lesions includes bisphosphonate therapy, with surgery reserved for cases of fracture, joint degeneration, or compromise of neural structures.[4] New or changing pains, or a change in radiographic appearance should raise suspicion for malignant degeneration or Paget's sarcoma.

Reactive and Inflammatory Disorders

Autoimmune, reactive, and inflammatory nodules can produce bone and soft-tissue lesions with marked contrast enhancement on MRI, often indistinguishable from true neoplasms. Although many lesions are associated with known medical conditions, a biopsy is often frequently necessary for diagnosis.

Sarcoidosis

Sarcoidosis is a granulomatous disease of unknown etiology that most commonly involves lymph nodes, lungs, and skin, but can manifest noncaseating granulomas in the bone or soft tissue. Lesions of the small bones of the hands and feet should prompt investigation for pulmonary lesions.

Gout

Gout is the deposition of monosodium urate crystals in the joint and periarticular tissues. When chronic, urate crystal deposition and its associated inflammatory changes can accumulate into tophaceous deposits that may produce lytic bone lesions and soft-tissue nodules in juxta-articular locations. This can be recognized radiographically when erosive changes of the joint are seen in association with a soft-tissue mass with or without mineralization (Figure 5-7). Management of gout includes medical optimization of serum uric acid and removal of tophaceous lesions that cause pain or mechanical symptoms.

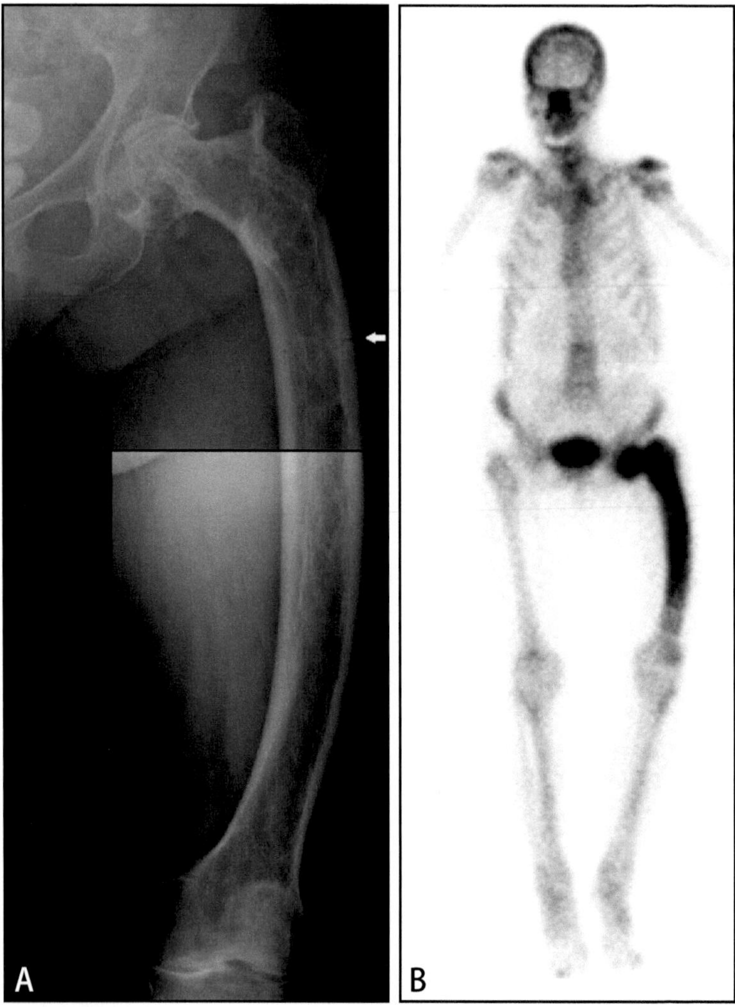

Figure 5-6. A 74-year-old woman presents with aching pain in the left thigh for the past 2 years, recently worsening with ambulation. (A) Anteroposterior radiographs demonstrate bowing deformity of the left femur with cortical thickening and coarsening trabecular markings consistent with Paget's disease of bone. A radiolucent line can be seen at the lateral cortex of the proximal femur (white arrow), consistent with pagetic pseudofracture. (B) Bone scintigraphy shows characteristically intense and diffuse uptake in the involved bone.

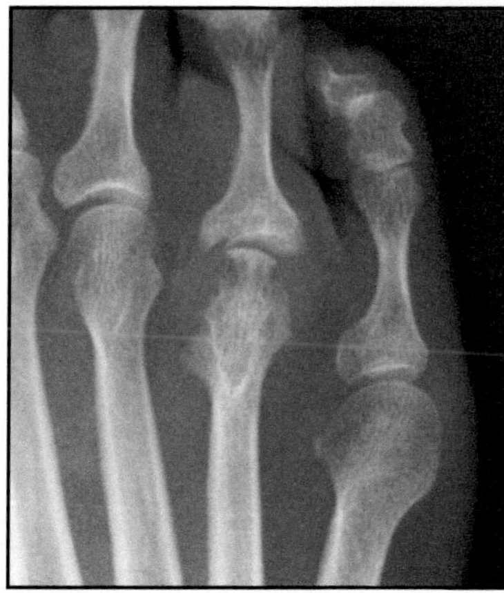

Figure 5-7. A 50-year-old woman presents with painful, firm swelling over the right fourth metatarsophalangeal joint. Plain radiographs demonstrate erosions of the metatarsal head. Biopsy confirmed tophaceous gout.

Nodular Fasciitis

Nodular fasciitis is a self-limiting reactive process that produces benign nodules of infiltrative, highly mitotic fibrous material that is easily mistaken for malignancy when not recognized clinically. These lesions are classically found in the upper extremities of young adults, often with bilateral or multifocal involvement, which suggests a non-neoplastic process. Biopsy is often warranted, and marginal excision is typically curative (Figure 5-8).

Wear Debris Pseudotumors

Wear debris pseudotumors should be suspected when a cystic mass communicates with a prosthetic joint (Figure 5-9). Chronic inflammation from particulate matter can induce substantial bony lysis, producing aseptic loosening of prosthetic components and progressive stripping of soft-tissue structures. Metal-on-metal articulations are at particular risk, and elevated serum metal ions may support the diagnosis. Treatment involves revision of the compromised joint.[5]

Take-Aways

1. Tumor mimickers can be organized into a few broad categories that are included or excluded from the differential by a thorough history-taking and physical examination.

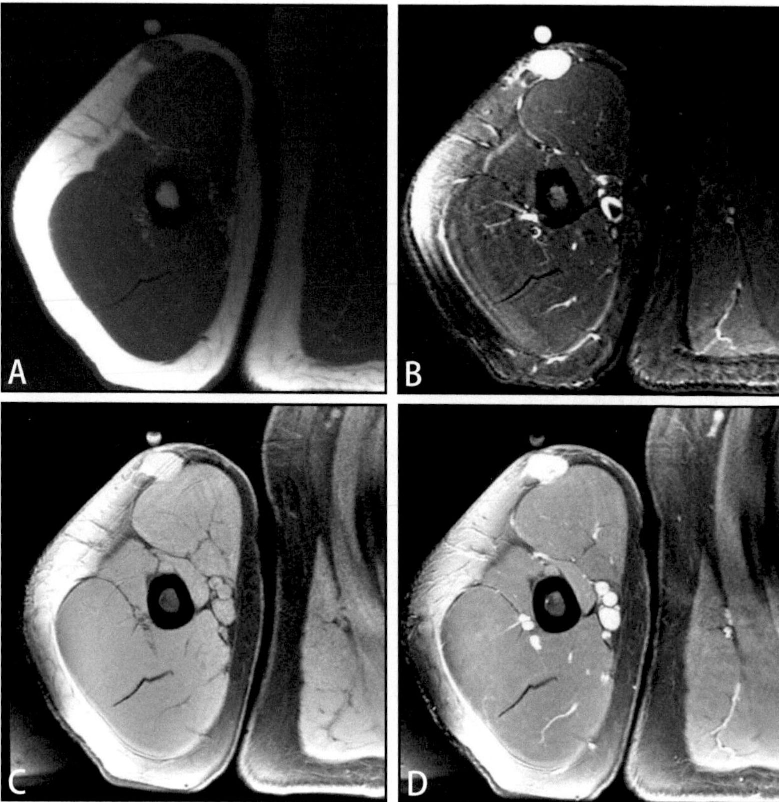

Figure 5-8. A 15-year-old boy presents with a tender nodule over the right upper arm. Axial MRI demonstrates a subcutaneous mass abutting the fascia of the anterior compartment that is hypointense on (A) T1 and hyperintense on (B) T2 sequences, with intermediate signal on (C) T1 fat-suppression sequencing and (D) marked enhancement on postcontrast sequencing. Biopsy confirmed a diagnosis of nodular fasciitis.

2. Stress fractures can be best diagnosed clinically by a pattern of activity-related pain. MRI findings can be concerning as well as discordant, with normal radiographs and intensely high T2 signal with near-normal T1 signal.
3. Infection is the most common and most effective tumor mimicker and should be actively ruled out during work-up. Unless definitively excluded, biopsy material should always be sent for tissue culture.
4. Systemic complaints, significant comorbid medical conditions, and diffuse skeletal involvement warrant consideration for metabolic bone disease in addition to the oncologic work-up.

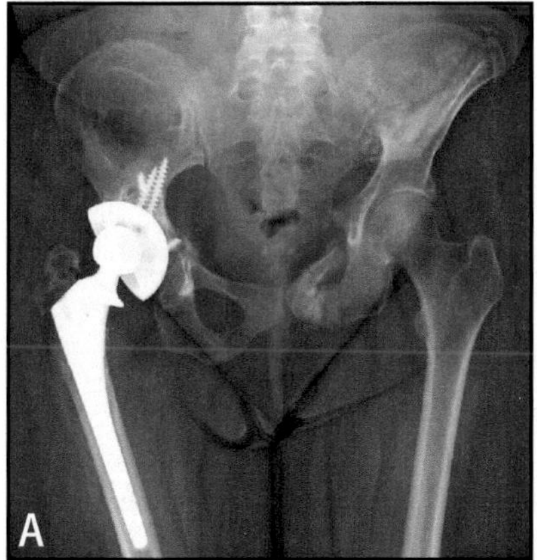

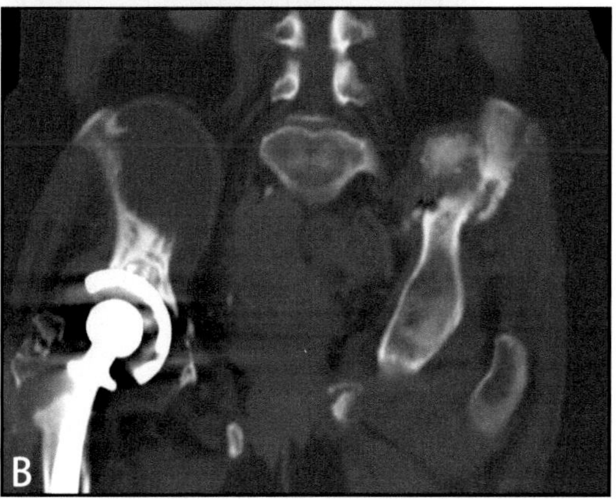

Figure 5-9. A 47-year-old woman with rheumatoid arthritis and drug-induced osteomalacia presents with worsening right hip pain. (A) Anteroposterior radiograph and (B) coronal computed tomography demonstrate a right total hip arthroplasty with vertical cup positioning, superior migration of the prosthetic head, osteolysis of the intertrochanteric femur, and a large, cystic, intrapelvic mass with effacement of the inner table of the iliac wing. An asymptomatic lateral-compression–type pelvic fracture is noted on the left. Biopsy of the mass confirmed wear debris pseudotumor.

Commonly Tested Topics for Trainees

- A history of injury or pain that is reproducible with mechanical loading or provocative musculotendinous maneuvers is suggestive of a traumatic or degenerative disorder.
- Musculoskeletal infection can have a variable radiological presentation, and the diagnosis should be considered during every work-up. Pain, tenderness, fever, and elevated inflammatory serologies should be carefully assessed.
- Bone infarcts can be recognized in patients with specific risk factors by their characteristic sclerotic margins and "double-line sign" on MRI.

- Paget's disease can be recognized radiographically by thickening and expansion of the bone and coarsening of trabecular markings. Elevated alkaline phosphatase levels and increased uptake on bone scan are typical.
- Heterotopic ossification can be identified radiographically by its zonal pattern, with a well-defined and mineralized periphery and relatively lucent center.

References

1. Nauth A, Giles E, Potter BK, et al. Heterotopic ossification in orthopaedic trauma. *J Orthop Trauma.* 2012;26(12):684-688. doi:10.1097/BOT.0b013e3182724624.
2. McGrory JE, Pritchard DJ, Unni KK, Ilstrup D, Rowland CM. Malignant lesions arising in chronic osteomyelitis. Clin Orthop Relat Res. 1999;(362):181-189.
3. Lakhanpal S, Ginsburg WW, Luthra HS, Hunder GG. Transient regional osteoporosis. A study of 56 cases and review of the literature. *Ann Intern Med.* 1987;106(3):444-450. doi:10.7326/0003-4819-106-3-444.
4. Ralston SH, Langston AL, Reid IR. Pathogenesis and management of Paget's disease of bone. *Lancet.* 2008;372(9633):155-163. doi:10.1016/S0140-6736(08)61035-1.
5. Pandit H, Glyn-Jones S, McLardy-Smith P, et al. Pseudotumors associated with metal-on-metal hip resurfacings. *J Bone Joint Surg Br.* 2008;90(7):847-851. doi:10.1302/0301-620X.90B7.20213.

Section **II**

Pediatric and Young Adult Bone Tumors

6

Latent Bone Lesions in Children

Overview

Latent bone lesions are common benign findings in the growing skeleton. Any clinician providing musculoskeletal care to the pediatric population should be familiar with the most common latent and incidental bone lesions so that prompt recognition can help avoid expensive testing and unnecessary interventions. We will discuss the most common latent bone lesions in children and identify treatment algorithms for deciding which lesions to observe and those that require more aggressive interventions.

Bone lesions that are termed "latent" display no aggressive behavior or tendency toward unrestricted growth. They are commonly developmental anomalies that are discovered incidentally, and typically have a favorable, quiescent natural history of stability or resolution over time. A small percentage of these lesions may present with pain or fracture when they affect growth or undermine the structural stability of the bone. Because of their non-neoplastic nature, operative treatment of latent lesions can present unique challenges, particularly when the biology of normal bone remodeling is absent.

For lesions with limited to no growth potential in locations that do not risk structural compromise of the bone, observation is generally appropriate. These lesions will either remain stable or resolve over time, usually after skeletal maturity. Lesions at a high risk for fracture, such as large lesions in the lower extremities, may warrant intralesional resection and structural augmentation. Developmental anomalies that affect normal growth may require treatment to prevent deformity.

Wallace, MT
Handbook of Musculoskeletal Tumors (pp 77-90).

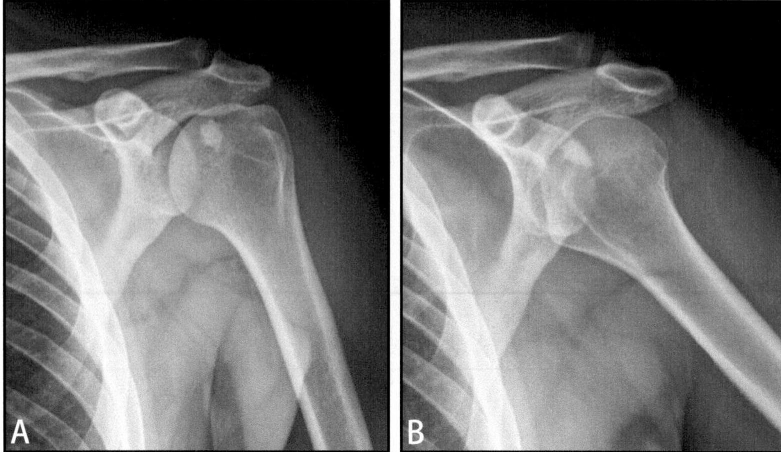

Figure 6-1. A 40-year-old man presents with an incidentally discovered lesion in the left proximal humerus discovered on chest x-ray. (A) Anteroposterior and (B) lateral radiographs demonstrate a well-defined intramedullary lesion in the proximal humeral epiphysis, isodense to cortical bone with normal surrounding trabecular markings, diagnostic of an enostosis, or bone island.

Bone Islands—Enostosis and Osteopoikilosis

Bone islands are asymptomatic areas of densely sclerotic bone formation within the medullary space. They are likely developmental anomalies due to abnormal endochondral bone formation and ossification.[1] Enostoses are recognized by determinate imaging features. Solid bone that is isodense to cortical bone with normal surrounding trabecular markings is typical. Bone islands will further display absent (dark) signal on T1 and T2 magnetic resonance imaging (MRI) sequences, with no perilesional edema or other reactive changes. These lesions can display modest to little uptake on bone scintigraphy, so technetium-99 medronic acid (Tc-99m) scans can be confirmatory only when negative.

Enostoses have no growth or invasive potential, and as such should be asymptomatic. Pain in the area of a discovered enostosis should suggest either an alternative source of pain such as degenerative joint disease, tendinopathy, or other inflammatory disorder, or an alternative diagnosis for the lesion such as blastic metastatic bone disease, sclerosing osteosarcoma, or a sclerosing form of multiple myeloma in association with POEMS (polyneuropathy, organomegaly, endocrinopathy, M component, and skin changes) syndrome.

There is no treatment necessary for bone islands beyond recognition. Large, asymmetric, lesions in areas of locoregional pain may be observed with serial radiographs until stability of the lesion is confirmed (Figure 6-1).

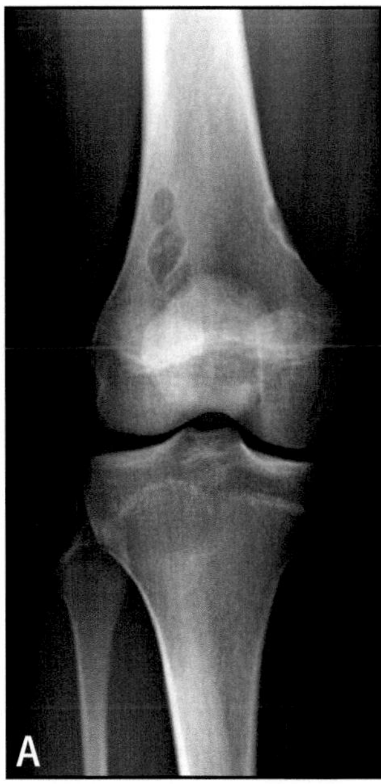

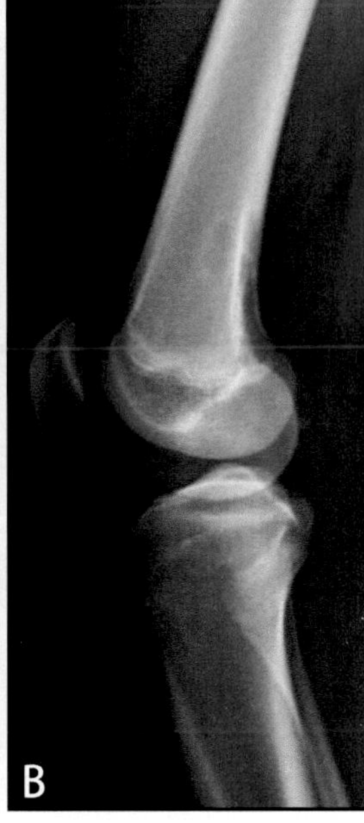

Figure 6-2. A 13-year-old boy presents after a soccer injury with no complaints. (A) Anteroposterior and (B) lateral radiographs demonstrate 2 well-defined, lobular, cortically based lucent lesions typical of nonossifying fibroma. Observation was recommended.

Nonossifying Fibroma—Fibrous Cortical Defect

Known by many names, the nonossifying fibroma (NOF) is the most common latent skeletal lesion observed in children. These are thought to represent developmental abnormalities in subperiosteal bone, in which fibrous and histiocytic tissue proliferates instead of bone. As a result, these lesions are classically eccentric, metaphyseal, and cortically based, with well-defined areas of rounded or lobular cortical bone replacement and minimal expansion of the cortex (Figure 6-2). Tc-99m scans may show mild to no activity.

NOFs are thought to be present in as many as 30% to 40% of children, though most of these never present clinically.[2] They are often identified incidentally on plain radiographs, but larger lesions may create weakened areas of the bone that present with insufficiency or completed pathologic fractures (Figure 6-3). When multiple lesions are discovered, the clinician should pursue evaluation for Jaffe-Campanacci syndrome.

Features of Jaffe-Campanacci syndrome include the following:

- Café-au-lait spots
- Multiple, bilateral NOFs
- Mental retardation

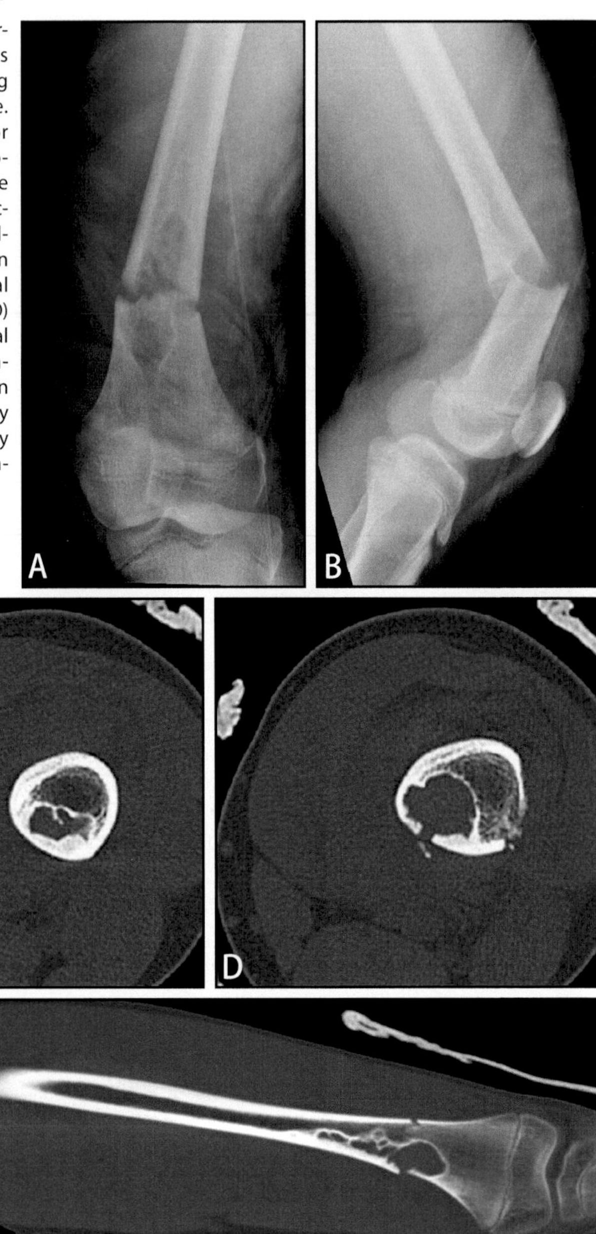

Figure 6-3. A 12-year-old boy presents with pain after falling onto his left knee. (A) Anteroposterior and (B) lateral radiographs demonstrate a transverse fracture through a well-defined lucency in the distal femoral metaphysis. (C and D) Axial and (E) coronal computed tomography demonstrates an eccentric, cortically based lobular lucency consistent with non-ossifying fibroma.

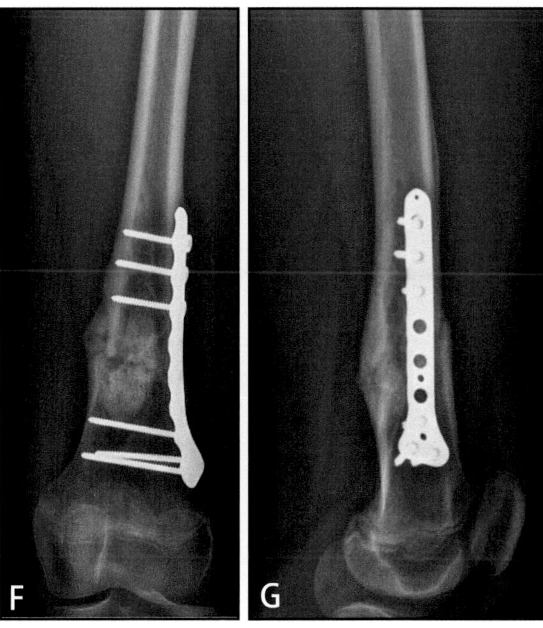

Figure 6-3 continued. (F and G) The patient underwent curettage, internal fixation, and synthetic bone void filling.

- Hypogonadism/cryptorchidism
- Ocular malformations
- Cardiovascular malformation

NOFs generally require no treatment other than observation. After skeletal maturity, NOFs can be expected to ossify and resolve. Lesions that are painful, or lesions with impending or completed pathologic fracture, may be treated with curettage and bone grafting, with or without hardware augmentation. The risk of fracture is related to the specific anatomic location of the lesion, and is thought to increase when the lesion exceeds 50% of the cross-sectional area of the involved bone.[3]

Fibrous Dysplasia

Fibrous dysplasia is a developmental disorder of bone caused by a mutation in the alpha subunit of the membrane protein G. This prevents deactivation of protein G, which couples hormone receptors to cyclic adenosine monophosphate production, leading to an increase in stromal cyclic adenosine monophosphate levels. The end result of this process in bone is increased fibro-osseous tissue proliferation with abnormal differentiation, creating metaphyseal and diaphyseal lesions with abnormal strength and structural characteristics.

The monostotic form of fibrous dysplasia is often discovered incidentally and is observed most commonly in the femur, followed by the tibia, pelvis, foot, ribs, and craniofacial bones. Lesions that are broad or extensively involving bone may present with pain, limp, stress fracture, or deformity (Figure 6-4). Polyostotic fibrous dysplasia may diffusely involve the skeleton, or may be restricted to one extremity, such as the ipsilateral pelvis, femur, tibia, fibula, and foot. Multiple areas of fibrous dysplasia involvement should be examined further for McCune-Albright syndrome or Mazabraud syndrome.[4]

Syndromes Associated With Polyostotic Fibrous Dysplasia

McCune-Albright Syndrome

- Irregular brown macular "coast-of-Maine" patches
- Precocious puberty
- Multiple bone lesions

Mazabraud Syndrome

- Multiple bone lesions
- Soft-tissue myxomas overlying areas of skeletal involvement

Endocrinopathies

- Hyperthyroidism
- Acromegaly/Growth hormone excess
- Cushing Disease/Hypercortisolism
- Oncogenic osteomalacia: FGF23 renal phosphate wasting or "phosphate diabetes"

Incidentally discovered lesions of fibrous dysplasia may be observed, but painful lesions and those causing deformity, fracture, or nonunion may require surgery. Intramedullary devices are preferred over plates and external fixators, and cortical strut allograft is a preferable bone graft material because autograft and particulate grafts will produce the same dysplastic bone on healing and remodeling (Figure 6-5). Excision of the lesions is generally unnecessary. Bisphosphonates may be useful for painful lesions that do not require surgery. There is a small but notable risk of malignant transformation of fibrous dysplasia, between 0.5% and 5%. Polyostotic disease and radiated lesions appear to be at an elevated risk.[5]

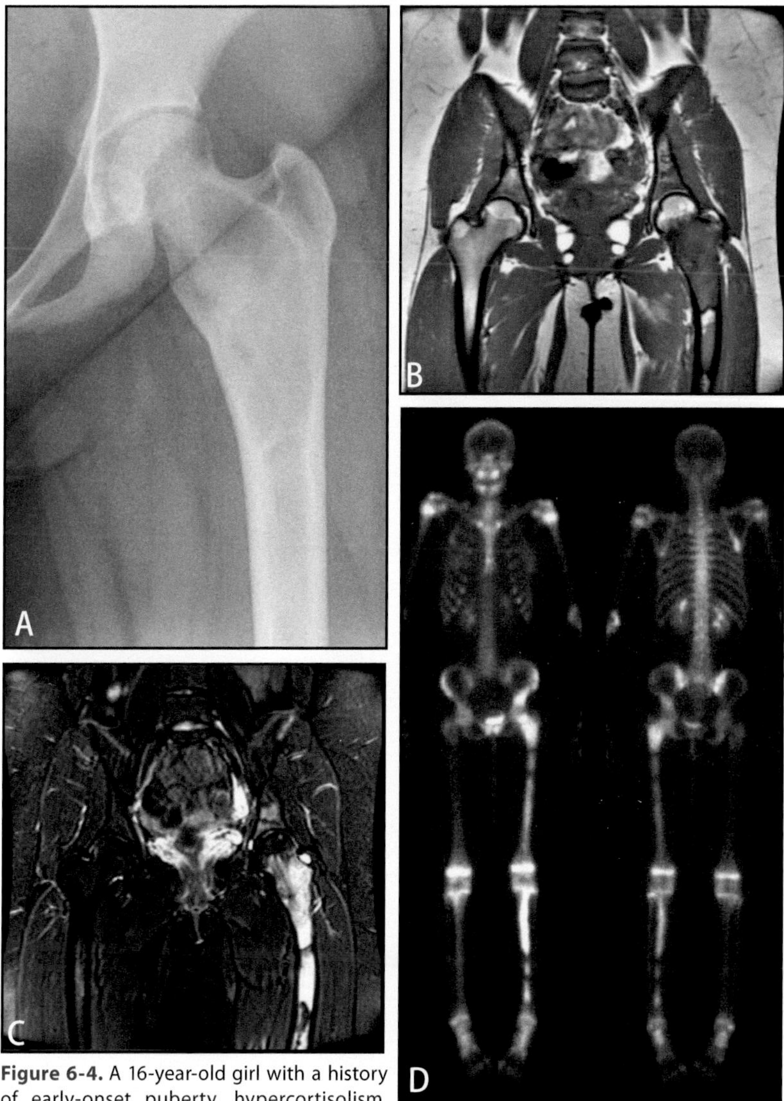

Figure 6-4. A 16-year-old girl with a history of early-onset puberty, hypercortisolism, and multiple guided-growth procedures of the knees presents with left hip pain. (A) Anteroposterior radiograph demonstrates expansion and mild bowing deformity of the proximal femur, with ground-glass opacification of the proximal femur consistent with fibrous dysplasia of bone. (B) T1 and (C) T2 MRI demonstrate diffuse and extensive marrow dysplasia, and (D) bone scintigraphy demonstrates involvement of the entire left hindquarter.

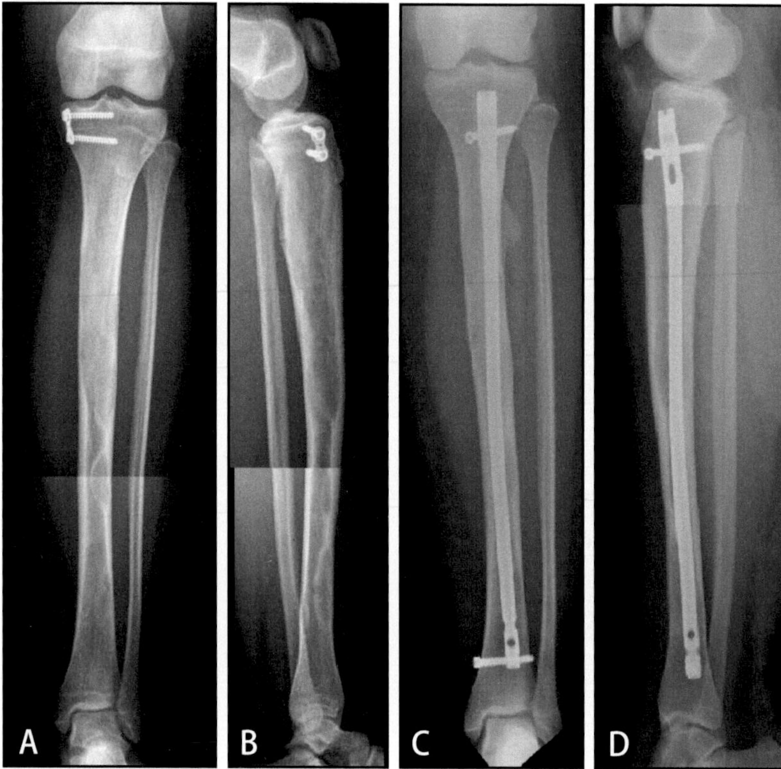

Figure 6-5. A 14-year-old girl presents with left lower leg pain. (A) Anteroposterior and (B) lateral radiographs demonstrate mild bowing of the tibia with multiple ground-glass lesions consistent with fibrous dysplasia. Guided growth of the proximal tibia was able to facilitate (C and D) intramedullary nail placement.

Unicameral (Simple) Bone Cyst

The simple bone cyst (UBC) is a non-neoplastic cavitation of the bone most commonly seen in the metaphyseal region of long bones in the growing skeleton. Though incompletely understood, it is theorized that a decrease in intraosseous drainage causes an increase in interstitial pressure, a decrease in local oxygen tension and pH, and elaboration of osteoclastogenic cytokines, interleukins, and prostaglandins. Regional bony lysis then creates cystic accumulations that further exacerbate this drainage impairment.[6]

UBCs can occur in any location, but are most common in the proximal humerus and proximal femur. They are classically well-defined lucencies that thin the overlying cortices and may expand the bone slightly, generally

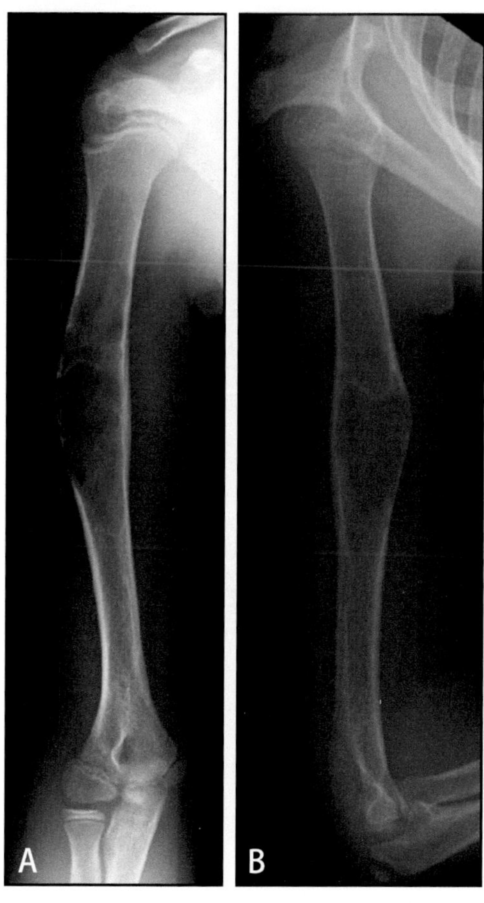

Figure 6-6. A 12-year-old boy presents with occasional right shoulder pain during overhead throwing. (A) Anteroposterior and (B) lateral radiographs demonstrate a well-defined, slightly expansile lesion of the right humerus with cortical thinning, consistent with unicameral bone cyst. This lesion has migrated away from the proximal humeral physis, and the lesion was observed.

no more than the width of the adjacent physis. At early onset, they typically extend to the physis, but may migrate away from the growth plate with longitudinal growth (Figure 6-6). Minimally displaced pathologic fractures or a cortical fragment within the cyst, termed a *fallen leaf,* may be observed. MRI will demonstrate a single fluid-filled cavity with rim enhancement and no internal enhancement or solid component.

Most UBCs are discovered incidentally but may present acutely with pain suggestive of fracture. Lesions abutting the physis are considered to be in an "active" phase of growth, propagating at the same rate as the growth of the bone. Lesions that have migrated away from the physis are more likely to be latent in nature. The natural history of the UBC is persistence until skeletal maturity, after which drainage through epiphyseal perforators may relieve the impairment in drainage and the cyst can be expected to resolve.

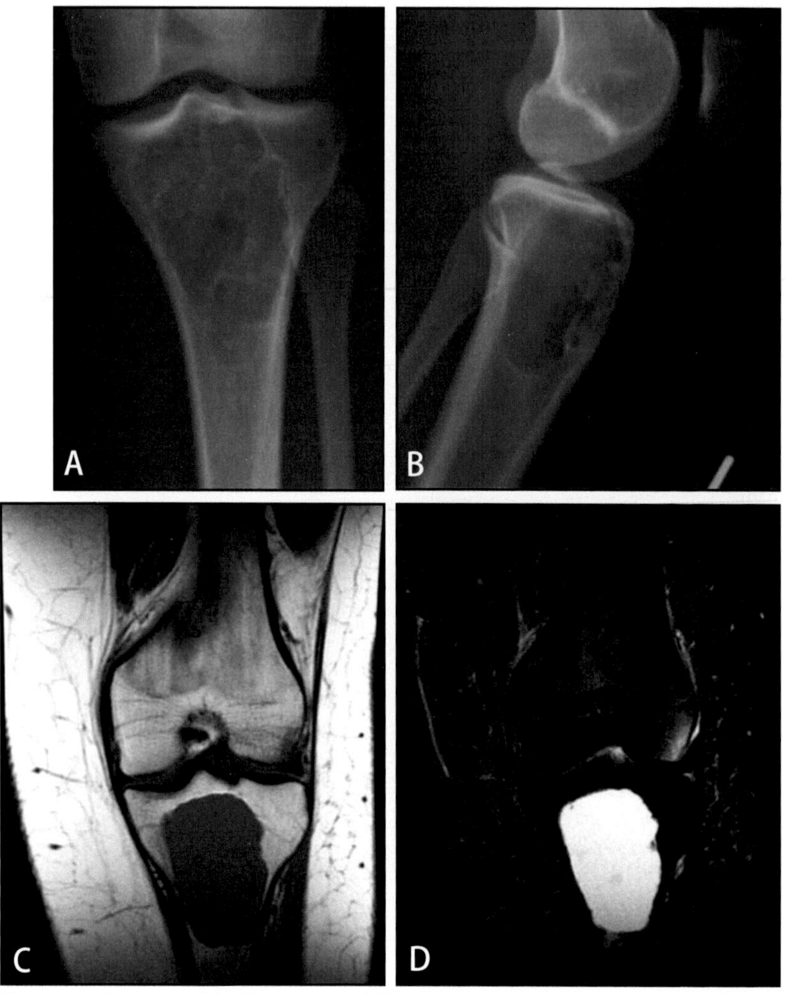

Figure 6-7. A 16-year-old girl presents with left knee soreness. (A) Anteroposterior and (B) lateral radiographs demonstrate a well-defined lucency in the metaphysis and epiphysis of the proximal tibia. (C) T1, (D) T2, and (E) postgadolinium fat-suppressed MRI demonstrate a fluid-filled cavity with a rim enhancement pattern diagnostic of unicameral bone cyst.

Asymptomatic lesions can therefore be observed, and painful lesions or those at risk of fracture may require surgery (Figure 6-7). Multiple methods of percutaneous and open treatment of unicameral bone cysts have been described, none with predictable or superior results. Figure 6-8 depicts an algorithm for recommending treatment of unicameral bone cysts.

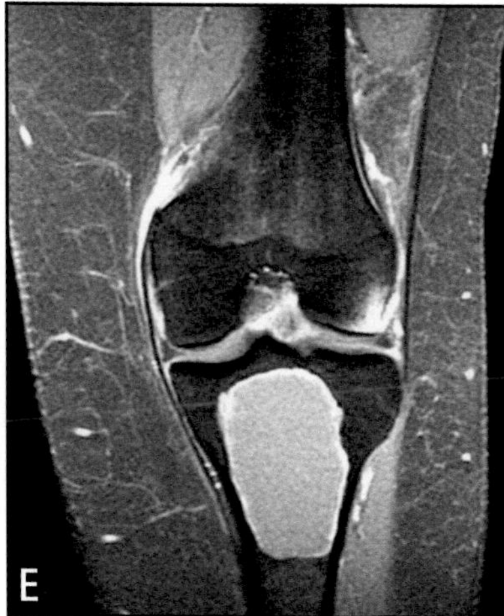

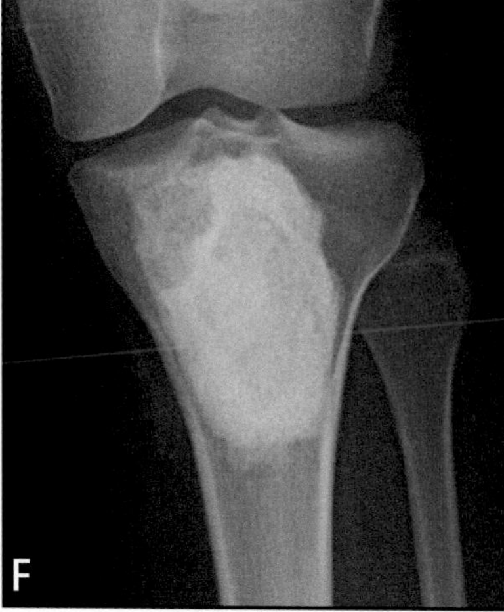

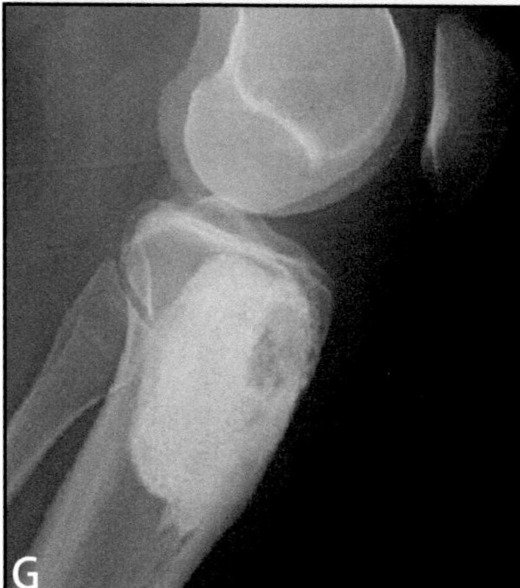

Figure 6-7 continued. (E) Postgadolinium fat-suppressed MRI demonstrates a fluid-filled cavity with a rim enhancement pattern diagnostic of unicameral bone cyst. Stability of the lesion is confirmed on (F) anteroposterior and (G) lateral radiographs at 1 year after curettage and synthetic bone void filling.

Enchondroma

Solitary enchondromas are lobulated lesions of hyaline cartilage. They are thought to develop from nests of cartilage left behind during endochondral ossification in the growing skeleton. The majority of enchondromas develop in the tubular bones of the hands and feet, followed by the metaphyseal areas of the long bones. Solitary enchondromas are usually centrally located and well defined, with stippled areas of chondroid matrix, although in the young patient they may be completely lucent. Similar to other latent lesions, enchondromas may migrate away from the growth plate with skeletal growth (Figure 6-9).

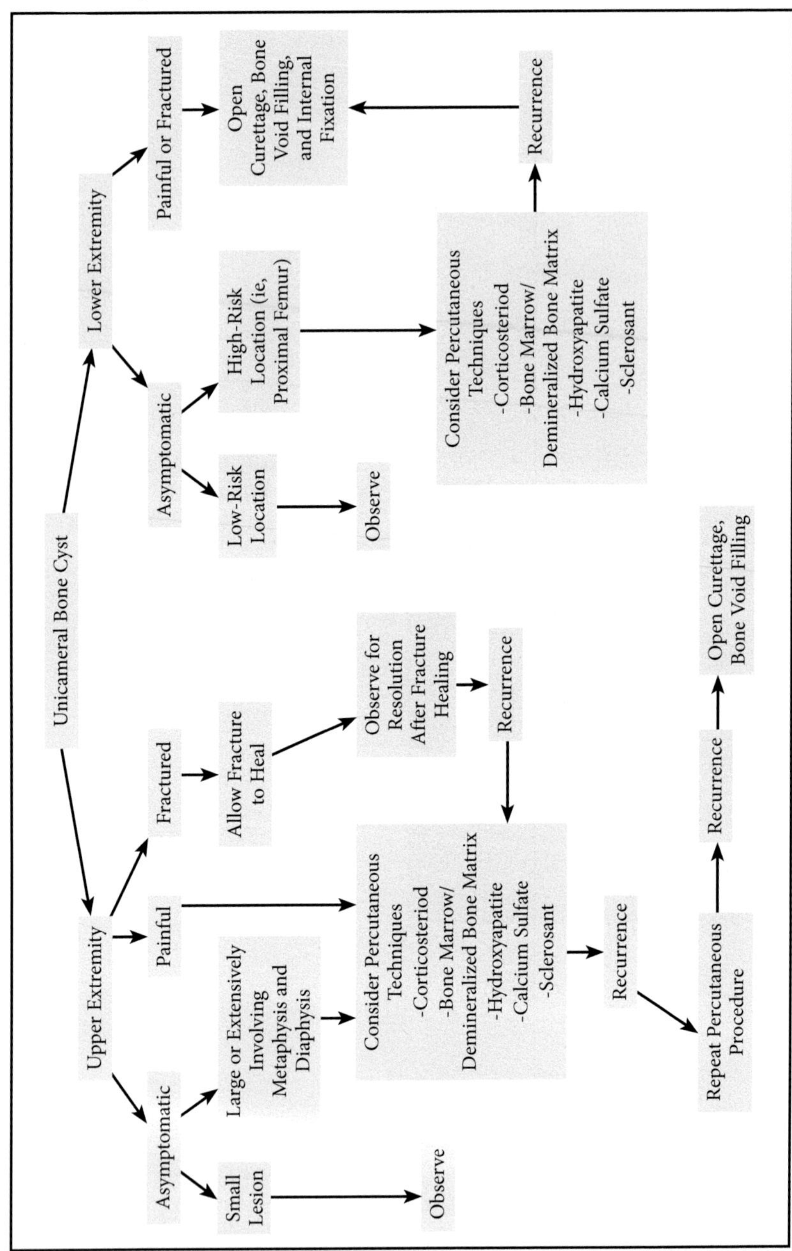

Figure 6-8. Algorithm for treatment of unicameral bone cysts.

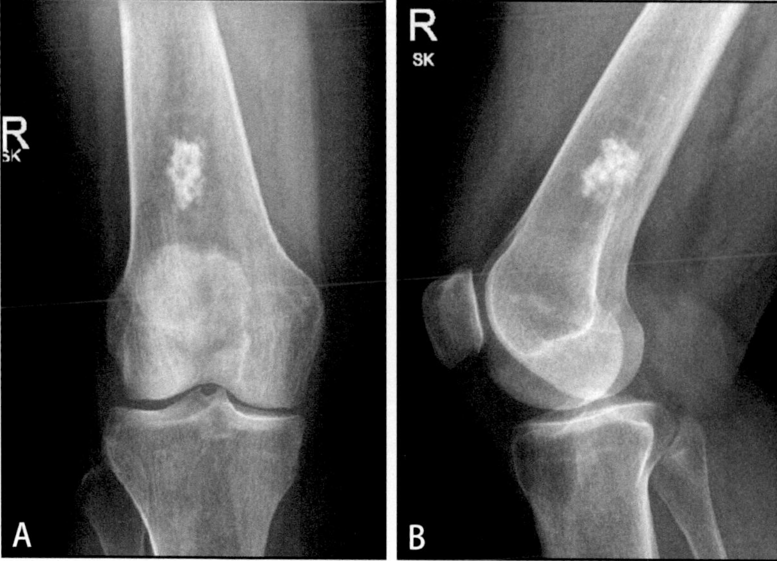

Figure 6-9. A 68-year-old woman presents with painful episodes of catching in the right knee. (A) Anteroposterior and (B) lateral radiographs demonstrate a well-defined, centrally located lesion in the right distal femoral metaphysis, with a lobular pattern of mineralization without secondary bony changes, confirming the diagnosis of benign enchondroma. Though typically lucent during childhood, these lesions may demonstrate dense mineralization with advancing age. This lesion was discovered incidentally during a work-up for her unrelated meniscal pathology.

Most enchondromas are discovered incidentally, and require little more than observation to confirm stability of the lesion. Lesions in the hands and feet and those that present with stable pathologic fractures should be allowed to heal before curettage and bone grafting. Prophylactic resection is generally unwarranted. Patients who present with pain in the area of a definitively benign enchondroma should be evaluated for alternative etiologies of pain.

Take-Aways

1. Latent bone lesions are often determinant on imaging, do not require biopsy, and rarely require treatment beyond observation.
2. Multiple fibrous lesions are commonly associated with genetic syndromes that affect bone differentiation and development, often with other associated endocrinopathies.

3. Unicameral bone cysts will typically persist until skeletal maturity, so painful lesions, fractured cysts, and lesions at risk for future fracture may require intervention.

Commonly Tested Topics for Trainees

- NOFs are very common in children and rarely require treatment. The risk of pathologic fracture is elevated when the lesion occupies more than half the cross-sectional area of the bone.
- Surgical management of fibrous dysplasia should focus on deformity correction, stabilization with intramedullary devices, and structural augmentation with cortical allograft.
- The fallen-leaf sign is pathognomonic for unicameral bone cyst.

References

1. Greenspan A. Bone island (enostosis): current concept—a review. *Skeletal Radiol.* 1995;24(2):111-115.
2. Dorfman HD, Czerniak B. Bone tumors. *Hum Pathol.* 1999;30:1269.
3. Arata MA, Peterson HA, Dahlin DC. Pathologic fractures through non-ossifying fibromas. Review of the Mayo Clinic experience. *J Bone Joint Surg Am.* 1981;63(6):980-988.
4. Collins MT, Singer FR, Eugster E. McCune-Albright syndrome and the extraskeletal manifestations of fibrous dysplasia. *Orphanet J Rare Dis.* 2012;7(suppl 1):4-14. doi:10.1186/1750-1172-7-S1-S4.
5. Ruggieri P, Sim FH, Bond JR, Unni KK. Malignancies in fibrous dysplasia. *Cancer.* 1994;73(5):1411-1424. doi:10.1002/1097-0142(19940301)73:5<1411::aid-cncr2820730516>3.0.co;2-t.
6. Chigira M, Maehara S, Arita S, Udagawa E. The aetiology and treatment of simple bone cysts. *J Bone Joint Surg Br.* 1983;65(5):633-637. doi:10.1302/0301-620X.65B5.6643570.

7

Active and Aggressive Benign Bone Lesions in Children and Young Adults

Overview

Benign bone tumors with a propensity to grow and adversely affect the bone are termed active lesions. These tumors generally have a favorable prognosis, but still require an accurate diagnosis and prompt and effective management. We will discuss the most common active benign bone lesions in children and adults younger than 40 years, and present and discuss treatment algorithms and strategies for managing locally destructive benign bone tumors.

Active and aggressive bone tumors are neoplastic proliferations with a natural history of continued activity with or without progressive bony destruction. Active lesions are typically painful, and often occur around the physes in the growing skeleton. Active lesions can grow quickly and compromise the stability of bone. Pathologic fractures may be a common presentation. Some lesions can penetrate the growing physis, and may contribute to growth arrest or deformity. Treatment options vary depending on the tumor's potential for growth, but some form of local treatment is required. Owing to the overall favorable prognosis with benign bone lesions, intralesional treatment such as ablation or curettage is generally acceptable. Recognition of characteristic defining features and an accurate diagnosis of these lesions are important because some imaging and histological findings can overlap with more serious diseases. After treatment, regular clinical and radiographic follow-up are required to monitor for locally recurrent disease.

Wallace, MT
Handbook of Musculoskeletal Tumors (pp 91-104).

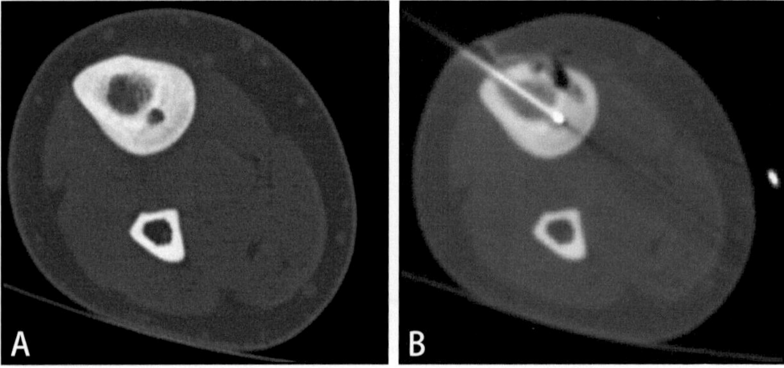

Figure 7-1. A 15-year-old boy presents with right lower leg pain at rest and at night, with substantial relief with nonsteroidal anti-inflammatory drugs. (A) Axial computed tomography demonstrates a cortically based lucent nidus with surrounding hyperostosis of the posterior cortex of the tibial diaphysis. After a core sample of the hypertrophic bone was obtained to confirm no neoplastic involvement, (B) radiofrequency ablation was performed, with immediate relief of the patient's symptoms.

Osteoid Osteoma and Osteoblastoma

Osteoid Osteoma

Osteoid osteomas are small, bone-forming benign tumors generally limited to 5 to 15 mm in size. They are defined radiographically by a lytic nidus surrounded by a rim of sclerotic bone and central ossification, with a predilection for the cortices of long bones, the spine, pelvis, and small bones of the hands and feet. Pain at rest and night pain are caused by prostaglandin secretion within the nidus, which is characteristically relieved with cyclooxygenase inhibitors.[1] Osteoid osteomas are limited in size potential, but may cause painful scoliosis, joint contractures, or growth disturbances when adjacent to a physis.

When combined with a convincing clinical presentation, osteoid osteoma can be diagnosed based on characteristic imaging features, and biopsy is usually not necessary. Significant uptake on bone scintigraphy is typically present, but fine-cut computed tomography is the imaging modality of choice. Lesions can burn out with years of observation and nonsteroidal anti-inflammatory drug therapy, but the toxicity of this treatment can be limiting. Radiofrequency ablation is an effective, minimally invasive treatment for most lesions, but it can be risky when performed around neural elements or in subcutaneous locations (Figure 7-1). Burr-down curettage and en bloc resection are options when surgery is required.

Table 7-1

Commonly Used Local Adjuvants in Benign Bone Tumor Treatment

ADJUVANT	MECHANISM OF ACTION	COMPLICATIONS
Radiofrequency ablation	Thermal denaturing: cycles of 4 minutes at 45°C to 80°C	Skin necrosis, nerve and spinal cord injury
Cryotherapy	Ice crystal damage: freeze-thaw cycles to −75°C to −20°C with cryoablation probe, −196°C with liquid nitrogen	Soft-tissue injury, fracture, delayed reossification, joint/articular cartilage injury
Phenol/Alcohol	Chemical denaturization: low (6%) or high (60%) phenol solution for 3 minutes	Tissue burns, leakage of chemical
Acrylic cement	Thermal denaturization at 48°C to 90°C	Altered Young's modulus, articular stress/cartilage damage
Argon beam coagulation	Tissue vaporization, carbonization, and necrosis: 50 to 150W electrical current applied to ionize argon gas into plasma	Tissue necrosis
Adapted from Di Giacomo G, Ziranu A, Perisano C, Piccioli A, Maccauro G.[2]		

Osteoblastoma

Osteoblastoma is a benign, bone-producing lesion similar to osteoid osteoma histologically, with much more aggressive biological potential for growth and recurrence. More than half occur within the posterior elements of the spine. Simple intralesional resection is associated with a 1-in-4 recurrence rate, so extended curettage with high-speed burring and local adjuvant use is recommended when en bloc resection is not feasible. Table 7-1 lists local adjuvants commonly used in benign bone tumor resection.

Aneurysmal Bone Cyst

Aneurysmal bone cysts (ABCs) are expansile, metaphyseal lesions of bone that may occur as primary bone lesions, or secondary to other underlying disorders, including giant cell tumor of bone, chondroblastoma, osteoblastoma, or osteosarcoma. Though a precise etiology is unknown, ABCs may develop as a reactive process in areas of intraosseous blood flow alteration from tumor, trauma, etc. As a result, ABC changes in the bone must be carefully evaluated and biopsied to exclude a more aggressive process.

Unlike unicameral (simple) bone cysts, aneurysmal cysts are not size limited. Bony expansion wider than the adjacent physis is often observed, with a well-defined, geographic rim of bone and internal septations. Magnetic resonance imaging (MRI) will demonstrate multiple cystic chambers with fluid-fluid levels (Figure 7-2). A biopsy is mandatory for confirmation of an accurate diagnosis. Aneurysmal bone cysts can be difficult to distinguish from telangiectatic osteosarcoma on imaging alone, and an open biopsy is recommended to ensure the correct diagnosis.

Intralesional resection of ABC is appropriate, with complete saucerization of the cavity preferred. Children with open physes and incomplete initial resection are at increased risk of recurrence. Percutaneous sclerotherapy with doxycycline foam and other sclerosing agents is a more recent development. This can be effective for smaller lesions and for lesions with fewer chambers, but only in experienced hands. This may be preferable in anatomical areas that are difficult to access surgically. The rate of retreatment with percutaneous techniques is high.[3]

Giant Cell Tumor of Bone

Giant cell tumor (GCT) of bone is one of the most common, most aggressive benign bone lesions in young adults age 20 to 40 years, with an average age of presentation of 33 years. They are classically metaphyseal, with extension toward the adjacent articular surface through the epiphysis. GCTs are often completely lytic, with an indistinct margin, cortical destruction, and adjacent soft-tissue extension. ABC changes may also be present. The most common locations of GCTs are the distal femur, proximal tibia, and distal radius.

GCTs demonstrate an aggressive pattern of local growth, and compromise of the adjacent joint may occur rapidly (Figure 7-3). Surgical resection remains the mainstay of treatment, but the procedure of choice depends on whether the joint can be effectively salvaged (Figure 7-4). Intralesional curettage is appropriate for joint salvage but must be extended with high-speed burring and local adjuvant. The recurrence rate with this approach remains high at 15% to 25%.

Growth and bony destruction in GCT is driven by the receptor activator of nuclear factor kappa-B ligand (RANKL)-mediated development of osteoclast-like macrophages. Medical management with bisphosphonates and denosumab, a monoclonal antibody to RANKL, has been shown to have

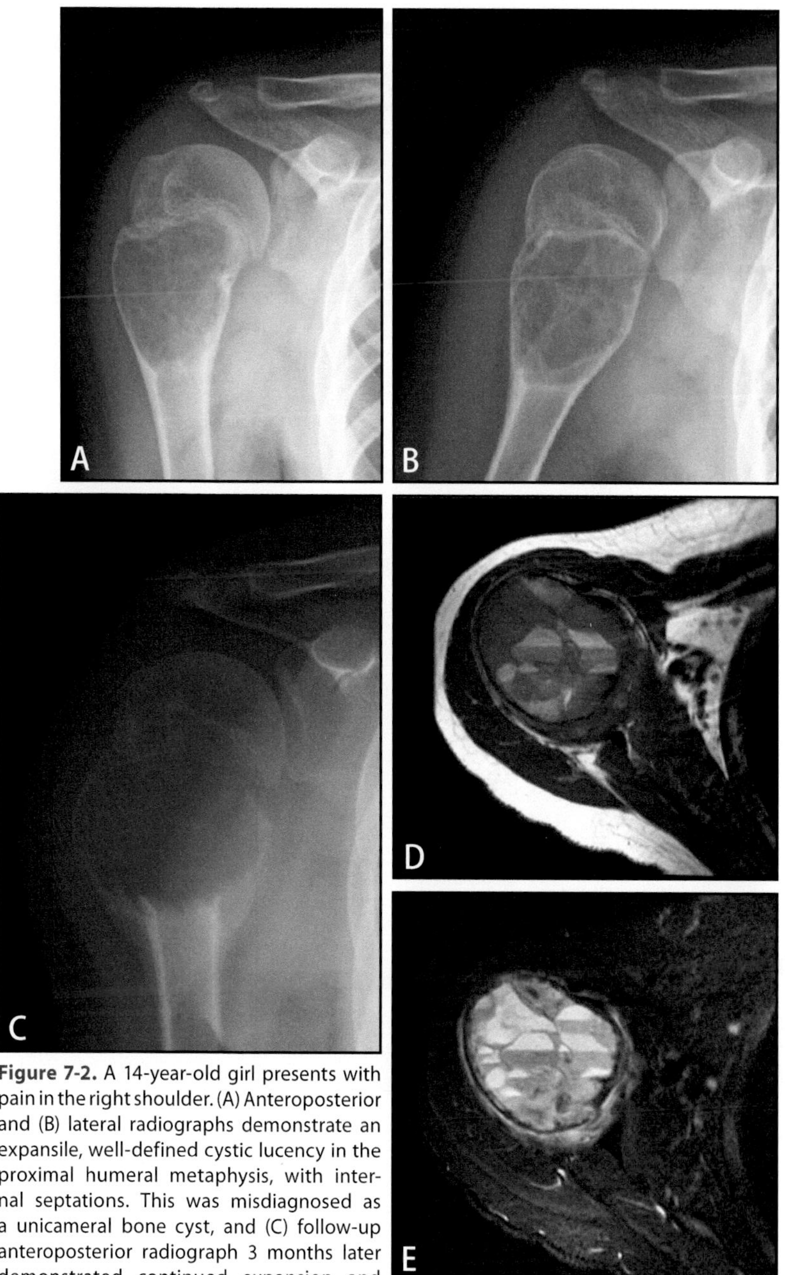

Figure 7-2. A 14-year-old girl presents with pain in the right shoulder. (A) Anteroposterior and (B) lateral radiographs demonstrate an expansile, well-defined cystic lucency in the proximal humeral metaphysis, with internal septations. This was misdiagnosed as a unicameral bone cyst, and (C) follow-up anteroposterior radiograph 3 months later demonstrated continued expansion and bony lysis. Axial (D) T1 and (E) T2 MRI sequences demonstrated multiple characteristic fluid-fluid levels. A biopsy confirmed the diagnosis of aneurysmal bone cyst.

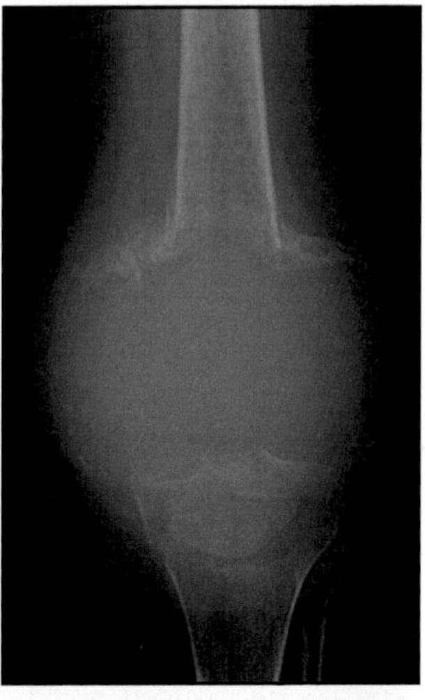

Figure 7-3. A 22-year-old woman presents with 9 months of painful swelling, flexion posturing, and inability to bear weight on the left knee. Anteroposterior radiograph demonstrates aggressive lysis of the distal femur, with significant expansion of the bone and sparse areas of rimming bone. Biopsy confirmed a diagnosis of giant cell tumor of bone.

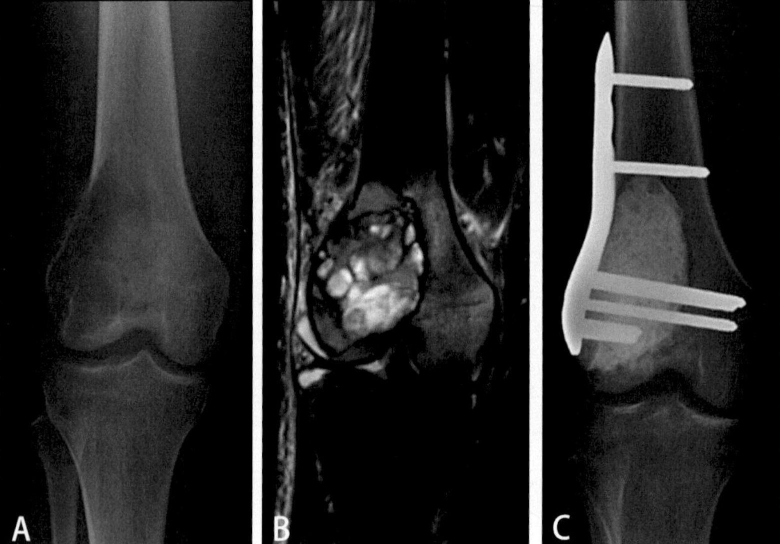

Figure 7-4. A 31-year-old man presents with progressive right lateral knee pain that is present at rest, at night, and with weight-bearing. (A) Anteroposterior radiograph demonstrates a lytic lesion of the lateral metaphysis of the distal femur with extension toward the articular surface. The margin is indistinct but with a pattern of geographic lysis without surrounding sclerosis, and cortical destruction is present. (B) Coronal T2-weighted MRI demonstrates a marrow-replacing lesion of the lateral femoral metaphysis, with areas of solid tumor mixed with aneurysmal cystic changes and surrounding perilesional edema. A biopsy confirmed giant cell tumor of bone, and (C) joint salvage with extended intralesional curettage, argon beam coagulation as local adjuvant, and cement reconstruction with internal fixation was performed.

a static effect on GCT of bone. Although there is great enthusiasm for adjuvant systemic treatment of GCT, it has not been shown to reduce the rate of local recurrence for otherwise resectable disease.[4]

Indications for Denosumab Use in Giant Cell Tumor of Bone

- Metastatic GCT
- Unresectable lesions, such as the axial skeleton
- Resectable lesions that require sacrifice of the adjacent joint, to increase the feasibility of joint salvage

Approximately 2% to 4% of patients with GCT will present with metastatic disease, most often within the chest. For this reason, screening of the lung fields with chest radiography should be performed for every patient with newly diagnosed GCT of bone. Figure 7-5 depicts an algorithm for the management of GCT of bone.

Chondroblastoma

Chondroblastoma is a benign, aggressive tumor of chondroblasts characteristically found in the epiphyses and apophyses of the young growing skeleton. Owing to their juxta-articular location, chondroblastomas commonly present with joint pain, swelling, stiffness, and decreased tolerance to weight-bearing. Long bones are most commonly affected.

Radiographically, chondroblastomas are sharply lytic, often with a well-defined rim of sclerosis and occasional stippled areas of mineralization. MRI will generally demonstrate substantial perilesional edema, and secondary ABC-like changes may be observed (Figure 7-6).

Chondroblastomas have a propensity for continued growth and compromise of the subchondral bone, which generally requires intralesional treatment both for local control and salvage of the joint surface. Extended intralesional curettage with or without local adjuvant is the recommended intervention with the lowest rate of local recurrence, but percutaneous radiofrequency ablation has been employed for smaller lesions that are not adjacent to weight-bearing surfaces. The high-risk location of chondroblastomas often requires subchondral bone grafting and structural augmentation to support the joint surface. Particular care must be taken with lesions that abut or penetrate the physis, as growth disturbances after treatment are known complications. Rates of local recurrence range from 8% to 25%, most commonly the result of inadequate initial resection.[5] In a small number of

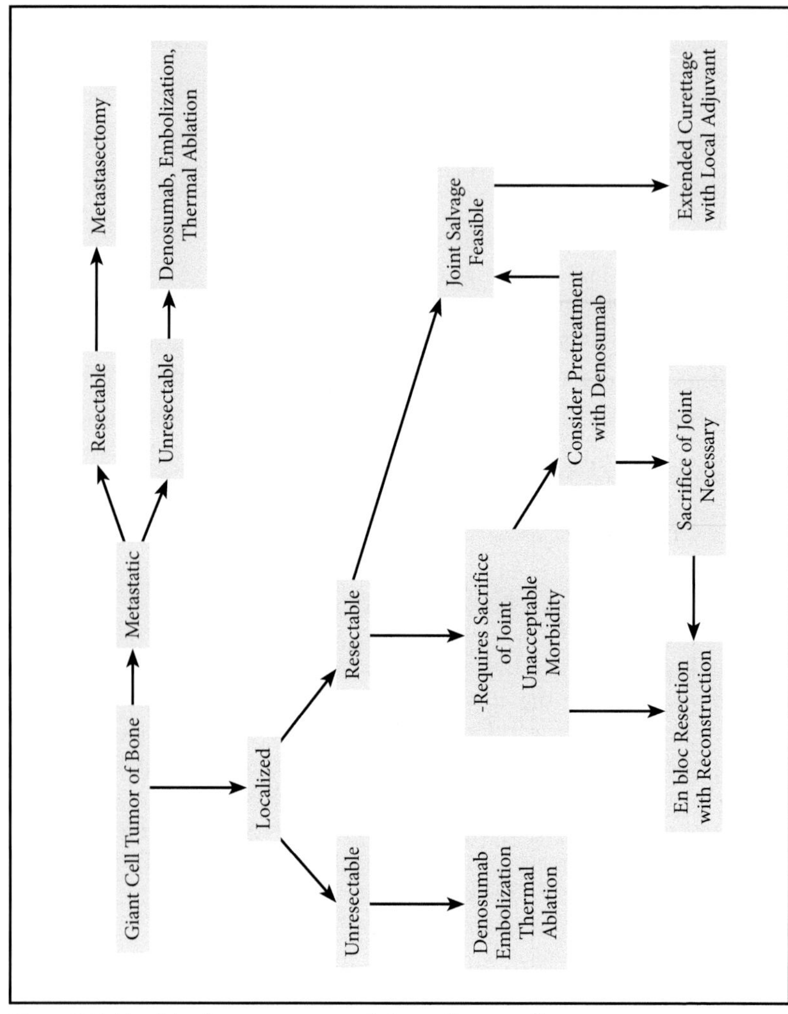

Figure 7-5. Algorithm for management of giant cell tumor of bone.

patients, pulmonary metastases may be identified. Therefore, as in GCT of bone, screening of the lung fields is indicated for a new diagnosis of chondroblastoma.

Chondromyxoid Fibroma

Chondromyxoid fibroma is a benign neoplastic proliferation of primitive chondroid lobules with fibrovascular stroma. Chondromyxoid fibromas

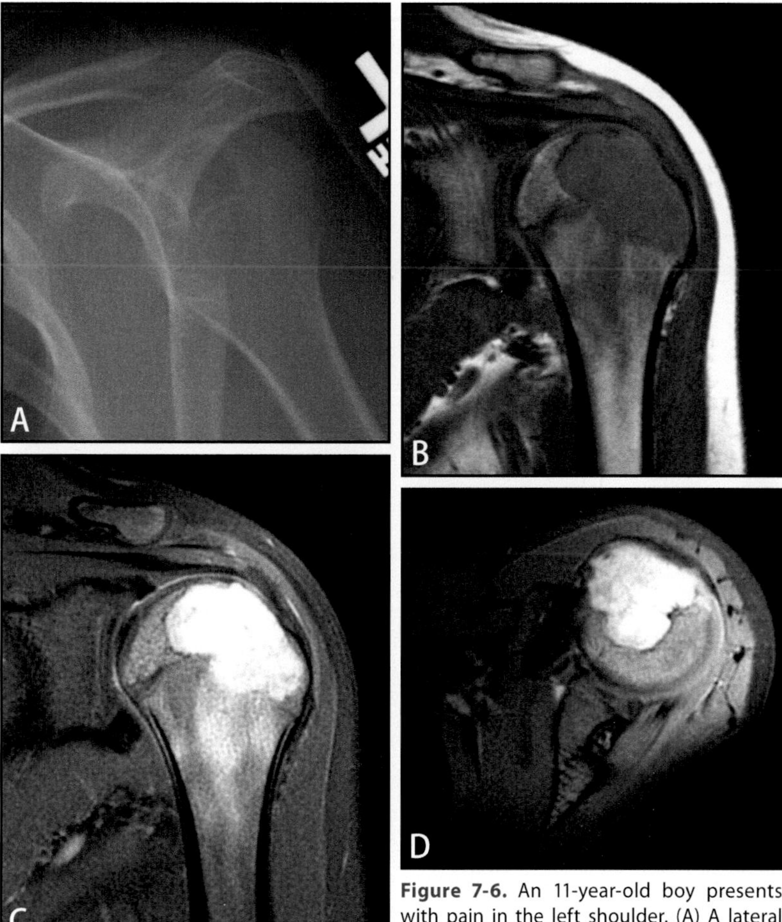

Figure 7-6. An 11-year-old boy presents with pain in the left shoulder. (A) A lateral radiograph of the shoulder demonstrates a lucent lesion of the proximal humeral epiphysis. Coronal (B) T1 and (C) T2, and (D) axial T2 MRI demonstrate a marrow-replacing lesion of the proximal humeral epiphysis with perilesional edema. Biopsy confirmed chondroblastoma.

may be slow-growing, indolent lesions, with a long duration of vague pain symptoms before discovery. Radiologically, these lesions are commonly metaphyseal and eccentric, with a scalloped or lobular appearance. The intramedullary border is often sharply demarcated and sclerotic, and thinning or loss of the overlying cortex is often present. T2-weighted MRI sequences may demonstrate heterogeneity within the lesion because hyperintense myxoid and chondroid areas are juxtaposed to hypointense fibrous areas (Figure 7-7).

As with other benign active lesions, intralesional resection with curettage and grafting is acceptable, with a local recurrence rate of 5% to 15%.

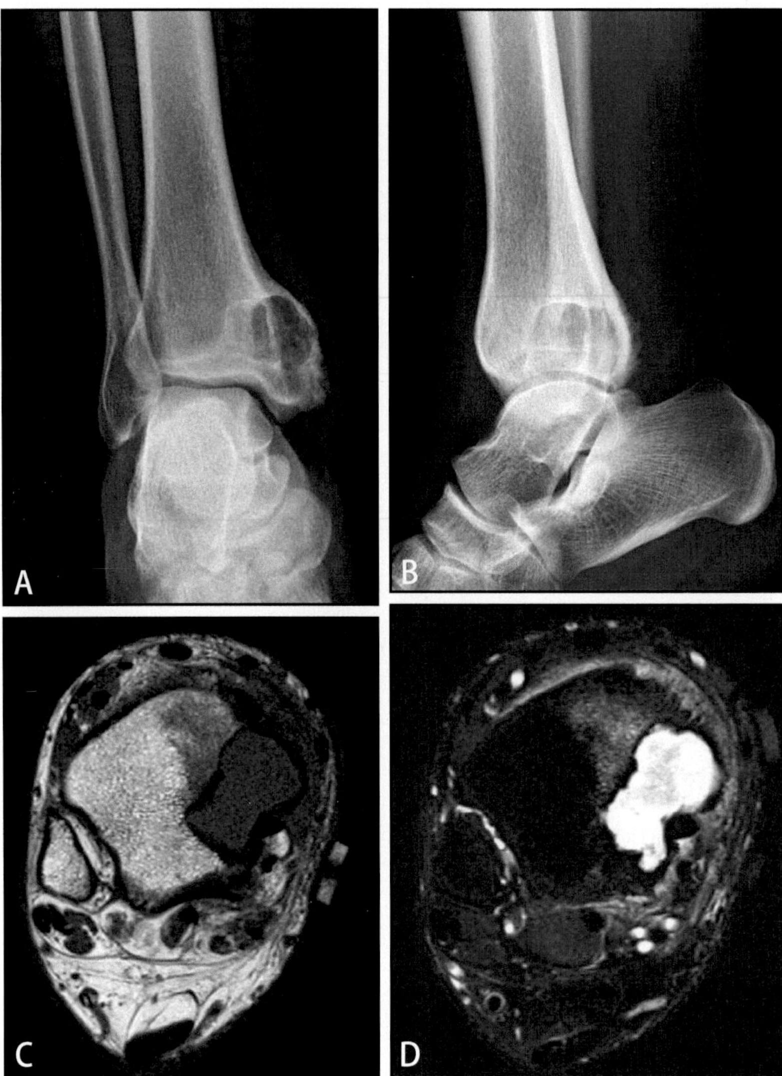

Figure 7-7. A 29-year-old man presents with 16 months of slowly progressive right ankle pain. (A) Anteroposterior and (B) lateral radiographs demonstrate a well-defined, lobular lesion of the distal tibial metaphysis, extending to the physeal scar, with expansion of the bone. Axial (C) T1 and (D) T2 magnetic resonance sequences demonstrate a marrow-replacing lesion with mild heterogeneity, with areas of intense fluid/myxoid signal admixed with more intermediate signal tumor. Biopsy confirmed a diagnosis of chondromyxoid fibroma.

Principles of Intralesional Resection

Preoperative Planning

An intralesional margin as definitive resection is acceptable only for known benign lesions, but the approach should be planned and performed by experienced practitioners similar to the approach for an open surgical biopsy, in the event that an unwelcome surprise or change in diagnosis is encountered (for example, the aneurysmal bone cyst that turns out to be a telangiectatic osteosarcoma).

Approach

A longitudinal incision should be made in line with the approach of definitive resection should conversion or revision to a more aggressive margin of resection be required. An oval opening is made in the bone, typically in the area of thinnest bone or soft-tissue extension. This window must be large enough to permit visualization of the entire lesional cavity. A headlamp or dental mirror can be useful. Visualization of the entire lesion is important because the risk of disease recurrence is inextricably linked to the adequacy of the resection. Areas of the cavity that cannot be seen cannot be curetted effectively. To that end, limited curettage through a keyhole or fenestration in the cortex is discouraged.

Resection

Large curettes and other instruments are used to remove the bulk of visible disease from the lesional cavity. This material should be processed for all appropriate diagnostic tests. Progressively smaller curettes are then used to clear out the crevices and corners of the cavity and scrape the walls free of bulky disease. Extremely thin or fragmented areas of cortex should be sacrificed with the resection because they are likely involved with disease, are unlikely to withstand extension of the curettage margin, and will not contribute significantly to the strength of the final reconstruction.

Extending the Resection Margin

High-speed burring of the walls of the cavity is performed to open and expose any small nooks and crannies within the bone, to smoothen the borders of the resection, and to fenestrate the margin of the lesion to reestablish continuity with the medullary space and intraosseous perfusion. This may be combined with a local adjuvant of choice for more aggressive lesions. Liquid adjuvants should be avoided if the defect is uncontained. Several cycles of

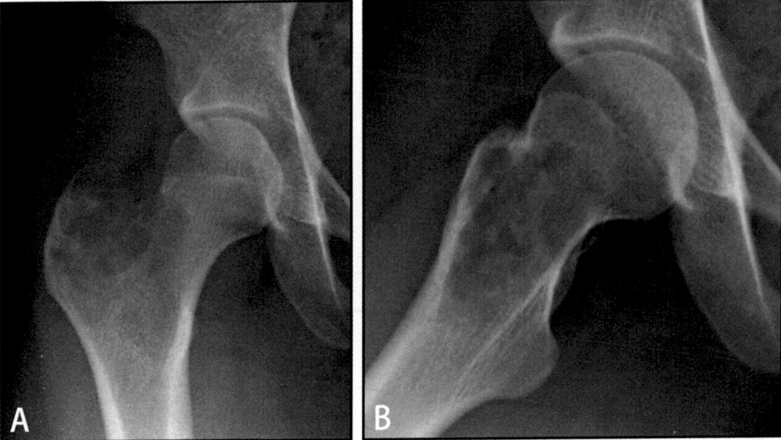

Figure 7-8. A 22-year-old woman presents with a painful limp and right hip discomfort. (A) Anteroposterior and (B) lateral plain radiographs demonstrate a lobular, lucent lesion extending from the greater trochanter into the proximal femoral metaphysis.

alternating argon beam coagulation of the cavity followed by high-speed burr removal of the carbonized material are a commonly employed method to safely extend the resection margin.

Filling the Defect and Mechanical Augmentation

There are numerous options for bone void filling after intralesional resection. Autograft bone provides immediate restoration of viable bone to the resection site, at the risk of donor site morbidity. Allograft bone and absorbable synthetics are available scaffolds for bone reconstruction, but are subject to graft resorption over the first few postoperative years, during which radiographic monitoring for local recurrence is important. Methyl methacrylate cement provides immediate structural augmentation of the bone but remains inert without the potential for reconstitution of bone stock. Often a hybrid approach may be appropriate, with grafting and rebuilding of the subchondral bone, followed by cementation of the structural defect with or without supplemental internal fixation (Figure 7-8).

Take-Aways

1. Osteoid osteomas are small but exquisitely painful lesions that are most effectively managed with percutaneous radiofrequency ablation.

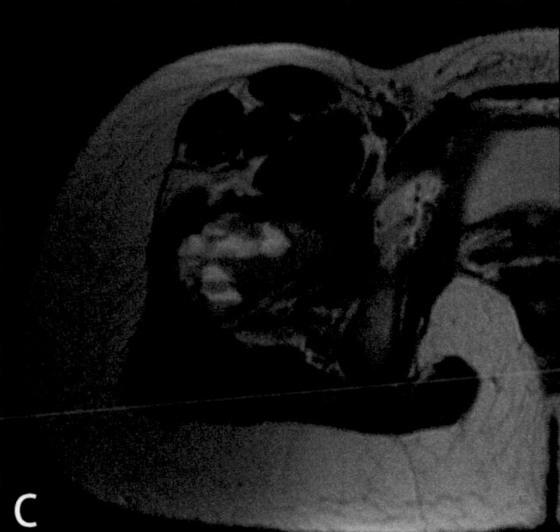

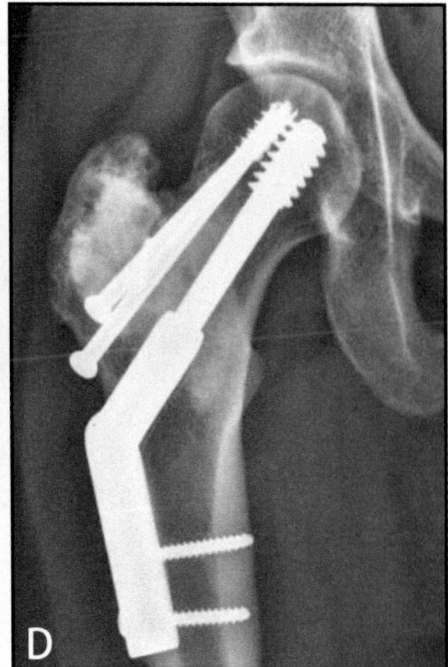

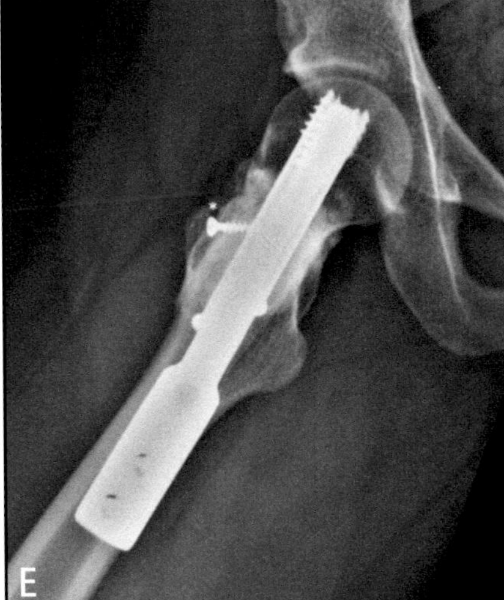

Figure 7-8 continued. (C) Non–fat-suppressed axial T2 MRI demonstrates fluid-fluid levels consistent with aneurysmal bone cyst, but biopsy confirmed a diagnosis of chondroblastoma of the greater trochanteric apophysis with secondary aneurysmal bone cyst features. An anterior cortical window was made to facilitate exposure of the intertrochanteric femur, through which extended intralesional curettage and argon beam coagulation was performed. (D and E) The defect was reconstructed with calcium phosphate cement and prophylactic internal fixation. After the cortical window was burred and treated with the argon beam, it was replaced and affixed with a single screw (white asterisk).

2. Aneurysmal bone cysts can occur as a primary bone tumor, but may also develop secondarily in other lesions. The possibility of an alternative underlying diagnosis must be considered in the management of ABCs.
3. GCT of bone and chondroblastoma are locally aggressive lesions with a small but notable incidence of pulmonary spread. These patients must be screened with chest imaging in addition to local treatment.
4. Intralesional curettage should not be approached as a "minimally invasive" surgical strategy. Local control of disease is most closely associated with the thoroughness and adequacy of the initial resection.

Commonly Tested Topics for Trainees

- A fine-cut computed tomography with a convincing clinical presentation for osteoid osteoma can be accepted as definitive, and referral for radiofrequency ablation is recommended. Osteoid osteoma can be recognized by 5 to 15 mm lucency within or adjacent to the bony cortex, surrounding sclerotic rim, and central ossification.
- The indications for denosumab in the management of GCT of bone are evolving. Current indications according to the Food and Drug Administration include unresectable lesions including metastatic disease, and lesions with unacceptable morbidity after surgical resection. Use of denosumab as a preoperative adjuvant to facilitate joint salvage is currently unproven and not within Food and Drug Administration guidelines.
- Apophyseal sites of appositional growth at tendon insertions are homologous to the epiphyses, and both are common locations for chondroblastoma.
- Aneurysmal bone cyst and telangiectatic osteosarcoma are very similar radiologically, and open biopsy is often the most reliable method to convincingly obtain a diagnosis.

References

1. Frassica FJ, Waltrip RL, Sponseller PD, Ma LD, McCarthy EF Jr. Clinicopathologic features and treatment of osteoid osteoma and osteoblastoma in children and adolescents. *Orthop Clin North Am.* 1996;27(3):559-574.
2. Di Giacomo G, Ziranu A, Perisano C, Piccioli A, Maccauro G. Local adjuvants in surgical management of bone lesions. *J Cancer Ther.* 2015;6(6):473-481. doi:10.4236/jct.2015.66051
3. Varshney MK, Rastogi A, Khan SA, Trikha V. Is sclerotherapy better than intralesional excision for treating aneurysmal bone cysts? *Clin Orthop Relat Res.* 2010;468(6):1649-1659. doi:10.1007/s11999-009-1144-8.
4. Errani C, Tsukamoto S, Leone G, et al. Denosumab may increase the risk of local recurrence in patients with giant-cell tumor of bone treated with curettage. *J Bone Joint Surg Am.* 2018;100(6):496-504. doi:10.2106/JBJS.17.00057.
5. Lin PP, Thenappan A, Deavers MT, Lewis VO, Yasko AW. Treatment and prognosis of chondroblastoma. *Clin Orthop Relat Res.* 2005;438:103-9. doi:10.1097/01.blo.0000179591.72844.c3.

8

Bone Malignancies in Children and Young Adults

Overview

Bone malignancies in young patients are uncommon but serious entities that can be missed by uninformed or inattentive practitioners. As with all malignancies, patient outcomes are optimized with early recognition, swift diagnosis, and prompt treatment. We will discuss ways to recognize the most common primary bone cancers in children and young adults, and present fundamentals of diagnosis, staging, and treatment. We will also touch on the peculiar entity of Langerhans cell histiocytosis.

Bone lesions that are painful, ill-defined, and destructive are worrisome in the young patient. Malignancies of bone in children are often ignored for weeks to months because symptoms may be wrongly attributed to growing pains or minor bumps and falls. Pain that is unilateral without a clear history of injury, persistent or unrelenting pain, or night pain that continues to be present by morning is generally inconsistent with growing pains and should be evaluated clinically. Skeletal pains associated with any swelling, limp, restricted range of motion, warmth or erythema, or tenderness to palpation should be evaluated radiographically. Any abnormal radiographic findings should then be pursued swiftly.

Approximately 5% to 10% of all pediatric malignancies arise in bone.[1] Any bone may be involved, but the long bones of the appendicular skeleton are favored sites. Advances in systemic treatment options have transformed the management of childhood cancers, and the prognosis is generally favorable

Wallace, MT
Handbook of Musculoskeletal Tumors (pp 105-123).

when diagnosed and managed properly. This requires close cooperation and regular communication between the musculoskeletal oncology specialist and other members of a multidisciplinary care team, including medical oncologists, radiation specialists, pain management, social work and support groups, and rehabilitation specialists including physical therapists and orthotists. For this reason, patients with primary bone malignancies are best managed at centers equipped to provide this broad range of services.

For primary bone malignancies that require surgical resection, a limb salvage strategy with wide resection and skeletal reconstruction is the recommended approach to treatment because functional outcomes are superior to limb ablation, and long-term survival outcomes are identical.[2] More than 90% of bone sarcomas can be effectively managed with limb salvage. Reconstructive options for limb salvage are numerous and include arthrodesis, vascularized autograft, distraction osteogenesis, rotationplasty, allograft, endoprosthesis, and composite reconstructions. These must be performed by experienced practitioners only, and it is not recommended to undertake management of primary bone malignancies outside a dedicated musculoskeletal oncology care center.

Osteosarcoma

Osteogenic sarcoma is the most common primary sarcoma of bone. The peak incidence of osteosarcoma is in the second decade of life, and this peak represents 3% of all pediatric malignancies. A second smaller peak occurs in the seventh decade of life, when osteosarcomas may occur secondary to preexisting conditions of bone.

Pathogenesis of Osteogenic Sarcoma

Pediatric Osteosarcoma (Most often de novo)

- Li-Fraumeni syndrome: inactivating mutation of *TP53* tumor suppressor gene
- Hereditary retinoblastoma: mutation of *RB1* tumor suppressor gene
- Rothmund-Thomson syndrome: mutation in *RECQL4* helicase gene
- Bloom syndrome: mutation in *BLM* gene *(RECQL3)*
- Werner syndrome: mutation in *WRN* gene *(RECQL2)*

Adult and Elderly Osteosarcoma (De novo)

- Paget's disease of bone
- Irradiated bone
- Fibrous dysplasia
- Chronic osteomyelitis
- Bone infarct

Osteosarcoma may develop in any bone, but the metaphyseal regions of the long bones are favored. The radiographic appearance of osteosarcomas can differ widely, with variable degrees of mineralization and bone destruction, but all osteosarcomas are defined by their ability to produce malignant osteoid. Table 8-1 presents the diagnostic and clinical features of the most common variants of osteogenic sarcoma.

Staging Studies to Order for Newly Diagnosed Osteosarcoma

- Whole-bone plain radiographs
- Whole-bone magnetic resonance imaging (MRI): evaluate for discontinuous tumor (skip metastases)
- Total-body technetium-99 medronic acid (Tc-99m) bone scan: evaluate for synchronous bone metastases
- Chest computed tomography (CT): evaluate for pulmonary metastases
- L-lactate dehydrogenase
- Alkaline phosphatase

The mainstay of management of lower-grade variants of osteosarcoma remains wide surgical resection with negative margins (Figure 8-1). Positive surgical margins after osteosarcoma resection are associated with near-certain rates of local recurrence, often with more aggressive clinical behavior at the time of recurrence.

Higher-grade osteosarcomas are managed with an aggressive protocol of high-dose multiagent chemotherapy and wide surgical resection. In the pre-chemotherapy era, treatment of nonmetastatic osteosarcoma with immediate amputation provided only a 15% to 20% rate of long-term survival, confirming that occult pulmonary micrometastatic disease is likely present at the time of diagnosis, undetectable by staging radiography. Multiagent chemotherapy has shown substantial improvement in rates of disease-free survival. Preoperative chemotherapy facilitates limb salvage by promoting ossification within the tumor, and histological examination of postchemotherapy response rates on the resected specimen has shown prognostic significance. A "good" chemotherapy response rate of greater than 90% tumor necrosis

Table 8-1

Osteosarcoma Variants

GRADE	OS SUBTYPE (%)	DEFINING FEATURES	TREATMENT	PROGNOSIS
Low	Parosteal (4%)	Surface based Radiodense Lobular, may encircle bone	Wide resection	95% survival
	Well-differentiated intraosseous (1%)	Fibroblastic	Wide resection	95% survival
Intermediate	Periosteal (2%)	Surface based "Sunburst" appearance Chondroblastic	Wide resection ± chemotherapy	85% survival
	Osteoblastoma-like (<1%)	Radiographically and histologically mimics osteoblastoma	Wide resection ± chemotherapy	67% survival
High	High-grade surface (<1%)	Surface based Variable osteoid production	1) Preoperative chemotherapy 2) Wide resection 3) Postoperative chemotherapy	60% to 70% survival
	Conventional (75%)	Intramedullary Variable osteoid production Heterogeneous differentiation (chondroblastic, fibroblastic, osteoblastic)	1) Preoperative chemotherapy 2) Wide resection 3) Postoperative chemotherapy	60% to 85% survival

(continued)

Table 8-1 (continued)

Osteosarcoma Variants

GRADE	OS SUBTYPE (%)	DEFINING FEATURES	TREATMENT	PROGNOSIS
	Telangiectatic (4%)	Expansile Mostly lytic Aneurysmal cystic changes on MRI "Bag of blood" gross appearance	1) Preoperative chemotherapy 2) Wide resection 3) Postoperative chemotherapy	60% to 80% survival
	Giant cell-rich (<0.5%)	Similar appearance and histology to GCT	1) Preoperative chemotherapy 2) Wide resection 3) Postoperative chemotherapy	60% to 70% survival
Aggressive	Small cell (1.5%)	Small round-cell tumor, similar to Ewing sarcoma	1) Preoperative chemotherapy 2) Wide resection 3) Postoperative chemotherapy	25% to 35% survival
	Postradiation (<0.5%)	Occurs within radiation field after minimum 3 years latency period	1) Preoperative chemotherapy 2) Wide resection 3) Postoperative chemotherapy	25% survival
	Paget's sarcoma (<0.5%)	Develops within pagetoid bone	1) Wide resection ± chemotherapy 2) Supportive care	0% to 10% survival

Abbreviations: GCT, giant cell tumor; MRI, magnetic resonance imaging; OS, osteosarcoma. (Adapted from Rougraff BT.[3])

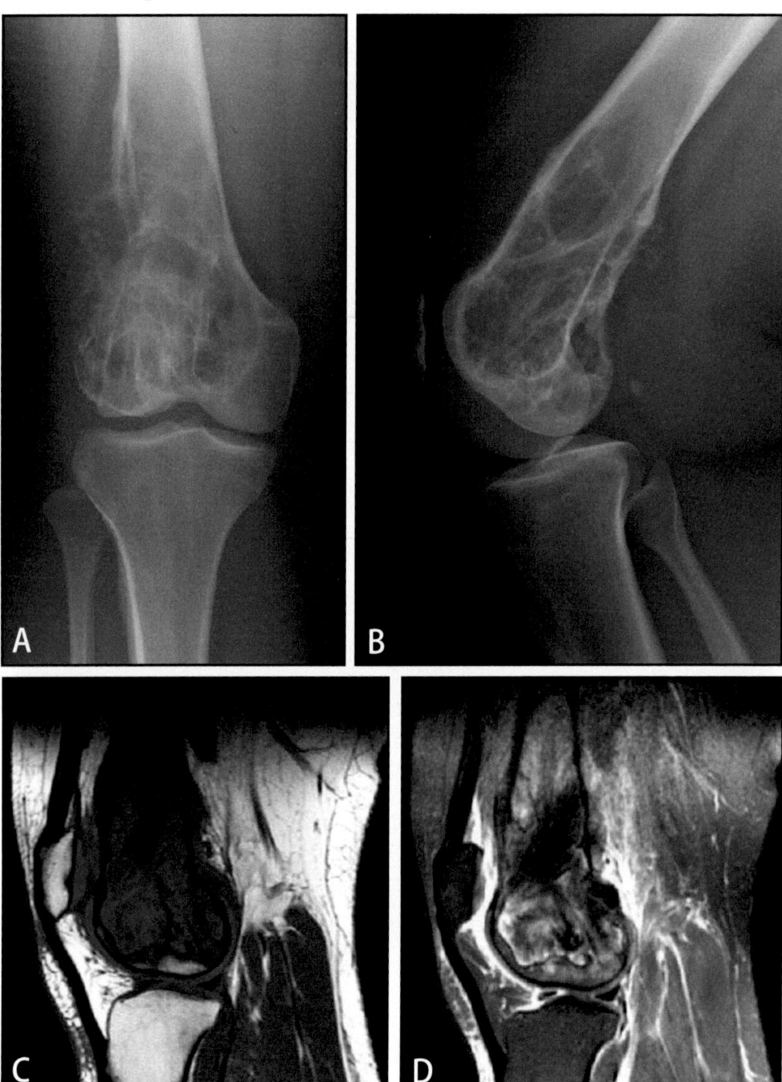

Figure 8-1. A 28-year-old woman presents with worsening right knee pain, stiffness, and a limp. (A) Anteroposterior and (B) lateral radiographs demonstrate a destructive lesion of the right distal femur with cortical breakout and extraosseous osteoid production. Sagittal (C) T1 and (D) T2 MRI demonstrates a marrow-replacing process involving the distal femur with associated soft-tissue extension.

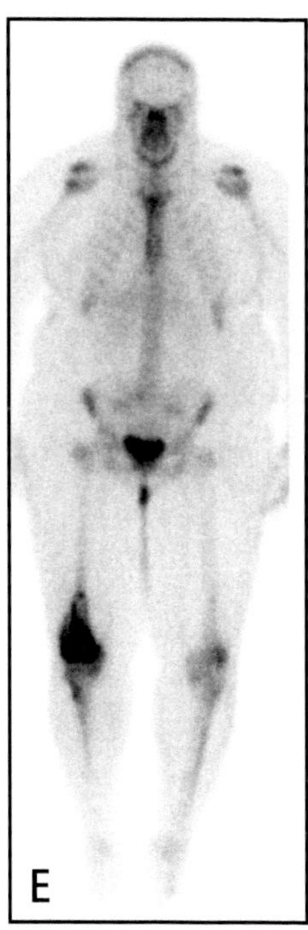

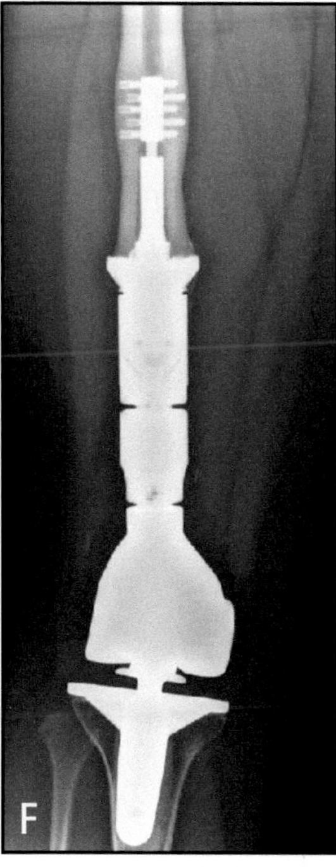

Figure 8-1 continued. Technetium-99 medronic acid (Tc-99m) bone scintigraphy (E) demonstrates intense uptake with no other sites of disease. Biopsy demonstrated a dense fibrous and bony lesion confirming a diagnosis of well-differentiated osteosarcoma. Limb salvage was performed with wide surgical resection and endoprosthetic replacement (F).

places the patient in an overall better prognostic category. Postoperative chemotherapy can then be planned based on this information. This chemo-surgery-chemo approach to treatment remains the standard of care for high-grade osteogenic sarcoma (Figure 8-2).

Chemotherapy Agents Used in Treatment of Osteosarcoma

- High-dose methotrexate
- Doxorubicin (adriamycin)
- Cisplatin
    - Ifosfamide
    - Etoposide

Figure 8-2. A 37-year-old man presents with pain and very firm swelling about the right clavicle. (A) Chest radiograph is largely unremarkable except for an indistinct superior border of the right clavicle. However, (B) axial and (C) coronal CT sequences demonstrate an ill-defined, bone-producing lesion of the right clavicle with soft-tissue extension. (D) Axial T2-weighted MRI shows circumferential soft-tissue involvement about the clavicle. A biopsy confirmed a diagnosis of high-grade conventional osteosarcoma. (E) After neoadjuvant chemotherapy, the patient underwent right claviculectomy followed by postoperative chemotherapy.

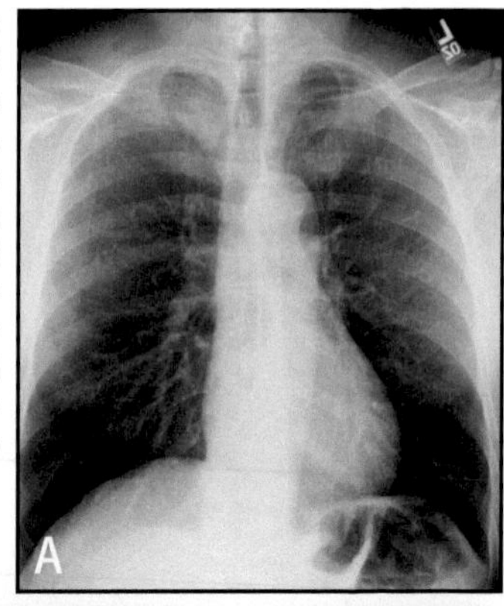

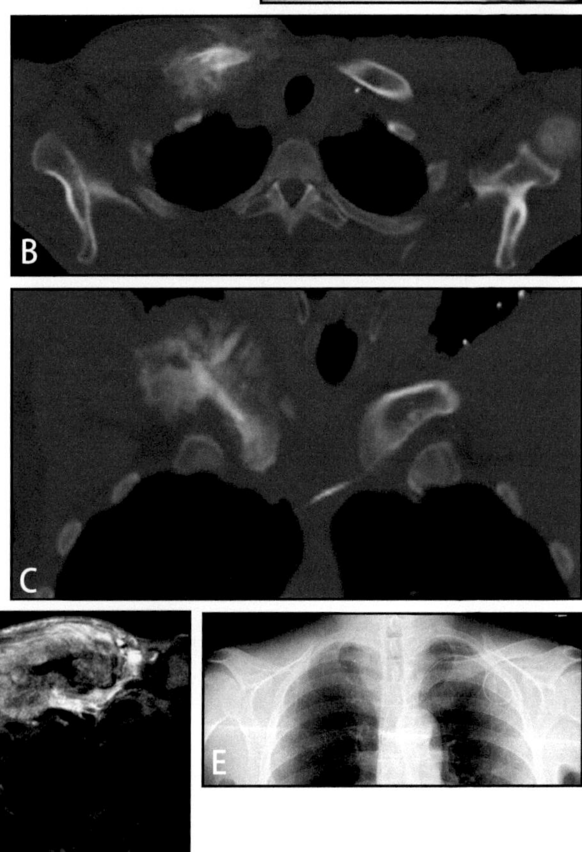

Ewing Sarcoma

Ewing sarcoma is the second-most common primary sarcoma of bone. Primarily a pediatric malignancy, the peak incidence of Ewing sarcoma is the second decade of life, representing 1% of pediatric malignancies. Ewing sarcoma is overwhelmingly more common in Caucasians. Ewing sarcoma presents with pain similar to other primary malignancies of bone, but soft-tissue swelling is often more pronounced, and unlike other sarcomas, systemic symptoms such as fever, fatigue, anorexia, and weight loss may be present.

Ewing sarcoma belongs to a family of malignancies known as small round-cell tumors, which includes primitive neuroectodermal tumor, rhabdomyosarcoma, non-Hodgkin lymphoma, retinoblastoma, neuroblastoma, and nephroblastoma/Wilms' tumor. Ewing tumor is differentiated from other small round-cell malignancies by immunohistochemical staining with CD99, and by cytogenetic identification of a translocation rearrangement of the *EWS* gene on chromosome 22q12. The t(11,22) EWS-FLI1 translocation is present in 90% of Ewing tumors, and an additional 5% of cases demonstrate a t(21;22) *EWS-ERG* rearrangement.

Although Ewing tumor is more common in the extremities, it displays a predilection for the flat bones of the pelvis and scapula. Radiographs frequently demonstrate subtle bony destruction with occasional layered periosteal reaction termed *onion skinning*. MRI is generally more impressive, with extensive marrow infiltration and an associated soft-tissue mass (Figure 8-3). A biopsy is always required for accurate diagnosis, and adequate tissue for specialized studies and cytogenetics should be obtained.

Staging Studies to Order for Newly Diagnosed Ewing Sarcoma

- Whole-bone plain radiographs
- Whole-bone MRI: evaluate for discontinuous tumor (skip metastases)
- Total-body Tc-99m bone scan: evaluate for synchronous bone metastases
- Chest CT: evaluate for pulmonary metastases
- L-lactate dehydrogenase
- Alkaline phosphatase
- Complete blood count
- Erythrocyte sedimentation rate, C-reactive protein
- Bone marrow evaluation: whole-body positron emission tomography-CT, whole-body MRI, or bone marrow aspiration

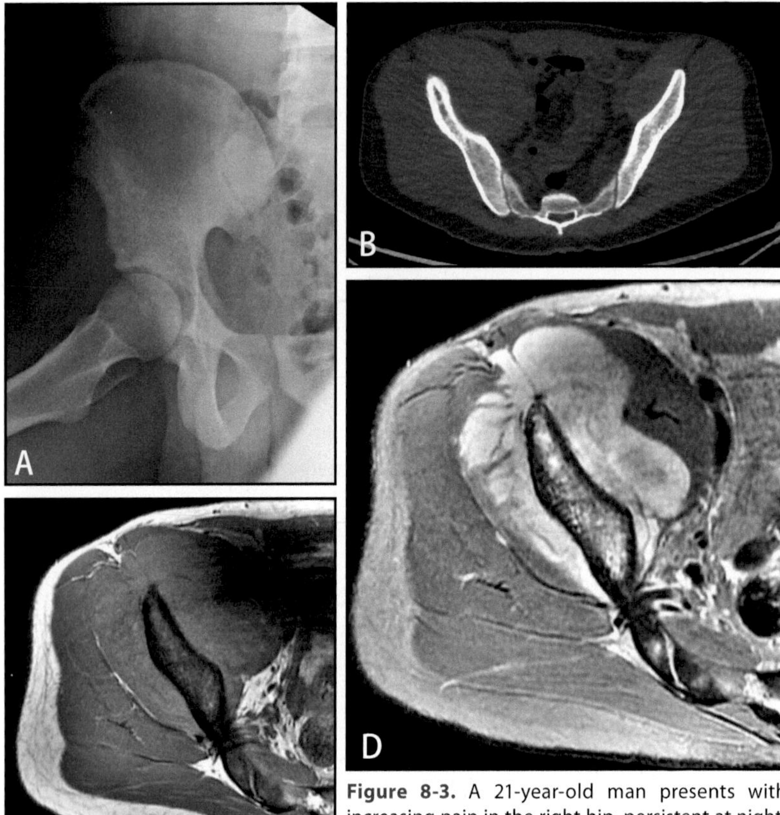

Figure 8-3. A 21-year-old man presents with increasing pain in the right hip, persistent at night. (A) Radiograph demonstrates very subtle, patchy sclerosis involving the anterior right ilium. CT demonstrates modest periosteal changes with a large soft-tissue mass in the right hemipelvis. Axial (C) T1 and (D) T2 MRI sequences demonstrate an infiltrative lesion of the right ilium with significant, circumferential soft-tissue extension. Biopsy confirmed a diagnosis of Ewing sarcoma.

Local control of Ewing sarcoma can be accomplished with either wide surgical resection with negative margins, or radiotherapy with a cumulative dose between 35 and 60 Gy. Owing to the complications of radiotherapy in the younger patient population, the recommended treatment for local control of Ewing sarcoma is surgical resection whenever feasible (Figure 8-4).

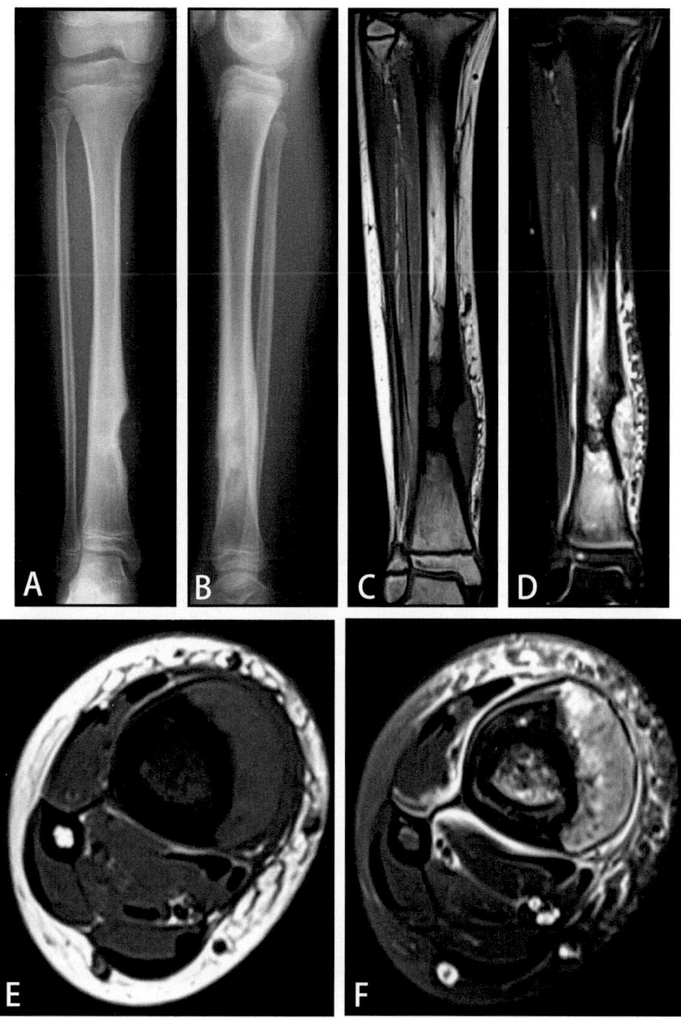

Figure 8-4. A 9-year-old girl presents with painful swelling in the right lower leg and pain at night. (A) Anteroposterior and (B) lateral radiographs demonstrate an ill-defined lesion of the distal tibial diaphysis, with cortical breakout and periosteal reaction. Coronal (C) T1, (D) T2, and axial (E) T1 and (F) T2 MRI sequences demonstrate a marrow-replacing lesion with notable soft-tissue extension.

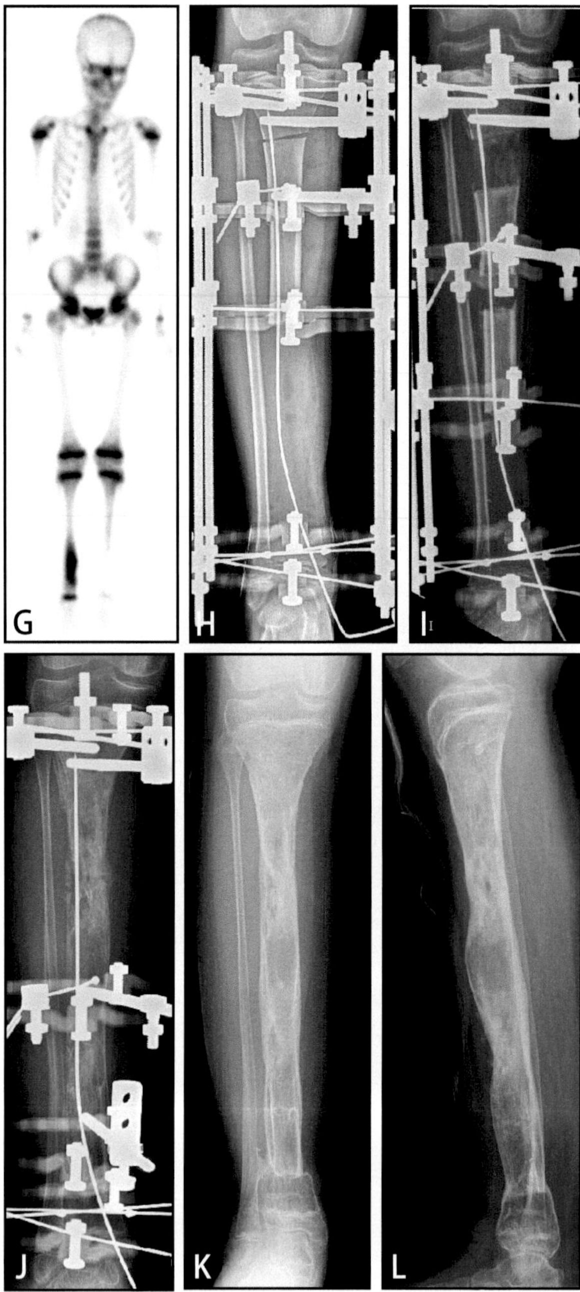

Figure 8-4 continued. (G) Technetium bone scan demonstrates an isolated lesion to the right tibia, and a biopsy confirmed Ewing sarcoma. (H-L) The patient underwent limb salvage with distraction osteogenesis.

Indications for Radiation Therapy as Definitive Local Treatment of Ewing Sarcoma

- Unresectable tumors: head and neck, spine and sacrum
- Metastatic disease
- Positive surgical margins
- Patient choice
- Palliation

Complications of Radiation Therapy for Ewing Sarcoma

- Higher risk of local recurrence (15% to 40%): viable cells likely left behind in tumors that are larger or with poor chemotherapy response[4]
- Postradiation malignancy (5% to 20% risk at 20 years posttreatment)[5]
- Tissue toxicity: fibrosis, atrophy, contracture
- Lymphedema
- Growth arrest or deformity
- Postradiation or insufficiency fractures with limited healing potential

Ewing sarcoma is a high-grade, aggressive malignancy, and is managed similarly to higher-grade osteosarcomas, with an aggressive regimen of preoperative chemotherapy, followed by local treatment with surgery or radiation, followed thereafter by an extended course of more chemotherapy. A chemotherapy response rate greater than 90% is considered "good," but ideal tumor necrosis is 99% to 100%, which provides the best prognostic stratification.[6]

Chemotherapy Agents Used in Treatment of Ewing Sarcoma

- Vincristine
- Doxorubicin (adriamycin)
- Cyclophosphamide
- Actinomycin D
- Ifosfamide
- Etoposide

Primary Lymphoma of Bone

Lymphomas represent 16% of all pediatric malignancies, and approximately 7% of primary bone malignancies. The majority of primary bone lymphomas are non-Hodgkin lymphomas, typically of the high-grade diffuse large B-cell type, followed by the more indolent follicular lymphoma. Lymphoma of bone can occur at any age, but should be considered in the young adult and middle-aged patient populations. Bone lymphomas present similarly to Ewing sarcoma, with significant pain, soft-tissue swelling, and systemic symptoms such as fever, fatigue, anorexia, and weight loss. Regional lymphadenopathy may also be present. Pain is often relieved with anti-inflammatories such as corticosteroids and nonsteroidal anti-inflammatories.

As with other small round-cell tumors, imaging of bone lymphomas will often demonstrate subtle, poorly defined bony destruction with an associated soft-tissue mass (Figure 8-5). Any bone may be involved, but flat bones are common sites. Lymphoma is differentiated from other small round-cell malignancies by immunohistochemical staining with CD20 and CD45, flow cytometry, and other cytogenetics. This requires aggressive lesional sampling for accurate diagnosis, and tissue should be sent in saline for initial processing so that specialized studies can be performed. For this reason, open biopsy may be preferable to percutaneous sampling.

Non-Hodgkin lymphoma can be definitively treated with systemic chemotherapy. After a thorough fracture risk assessment, patients should be referred for whole-body positron emission tomography-CT for staging, followed by prompt referral to a medical oncologist to begin treatment. Surgery for large, infiltrative lesions at risk of fracture is managed similarly to metastatic disease to bone. Localized disease is associated with long-term survival rates greater than 80%.[7]

Special Note: Histiocytosis

Langerhans cell histiocytosis, formerly known as histiocytosis X, is a disease of non-neoplastic proliferating histiocytes with a spectrum of severity ranging from focal, self-limiting lesions to disseminated fatal disease. Bony involvement is typically painful, and may present similarly to primary bone malignancy, including the presence of low-grade fevers. The axial skeleton, including skull, spine, ribs, and pelvis are favored sites, but extremity involvement is not unusual. Bony lesions can present in any location within the bone, and may be well defined and punched out, or more infiltrative with cortical and periosteal changes. For this reason, Langerhans cell histiocytosis is an effective mimicker both of benign and malignant bone tumors and

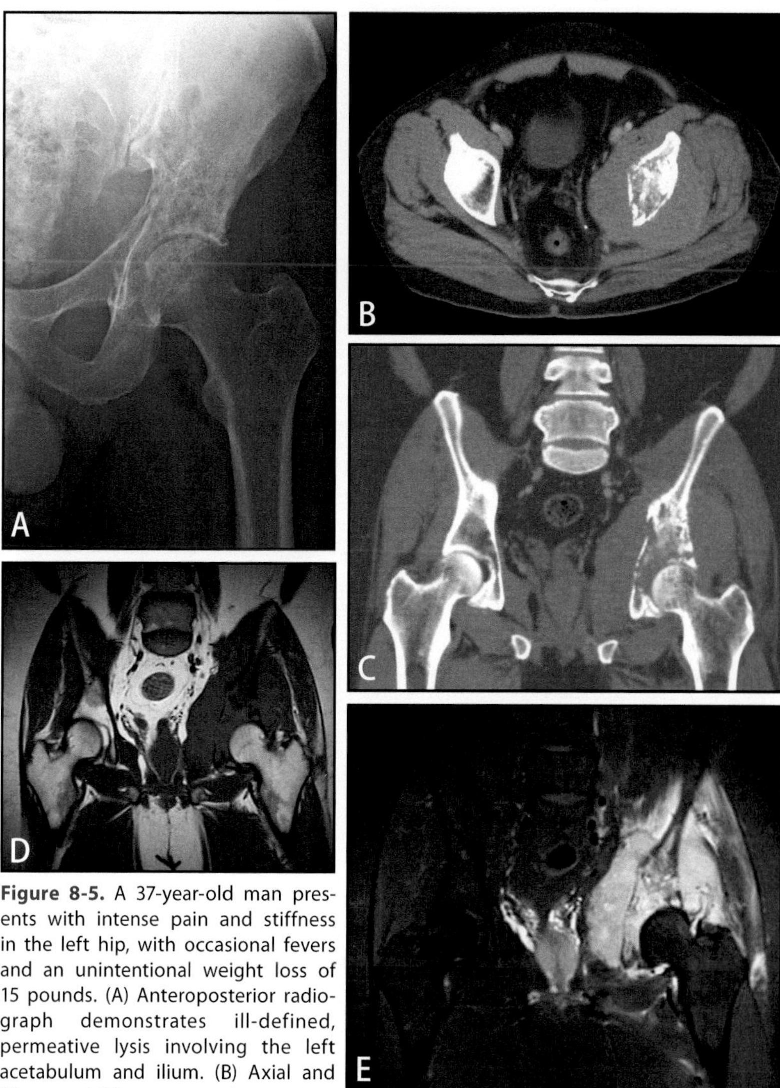

Figure 8-5. A 37-year-old man presents with intense pain and stiffness in the left hip, with occasional fevers and an unintentional weight loss of 15 pounds. (A) Anteroposterior radiograph demonstrates ill-defined, permeative lysis involving the left acetabulum and ilium. (B) Axial and (C) coronal CT sequences demonstrate lytic changes involving the left acetabulum with an associated soft-tissue mass. Coronal (D) T1 and (E) T2 MRI sequences demonstrate an extensive marrow-replacing process involving the left hemipelvis with circumferential soft-tissue involvement.

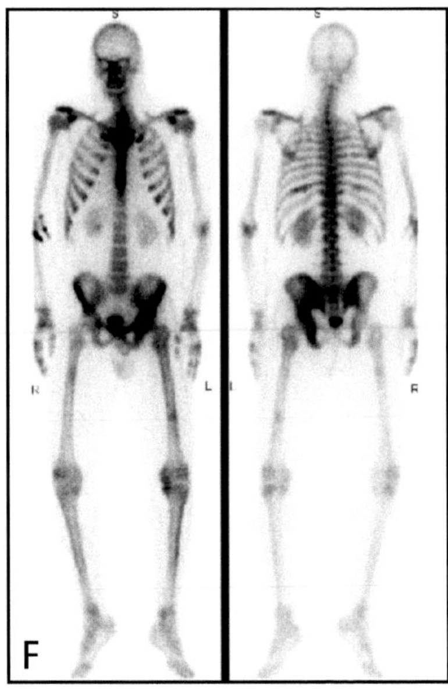

Figure 8-5 continued. (F) Bone scintigraphy demonstrates isolated involvement of the left pelvis. A biopsy confirmed diffuse large B-cell lymphoma, and the patient was managed with systemic chemotherapy only.

should be considered in the differential for bone lesions in any young patient (Figure 8-6).

Clinical Spectrum of Langerhans Cell Histiocytosis With Skeletal Involvement

- Eosinophilic granuloma: solitary, self-limited lesions confined to bone
- Hand-Schüller-Christian syndrome: clinical triad of multifocal bony disease, classically of the skull, exophthalmos, and diabetes insipidus from pituitary involvement
- Abt-Letterer-Siwe disease: multiorgan involvement with disseminated bony lesions, hepatosplenomegaly, skin lesions, and a poor prognosis

Biopsy is usually required for diagnosis, and newly diagnosed patients should be screened for cranial and visceral disease. Multifocal and systemic disease must be referred to a medical oncologist for systemic chemotherapy and possible radiotherapy. Isolated skeletal lesions are typically self-limiting, and are responsive to corticosteroid injection or observation if asymptomatic. Curettage and grafting of high-risk lesions in the extremities is also appropriate. Unifocal spinal involvement (vertebra plana) can be effectively managed with nonoperative bracing, but low-dose radiotherapy or surgery may be considered for patients with signs of compressive myelopathy or neuropathy.

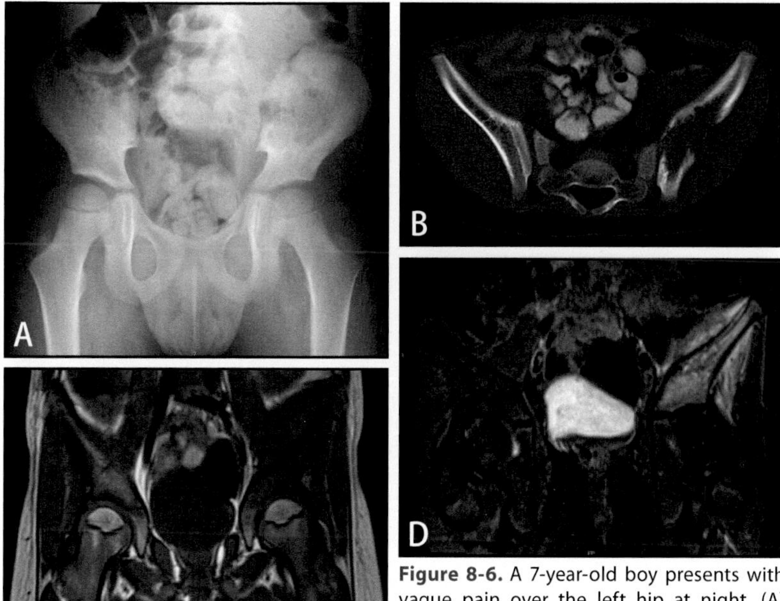

Figure 8-6. A 7-year-old boy presents with vague pain over the left hip at night. (A) Anteroposterior radiograph and (B) axial CT demonstrate an ill-defined destructive lesion within the superior left ilium. Coronal (C) T1 and (D) T2 MRI sequences demonstrate an infiltrative marrow-replacing process with involvement and edema in the adjacent soft tissues. Biopsy confirmed a diagnosis of eosinophilic granuloma.

The vertebral body can be expected to reconstitute to a height correlated to the age of onset; younger patients may demonstrate greater height recovery.[8] In the young patient, vertebra plana may be diagnosed without biopsy if there is collapse of the vertebral body, intact intervertebral disc spaces above and below the affected vertebra, and there is no associated soft-tissue mass.[9]

Take-Aways

1. An ill-defined or destructive bone lesion in a young patient should be evaluated and considered a potential primary bone malignancy until definitively diagnosed otherwise.
2. Osteosarcoma and Ewing sarcoma are the 2 most common pediatric bone cancers. Management generally consists of a combination of chemotherapy and wide surgical resection.

3. Lymphoma of bone is managed primarily with chemotherapy, with surgery reserved for lesions that have fractured or are at high risk of fracture.
4. Langerhans cell histiocytosis has several forms. Solitary lesions can be managed conservatively or with percutaneous injection. Multifocal forms are managed like malignancies.

Commonly Tested Topics for Trainees

- Low-grade variants of osteogenic sarcoma are managed with wide surgical resection, with excellent long-term prognosis. Intermediate-to-high grade lesions are managed with a chemo-surgery-chemo "sandwich."
- Ewing sarcoma is associated with a characteristic cytogenetic t(11:22) translocation in 90% of cases, which creates the gene-fusion product EWS-FLI1. EWS rearrangements are ubiquitous in mesenchymal malignancies.
- Surgery and radiation both are acceptable forms of obtaining local control for Ewing tumor, but surgical resection is recommended when possible because of the complication profile and elevated risk of recurrence with radiation therapy in young patients.
- Langerhans cell histiocytosis is a commonly tested and effective mimicker of benign as well as aggressive bone lesions.
- Langerhans cell histiocytosis of the spine (vertebra plana) can be effectively managed with bracing alone.

References

1. Hewitt M, Weiner SL, Simone JV. The epidemiology of childhood cancer. In: Institute of Medicine, National Research Council, National Cancer Policy Board, Hewitt M, Weiner SL, Simone JV, eds. *Childhood Cancer Survivorship: Improving Care and Quality of Life*. Washington, DC: National Academies Press; 2003.
2. Simon MA, Aschliman MA, Thomas N, Mankin HJ. Limb-salvage treatment versus amputation for osteosarcoma of the distal end of the femur. *J Bone Joint Surg Am.* 1986;68(9): 1331-1337.
3. Rougraff BT. Variants of osteosarcoma. *Curr Opin Orthop.* 1999;10(6):485-490.
4. Arai Y, Kun LE, Brooks MT, et.al. Ewing's sarcoma: local tumor control and patterns of failure following limited-volume radiation therapy. *Int J Radiat Oncol Biol Phys.* 1991;21(6):1501-1508. doi:10.1016/0360-3016(91)90325-x.
5. Fuchs B, Valenzuela RG, Petersen IA, Arndt CA, Sim FH. Ewing's sarcoma and the development of secondary malignancies. *Clin Orthop Relat Res.* 2003;(415):82-89. doi:10.1097/01.blo.0000093900.12372.e4.

6. Lin, PP, Jaffe N, Herzog CE, et.al. Chemotherapy response is an important predictor of local recurrence in Ewing sarcoma. *Cancer.* 2007;109(3):603-611. doi:10.1002/cncr.22412.
7. Ramadan KM, Shenkier T, Sehn LH, Gascoyne RD, Connors JM. A clinicopathological retrospective study of 131 patients with primary bone lymphomas: a population-based study of successively treated cohorts from the British Columbia Cancer Agency. *Ann Oncol.* 2007;18(1):129-35. doi:10.1093/annonc/mdl329.
8. Raab P, Hohmann F, Kühl J, Krauspe R. Vertebral remodeling in eosinophilic granuloma of the spine. A long-term follow-up. *Spine (Phila Pa 1976).* 1998;23(12):1351-1354. doi:10.1097/00007632-199806150-00011.
9. Garg S, Mehta S, Dormans JP. Langerhans cell histiocytosis of the spine in children. Long-term follow-up. *J Bone Joint Surg.* 2004;86(8):1740-1750. doi:10.2106/00004623-200408000-00019.

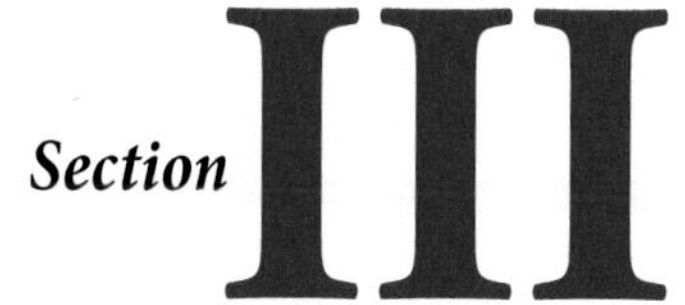

Bone Tumors in Older Adults

9

Myeloma and Metastatic Bone Disease

Overview

Millions of new cancer cases are diagnosed each year in the developed world. Advances in treatments continue to improve survivorship numbers to the point that a substantial percentage of these patients are surviving to later stages of disease. Myeloma and metastatic bone disease are the most common diseases encountered by musculoskeletal practitioners. We will discuss the evaluation and diagnosis of destructive bone lesions in older adults, review methods of predicting and preventing pathologic fracture, and present algorithms for management of lesions by anatomic location.

An ill-defined, destructive lesion in a patient older than 40 years is more often than not a complication of metastatic bone disease, myeloma, or lymphoma. The work-up of these lesions is therefore focused on accurate diagnosis, the determination of a primary site of origin, and identification of sites of skeletal involvement that require treatment.

Once confirmed, metastatic bone disease is no longer considered curable, and the goals of treatment shift to palliation. Surgical treatment should focus on pain relief, restoration of skeletal stability, maintaining ambulation, and optimization of functional mobility and independence. This requires communication and close coordination among surgical, medical, and radiation oncology practitioners to plan the timing of various treatments. As the role of personalized cancer care continues to expand and reach new frontiers, a secondary but important role of the surgeon is obtaining adequate tissue

Wallace, MT
Handbook of Musculoskeletal Tumors (pp 127-157).

not just for diagnosis, but for immunohistochemical staining, cytogenetic analysis, and tumor profiling. This is to assist the cancer team in identifying treatments with a reasonable likelihood of efficacy.

It is a statistical certainty that every musculoskeletal practitioner will encounter patients with metastatic bone disease and myeloma. Understanding the patterns of clinical presentation, key imaging features, and principles of diagnosis and management will ensure that these patients are diagnosed quickly, and that high-risk lesions can be managed safely, even outside musculoskeletal oncology specialty centers.

Evaluation of a Destructive Bone Lesion

Destructive bone lesions in older adults are usually discovered when they are painful or otherwise symptomatic, but occasionally are identified incidentally or during the staging work-up for a newly diagnosed malignancy. Unfortunately, many patients are not diagnosed until a lesion has progressed to the point of mechanical failure of the bone, and a pathologic fracture results.

Metastatic bone disease and lesions of myeloma typically present with deep and progressive bony pain. This pain may be poorly localized, present at rest, night-time, awakening, or with weight-bearing and use of the extremity. This pain is often unresponsive to oral analgesics, rest, and conservative measures. When spinal or neurological involvement is present, myelopathy and neuropathy may be presenting symptoms. Systemic complaints such fatigue, weight loss, anorexia, and symptoms of hypercalcemia may be present when disease is extensive.

Symptoms of hypercalcemia occur in 10% to 15% of patients presenting with metastatic bone disease and myeloma:

- Bones/moans: pain, arthralgias, myalgias, limp
- Groans: nausea, anorexia, constipation, abdominal pains, pancreatitis
- Stones: nephrolithiasis, cholelithiasis
- Psychiatric overtones: confusion, headache, depression, altered mental status

At extreme levels and when calcium levels escalate over a short period of time, hypercalcemia may cause renal shutdown, coma, and arrhythmia with cardiac arrest, and should be considered the most urgent medical threat to patients.

The most common carcinomas with a predilection for metastasis to bone can be remembered by the mnemonic device *"BLT with a Kosher Pickle,"* for Breast, Lung, Thyroid, Kidney, and Prostate cancer. This is far from a comprehensive list, however, because recent advances in systemic therapy and immunotherapy have prolonged the rates of survival for patients with gastrointestinal carcinomas and melanoma, which should also be considered. The work-up for a suspected metastatic lesion of unknown primary can be best facilitated by a thorough history and physical examination, followed by judiciously obtaining serological and imaging studies to screen for the aforementioned malignancies (Table 9-1).

A thorough history and physical examination will be able to identify a primary site of origin in 5% to 10% of cases. Adding appropriate laboratory and imaging studies increases this rate to 70% to 80%. A biopsy will be required in most cases to establish or confirm diagnosis.[1,2] Up to 3% to 5% of lesions will ultimately be diagnosed as carcinoma of unknown primary, and follow-up imaging studies or cytogenetic panels may be required to identify the most likely organ of origin.

Imaging Patterns Suggestive of Specific Diseases

- Solitary metastasis/few sites of disease (oligometastasis): renal cell carcinoma, but should be careful to rule out primary sarcoma of bone
- Blastic lesions of the spine and pelvis: prostate cancer (Figure 9-1)
- Mixed, diffuse lytic/blastic lesions: breast carcinoma, commonly receptor positive (Figure 9-2)
- Metastases distal to elbow or knee (acral metastases): lung carcinoma
- Painful metastases to soft tissue: lung carcinoma
- Numerous small, diffuse lesions: multiple myeloma (Figure 9-3)

Rationale for thorough prebiopsy evaluation:

- Blind biopsy without imaging is unable to render a diagnosis in more than 30% of cases.[1]
- Physical examination, serologies, or other studies may provide a definitive diagnosis and obviate the need for biopsy.
- Skeletal staging can help identify the lesion that is easiest and safest to biopsy, which may not be the most symptomatic lesion.
- Computed tomography (CT) may identify a tumor of origin associated with an elevated bleeding risk, for which needle biopsy and/or preoperative embolization should be considered.
- The clinician MUST exclude the possibility of a primary sarcoma of bone to avoid compromising later limb salvage.

Table 9-1

Data to Assist in the Work-Up of a Destructive Skeletal Lesion in an Adult

	METASTATIC CARCINOMA	MULTIPLE MYELOMA	SYSTEMIC NON-NEOPLASTIC
HISTORY	Smoking history Asbestos exposure Personal hx of cancer (be sure to obtain chemotherapy and radiation histories) Health screening tests (prostate exam, colonoscopy, mammogram, Papanicolaou smear) Immunosuppression Family hx	Immunosuppression Obesity MGUS/ Plasmacytoma Family hx	Metabolic bone disease • Renal insufficiency • Glucocorticoids • Anticonvulsants • MEN • Prior fractures • Malabsorption syndromes Infection • Immunodeficiency • Sepsis/ bacteremia • Invasive procedures/ trauma
PHYSICAL EXAMINATION	Breast exam Prostate exam Rectal exam/rectal blood Thyroid exam Abdominal exam Lymph node examination Skin check	Anemia/pallor Abdominal exam—organomegaly	Deformities Dentition Warmth, erythema, fluctuance Sinus/drainage

(continued)

- Identification of a suspected site of origin provides greater confidence in the biopsy material obtained. This increases the likelihood that a surgery can be performed as planned rather than aborting the procedure midcase to return at a later date.

Table 9-1 continued

Data to Assist in the Work-Up of a Destructive Skeletal Lesion in an Adult

	METASTATIC CARCINOMA	MULTIPLE MYELOMA	SYSTEMIC NON-NEOPLASTIC
LABORATORY	BMP, serum creatinine Serum calcium TSH, free T4 PSA CEA CA 125	CBC BMP, serum creatinine Serum calcium SPEP/UPEP β-2 microglobulin	Serum calcium, phosphorous PTH, TSH Alkaline phosphatase Vitamin D Inflammatory markers (ESR/CRP)
IMAGING	X-rays of involved bone and any other painful extremities Technetium-99m bone scan CT chest/abdomen/pelvis MRI if spinal involvement, +/- PET-CT	Skeletal survey ± PET-CT	Plain radiographs DEXA MRI as necessary

Abbreviations: BMP, basic metabolic panel; CBC, complete blood count; CEA, carcinoembryonic antigen; CRP, C-reactive protein; CT, computed tomography; DEXA, dual-energy x-ray absorptiometry; ESR, erythrocyte sedimentation rate; hx, history; MEN, multiple endocrine neoplasia; MGUS, monoclonal gammopathy of undetermined significance; MRI, magnetic resonance imaging; PET, positron emission tomography; PSA, prostate-specific antigen; PTH, parathyroid hormone; SPEP/UPEP, serum and urine protein electrophoresis; TSH, thyroid stimulating hormone.

If the primary tumor of origin is unknown or unconfirmed, if the lesion represents the first known site of skeletal involvement, or if internal fixation/violation of the tumor is planned, then a biopsy is MANDATORY to establish a tissue diagnosis BEFORE treatment is rendered.

- **It never hurts to know the diagnosis before treating the patient.**

The tissue confirmation must come before any other invasive intervention, so a needle biopsy or open biopsy should be considered the first stage of treatment. It is appropriate to obtain as much material as feasible for traditional histological staining, immunohistochemical staining, flow cytometry,

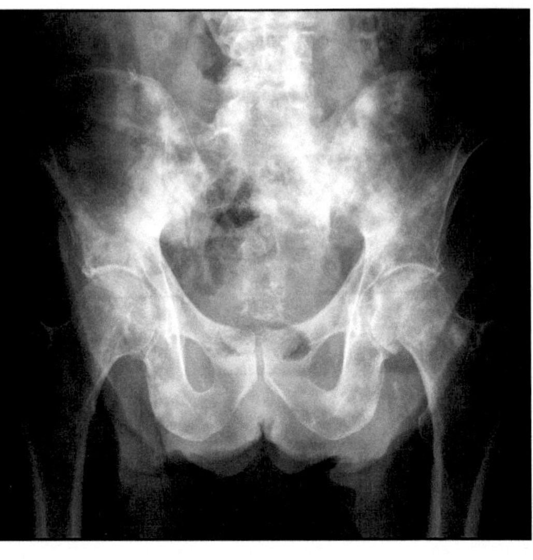

Figure 9-1. An 80-year-old man with known, stable metastatic prostate cancer to bone presents with left hip pain after a fall. Anteroposterior radiograph demonstrates numerous blastic lesions of the pelvis, spine, and proximal femora, as well as an impacted fracture of the left subcapital femoral neck. The stability of the patient's disease and clear mechanism of injury suggest that this fracture occurred as a result of impaired bone density rather than tumor involvement of the femoral neck. Impaired bone density is a risk with androgen-deprivation treatment for metastatic prostate cancer.

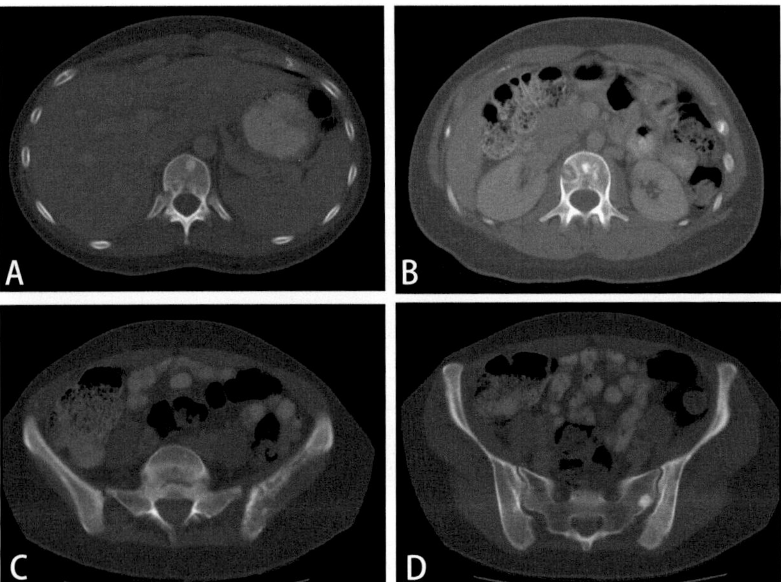

Figure 9-2. A 30-year-old woman presents with lower back and left-sided pelvic pain. (A through D) Axial CT demonstrates multiple lesions throughout the lumbar spine and pelvis, with areas of mixed lysis and sclerosis. Biopsy confirmed metastatic breast cancer.

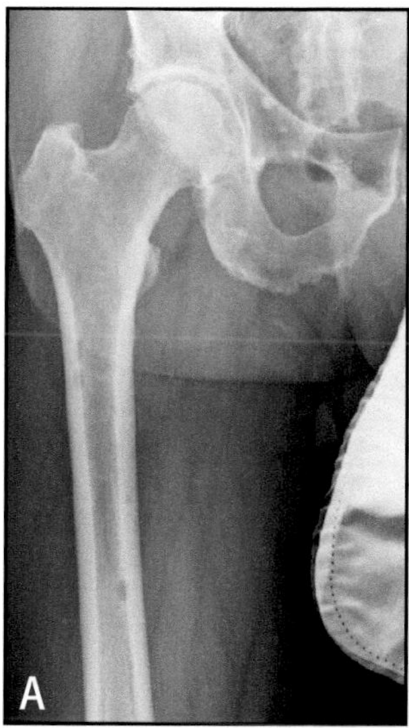

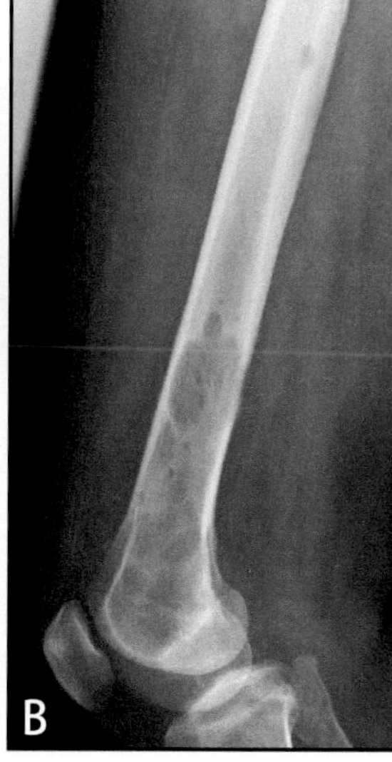

Figure 9-3. A 79-year-old man presents with increasing right lower-extremity pain with ambulation. Anteroposterior radiograph of the (A) right proximal femur and (B) lateral radiographs of the right distal femur demonstrate multiple, round, "punched-out" lucencies. Serological studies and biopsy were consistent with multiple myeloma.

cytogenetics and genomic profiling, and culture. Intramedullary reamings are not appropriate biopsy material. Reamings should be considered acceptable only when the diagnosis is already established, and the reamed material can be used for additional studies as previously stated.

Predicting Fracture Risk

Once the diagnosis has been established, specific treatment for each lesion is determined based on the severity of the patient's symptoms, the histology of the site of origin, the overall extent of disease, the performance status of the patient, and any history of favorable responses to prior treatments, including chemotherapy, hormone therapy, immunotherapy, and/or radiotherapy. Lesions that are asymptomatic and in low-risk anatomic locations are appropriate to observe on systemic treatment. Patients in poor health with severely limited life expectancy (patients actively dying or in hospice care) may be treated palliatively without surgery. Otherwise, painful lesions or lesions of the long bones and weight-bearing areas must undergo an assessment of fracture risk.

Identifying and preventing impending fractures is of critical importance for the musculoskeletal practitioner. Compared with patients treated after fracture, prophylactically stabilized patients are more likely to have shorter

Table 9-2

Mirels Scoring System for Diagnosing Impending Pathologic Fractures

CRITERIA	LOW RISK (1 POINT)	MODERATE RISK (2 POINTS)	HIGH RISK (3 POINTS)
Location	Upper extremity	Lower extremity	Peritrochanteric femur
Pain	Mild, manageable	Moderate, uncomfortable	Functional, reproducible with weight-bearing or mechanical loading
Radiographic pattern	Blastic/ sclerotic	Mixed lytic and blastic	Lytic
Size	<1/3 bone diameter	1/3 to 2/3 bone diameter	>2/3 bone diameter
Adapted from Mirels H.[5]			

postprocedure hospitalizations, are more likely to be discharged to home, return more quickly to previous functional level, and have a reduced risk of postoperative mortality.[3]

Pathologic bone fails most easily in torsion and bending. The overall size of the bony defect and the degree of cortical bone loss correlate to a loss of strength and subsequent risk of fracture that has been observed and validated statistically across many generations of risk-scoring criteria. Contemporary use of scoring systems has waned in favor of earlier intervention for painful lesions and the use of more predictive computer-based structural rigidity analysis, but these are not always readily available to the community practitioner.[4] The most common fracture risk-scoring system is that of Mirels, which estimates the risk of pathologic fracture based on 4 factors:

1. The location of the lesion
2. The character of the patient's pain
3. The pattern of radiographic involvement
4. The overall size of the lesion (Table 9-2, Figure 9-4)

If a lesion is fractured at presentation or is at a high risk of fracture, surgery to restore skeletal stability, alleviate pain, and restore function is appropriate. There are numerous options for stabilizing and/or reconstructing metastatic bone disease or myeloma, including internal fixation devices, prosthetic replacements, grafts, or a combination of options. The construct must be

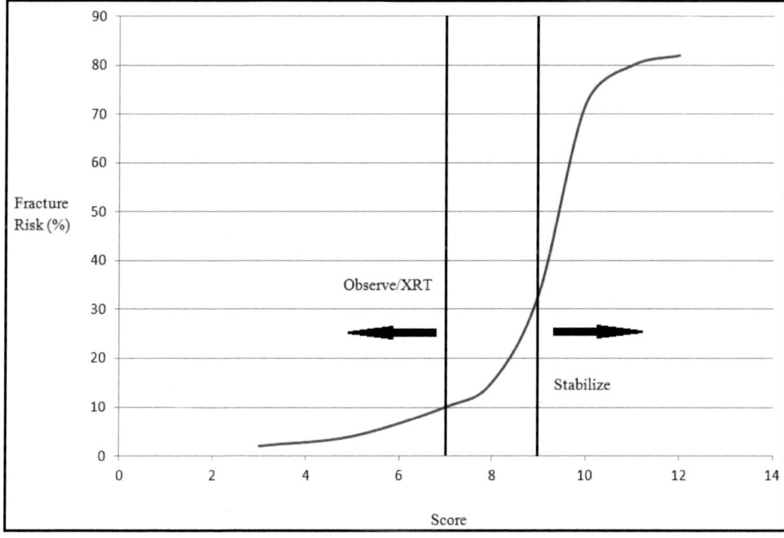

Figure 9-4. Probability of pathologic fracture as a function of Mirels' score. XRT indicates radiation therapy. (Adapted from Mirels H.[5])

planned to provide durable stabilization for the remainder of the patient's life, tolerate some local progression of disease, and protect as much of the bone as feasible. The origin of the primary tumor can suggest whether the lesion has a high likelihood of healing, or whether nonunion and local progression is expected. Myeloma, breast, and prostate cancers are more often responsive to systemic therapy and radiotherapy, and such lesions demonstrate greater healing potential than lung cancer, renal cell carcinoma, and metastatic melanoma, which tend to be more resistant to treatments.[6] As a general rule, the surgeon should not depend on expedient fracture healing to provide stability.

When to Resect Rather Than Stabilize

- Completed pathologic fractures with a low likelihood of healing, such as displaced femoral neck fractures
- Treatment-resistant tumors, including renal cell carcinoma, lung and gastrointestinal cancers, malignant melanoma, and metastatic sarcoma
- Lesions with extensive extraosseous disease/soft-tissue involvement
- Lesions with insufficient bone stock for fixation; do not expect reconstitution of bone stock after radiation therapy
- Solitary lesions with no other sites of skeletal disease
- Areas of failed prior internal fixation

- Postradiation fractures

When to Plan a Preoperative Embolization

- Hypervascular tumors: renal cell carcinoma, thyroid carcinoma, and pheochromocytoma
- Hemophilia or other bleeding diathesis
- Preoperative anemia or marrow suppression
- Jehovah's witnesses (The risk of life-threatening exsanguination should be frankly discussed with patients, and if a high probability of fatal blood loss can be expected even after embolization, nonoperative management should be strongly recommended.)

Management of Upper-Extremity Disease

The upper extremities are involved in 20% of patients with metastatic bone disease. Though not technically weight-bearing, the upper extremities may be required for support with assistive devices, and impairments in upper-extremity function can be significantly detrimental to self-care, functional independence, and activities of daily living. Upper-extremity disease should therefore be managed just as aggressively as lower-extremity disease.

Clavicle/Scapula

For oncologic indications, the clavicle is an expendable bone that can be resected in part or completely, with modest if any functional detriment. Lesions of the scapula generally do not contribute to skeletal instability, but pain and neurovascular compression can be no less limiting. Local treatment with radiotherapy and percutaneous thermal ablation techniques can provide effective relief of pain with favorable rates of local control.[7] Resection of selected lesions may be reserved for challenging cases.

Proximal Humerus

Surgical management of metastatic bone disease and myeloma of the proximal humerus should focus on restoring skeletal stability as well as glenohumeral joint stability. Figure 9-5 demonstrates an algorithm for management of proximal humerus disease. The primary diagnosis, likelihood of lesional healing, and remaining bone stock should be considered when choosing the method of reconstruction (Figures 9-6 and 9-7).

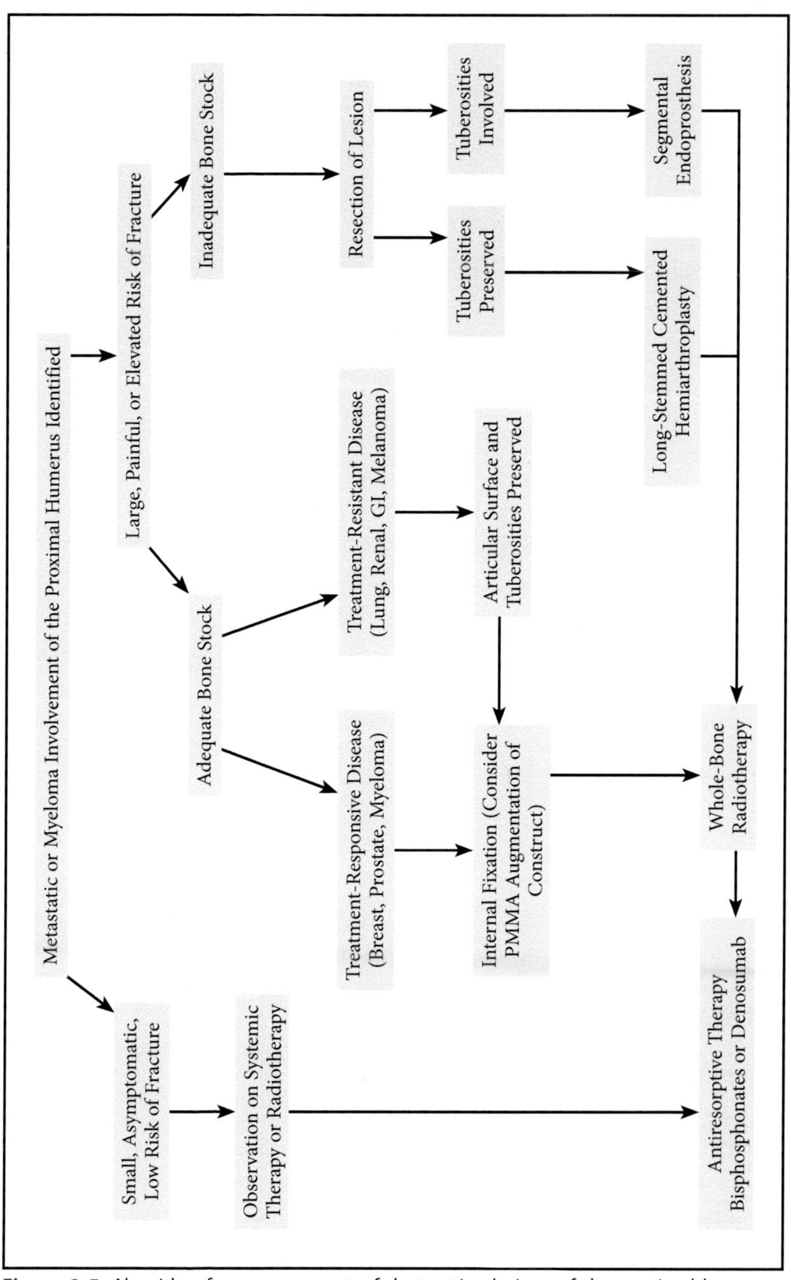

Figure 9-5. Algorithm for management of destructive lesions of the proximal humerus. Abbreviations: GI, gastrointestinal; PMMA, polymethyl methacrylate.

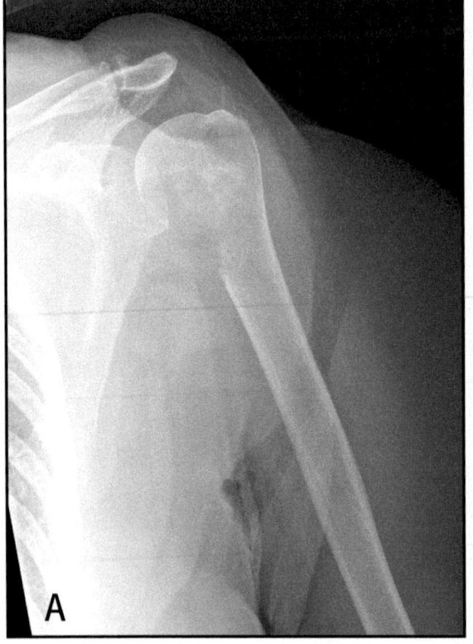

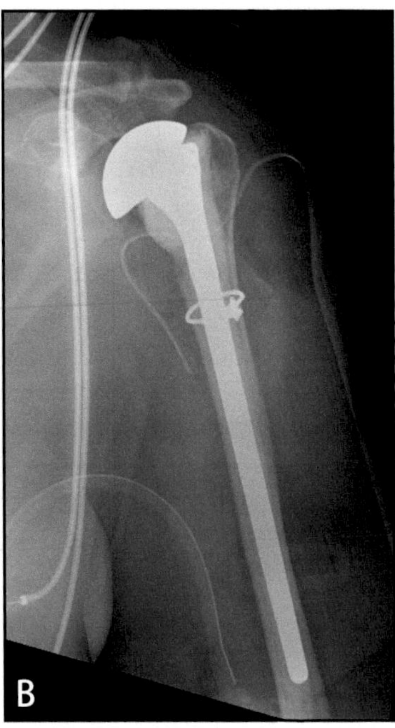

Figure 9-6. A 71-year-old female with metastatic non-small cell carcinoma of the lung presents with intense left shoulder pain. (A) Anteroposterior radiograph demonstrates a lytic, destructive lesion of the medial proximal humerus with extension to the articular surface, and relative sparing of the tuberosities. (B) Curettage resection of the lesion and reconstruction with a long-stemmed cemented arthroplasty implant was performed.

Humeral Shaft

Most diaphyseal lesions can be effectively managed with internal fixation devices that span the lesion. Lesions that meet indications for resection can be reconstructed with polymethyl methacrylate (PMMA) or an intercalary endoprosthesis (Figure 9-8).

Technical Tips for Intramedullary Nailing of Metastatic Disease of the Humerus

- Template nails preoperatively. Know the expected diameter and length of the implant to ensure that the implant is available, and have a slightly smaller implant in the room and on standby, so that if unexpected bleeding from the canal is encountered, the implant can be immediately inserted to provide tamponade
- Avoid attempting percutaneous nailing. Injury to the rotator cuff and reamings extruded into the joint can contribute to long-term rotator cuff

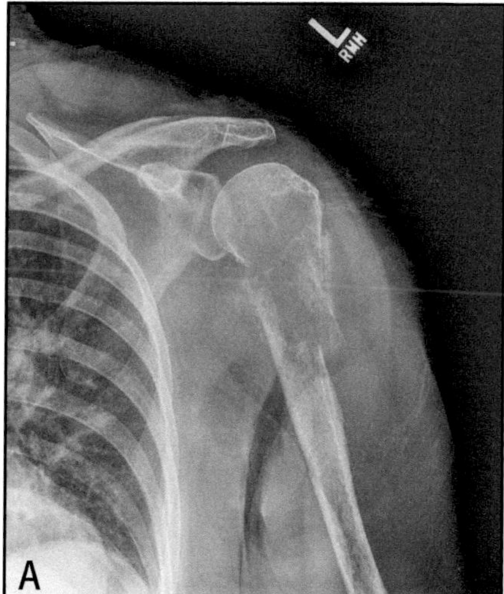

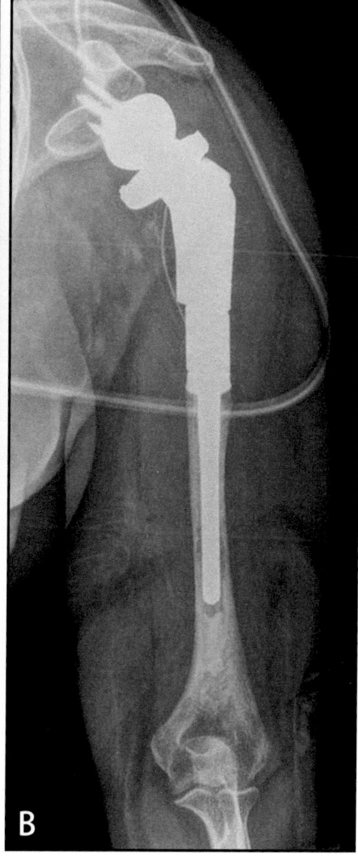

Figure 9-7. A 72-year-old woman with metastatic renal cell carcinoma presents with increasing pain and decreased tolerance to use of the left shoulder. (A) Anteroposterior radiograph demonstrates a pathologic fracture of the left proximal humerus through a lesion, with extensive bony lysis extending into the greater and lesser tuberosities. (B) Owing to poor expected healing potential, the decision was made to proceed with resection of this metastasis and reconstruction with an endoprosthetic proximal humeral replacement with reverse shoulder arthroplasty.

pain and shoulder dysfunction. A mini-open approach to the rotator cuff through a deltoid-splitting approach facilitates direct visualization and protection of the cuff and joint

- Perform a longitudinal tenotomy through the cuff tendon, and place the starting point of the nail well medial to the tip of the greater tuberosity. The cuff can then be easily repaired side to side at the end of the procedure without disruption of the insertional footprint of the cuff
- Be sure to radiographically confirm that the reamer reaches the end of the available canal. The canal of the humerus tapers distally, and insertion of an oversized implant will fracture the distal humerus at an unfavorable location
- Strongly consider a mini-open approach to the distal interlocking screw sites, so that dissection and drill bit placement can be performed directly

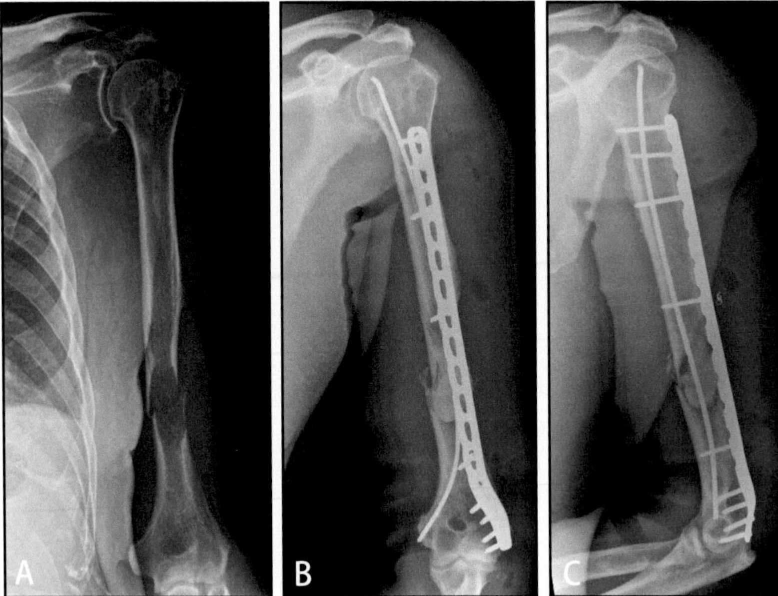

Figure 9-8. A 77-year-old man with metastatic renal cell carcinoma to bone presents with left upper arm pain after an audible snapping sound when rising from a chair. (A) Anteroposterior radiograph demonstrates a pathologic fracture through a radiolucent lesion of the distal third of the humeral shaft. (B and C) Curettage resection, polymethyl methacrylate reconstruction, telescoping, and internal fixation was performed.

onto the bone, and protection of the adjacent neurovascular structures, particularly the radial nerve, can be assured

Distal Humerus

Much like the proximal humerus, management of metastatic disease of the distal humerus can be accomplished with internal fixation devices, including flexible pediatric nails, plate fixation, PMMA, or in the case of segmental bone loss, resection with endoprosthetic reconstruction (Figure 9-9).

Forearm/Hand

The proximal radius and distal ulna are expendable and can be resected. Lesions in other locations may benefit from internal fixation devices with PMMA augmentation, particularly about the wrist or elbow. Options such as arthrodesis of the wrist or single-bone forearm transfer require union of an osteotomy site, and are generally reserved for resection of primary bone tumors, but can be considered in select cases. Acral metastases in the hand

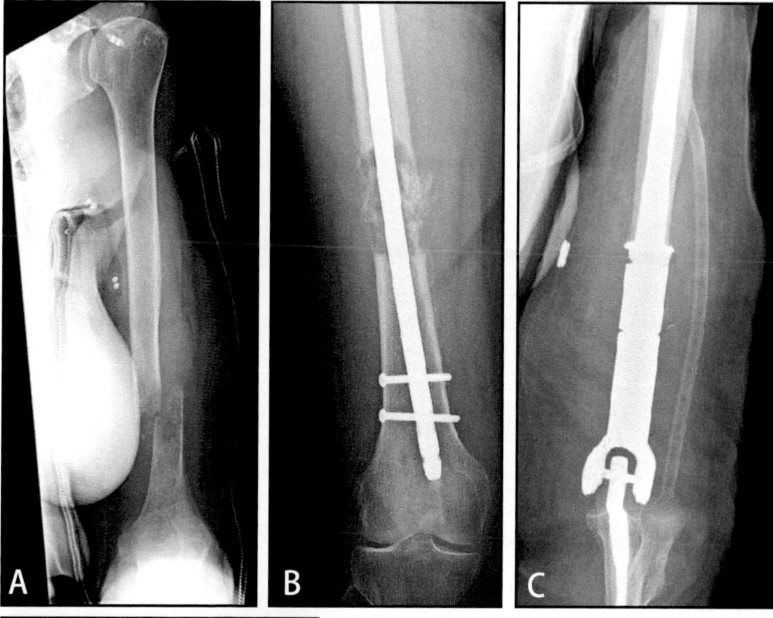

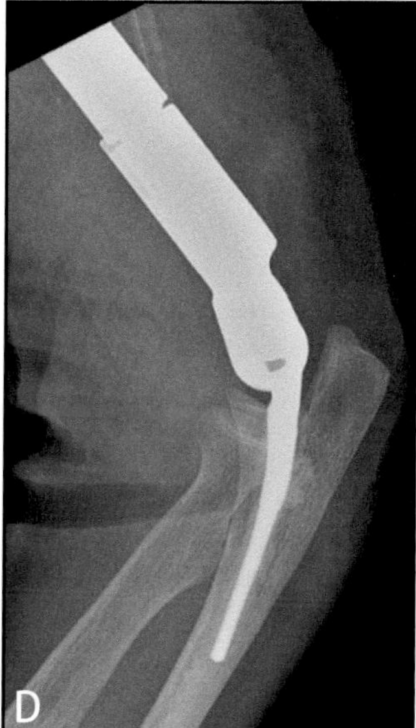

Figure 9-9. An 86-year-old woman with metastatic renal cell carcinoma presents with pain and inability to use the left upper arm. (A) Anteroposterior radiograph of the humerus demonstrates a pathologic fracture of the left distal humerus with permeative changes into the medial and lateral columns of the distal humerus. (B) Prior stabilization of a right femoral lesion 6 months earlier demonstrates continued local disease progression and segmental bone loss. (C and D) The recommendation was made to proceed with resection of this treatment-resistant lesion with endoprosthetic distal humeral replacement.

and wrist are frequently preterminal events. PMMA reconstruction or amputation for palliation may be appropriate in select patients.

Management of Lower-Extremity Disease

More than 25% of metastatic bone disease and myeloma occurs in the lower extremities.[8] Owing to the weight-bearing nature of the lower extremities, the fracture risk is elevated, particularly in the peritrochanteric femur area. The importance of avoiding fracture and maintaining ambulatory function in the oncology patient population cannot be overstated. Complications of thromboembolism, deconditioning, and perioperative medical morbidity and mortality are increased in the cancer patient. The construct selected should permit immediate, full weight-bearing to facilitate mobility and minimize these risks.

Proximal Femur

Femoral head and neck lesions are best managed with resection and endoprosthetic replacement, typically by way of hemiarthroplasty (Figure 9-10). Cemented implants are historically favored, as there is a theoretical risk of impaired ingrowth into press-fit implants after radiation of the bone. The length of the stem required is somewhat controversial, as it is generally ideal to protect as much of the involved bone as possible in the setting of metastatic disease, but this is dogma that is not validated statistically.[9] If the femoral head/neck metastasis is an isolated lesion, or if there is no other discernable disease in the femur distally, a conventionally shorter stem may be appropriate. Unless significant degenerative changes are observed in the hip, or metastatic involvement of the acetabulum is present, resurfacing of the acetabulum is unnecessary.

Intraoperative hypotension, pulmonary insufficiency, cardiovascular collapse, and death are rare but known complications in this high-risk patient population and should be discussed with the patient and family preoperatively. Theories on contributing factors to "bone cement implantation syndrome" include:

- Pressurization-mediated intravasation of marrow fat and/or tumor emboli
- Hemodynamic effects of intramedullary reaming
- Air embolization during implant insertion
- Vasodilatation reaction to the methyl methacrylate monomer

Tips for Reducing Risk of Insertion of Long-Stemmed and Cemented Femoral Implants

- Consider preoperative placement of an inferior vena cava filter
- Template implants preoperatively

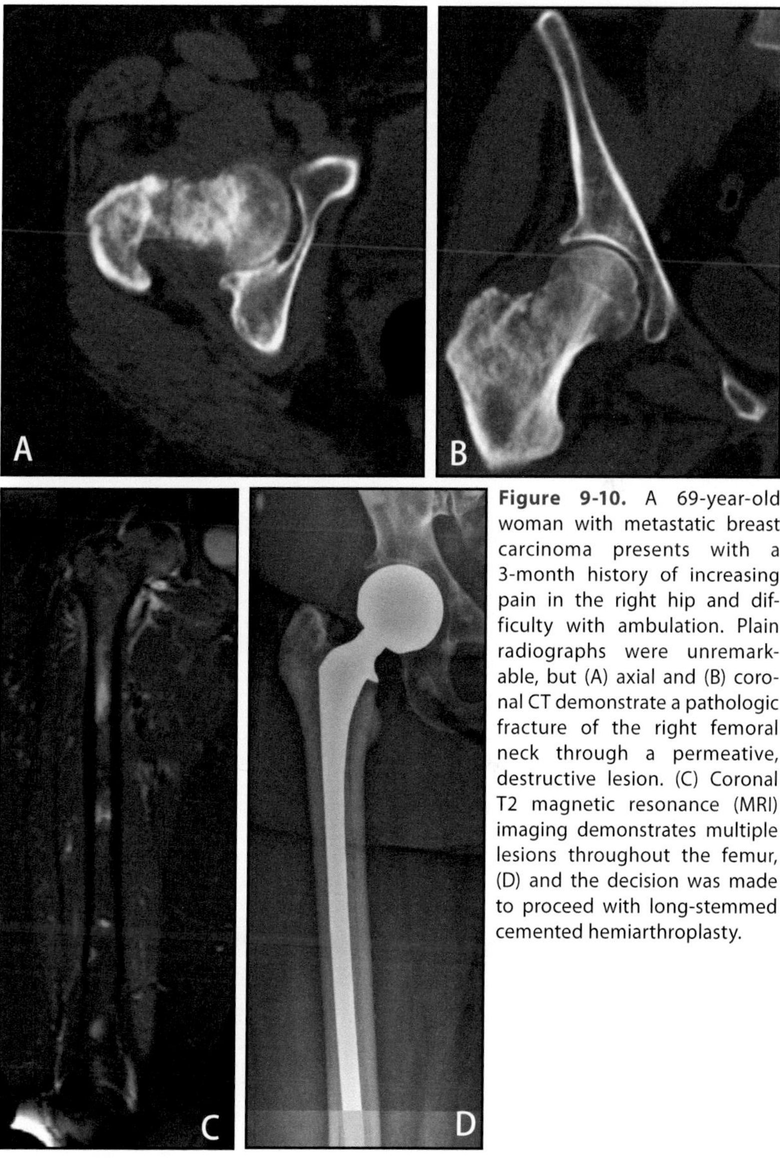

Figure 9-10. A 69-year-old woman with metastatic breast carcinoma presents with a 3-month history of increasing pain in the right hip and difficulty with ambulation. Plain radiographs were unremarkable, but (A) axial and (B) coronal CT demonstrate a pathologic fracture of the right femoral neck through a permeative, destructive lesion. (C) Coronal T2 magnetic resonance (MRI) imaging demonstrates multiple lesions throughout the femur, (D) and the decision was made to proceed with long-stemmed cemented hemiarthroplasty.

- Be mindful of the radius of curvatures of the bone and the implant. Do not hesitate to undersize or shorten the implant if excessive force must be used with the trial components. Intraoperative x-ray is useful to confirm implant sizing

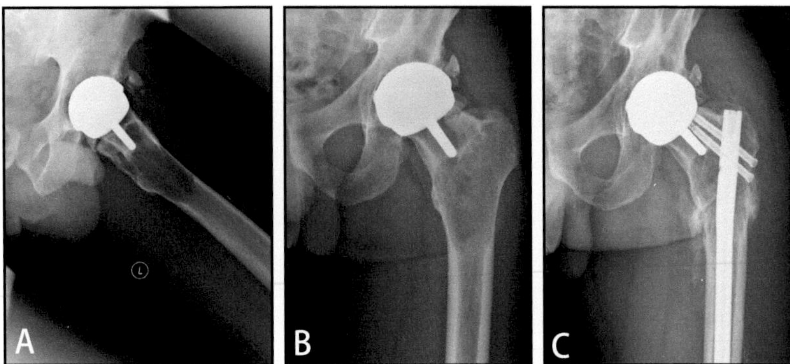

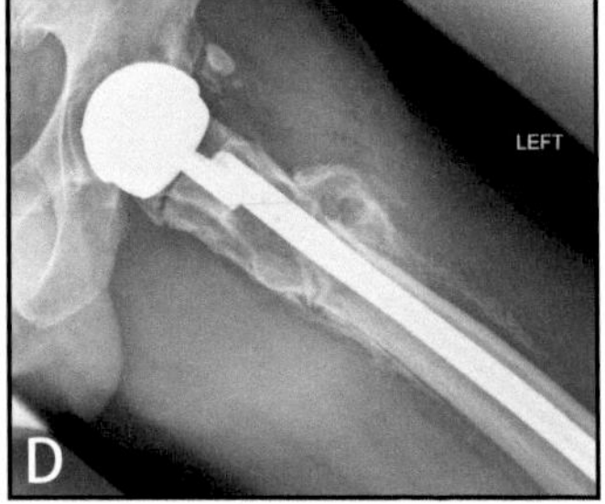

Figure 9-11. A 46-year-old man presents with worsening pain with ambulation on the left side 5 years after bilateral hip resurfacing procedures. (A) Anteroposterior and (B) lateral radiographs demonstrate a large lucency in the intertrochanteric femur. Differential includes metastatic bone disease, myeloma, or wear debris granuloma/ pseudotumor. Work-up and biopsy demonstrated plasmacytoma, an isolated plasma cell lesion that is commonly a precursor to multiple myeloma. (C and D) Owing to the favorable rates of healing of this lesion with radiotherapy, stabilization with an intramedullary recon nail and adjuvant radiotherapy provided definitive treatment.

- Inform anesthesia provider on the timing of cementation to ensure optimization of fluid status and blood pressure prior to insertion of cement
- Consider using a canal lavage/irrigator during reaming
- Consider suctioning or venting of the canal during cementation and implantation
- Use a low-viscosity cement and allow the cement to move from the liquid phase (a glossy, shiny appearance that will stick to the glove) to the early dough phase (matte appearance, compressible without adherence to the glove) before injecting into the canal. This allows more of the monomer to polymerize and/or elute, and reduces the amount of bioavailable monomer
- Insert the implant slowly and gently

Intertrochanteric and subtrochanteric lesions of the femur are subject to considerable mechanical stresses and are at a notably higher risk of fracture. Metastatic disease to the proximal femur is therefore treated more aggressively than lesions in other locations. Small lesions, lesions with appropriate bone stock, and favorable, treatment-sensitive histologies are treated with

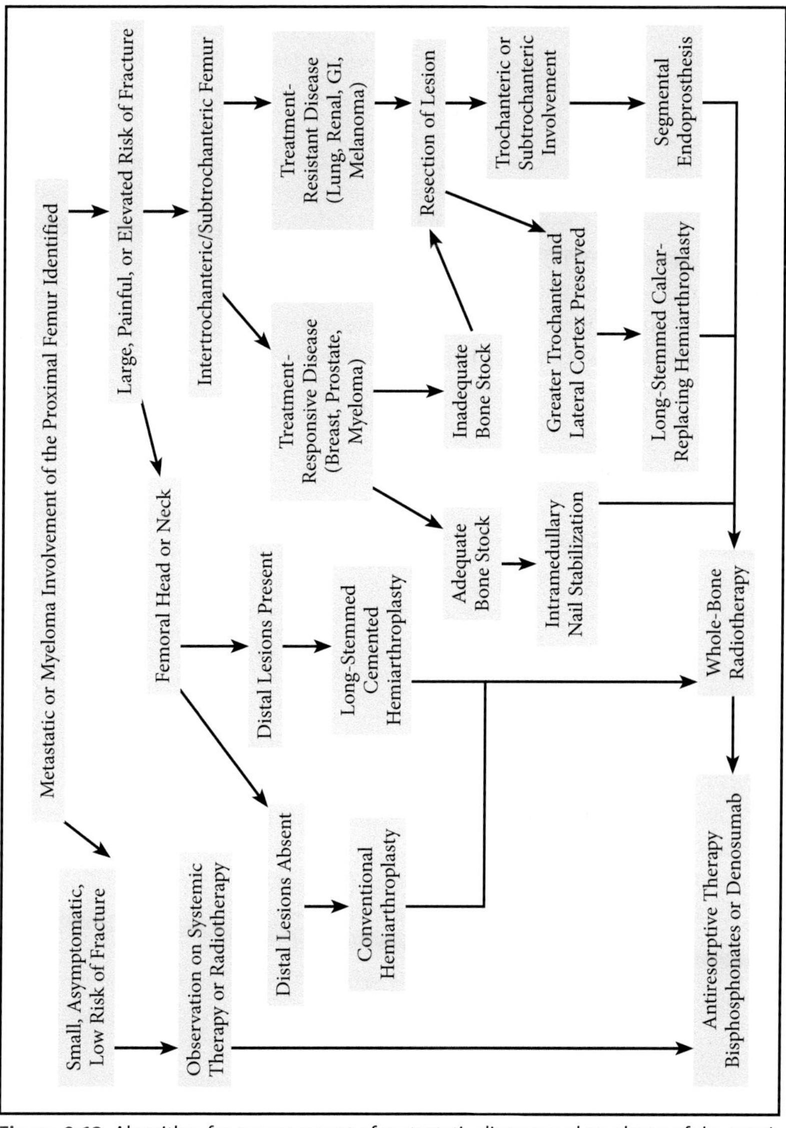

Figure 9-12. Algorithm for management of metastatic disease and myeloma of the proximal femur.

intramedullary nail devices (Figure 9-11). Endoprosthetic options include conventional arthroplasty stems, calcar-replacing implants, and segmental tumor prostheses. Figure 9-12 demonstrates an algorithm for management of proximal femoral disease. Resection of the proximal femur with prosthetic reconstruction should be performed by experienced practitioners, but stability and function of the prosthesis can be optimized by the following:

- Use of a hemiarthroplasty for the femoral head rather than resurfacing of the acetabulum
- Circumferential release of the joint capsule from the femoral insertion, with an inferiorly based T-incision of the capsule to permit dislocation of the femoral head and cerclage tightening around the neck of the prosthesis
- Sagittal osteotomy of the greater trochanter to preserve length and tension of the abductors with the origin of the vastus lateralis as a continuous soft-tissue sleeve, for later repair/tenodesis to the prosthesis
- Abduction braces and other devices are usually unnecessary

Femoral Shaft

With exceptions for lesions that are best treated with intercalary resection and reconstruction, metastatic bone disease and myeloma of the femoral shaft are best treated with large-diameter intramedullary nails of the femur. Implants with options for protection of the femoral neck are preferred.

Technical Tips for Intramedullary Nailing of Metastatic Disease of the Femur

- Consider preoperative placement of an inferior vena cava filter and/or embolization
- Determine the precise implant required, including the desired number of interlocking screws distally and proximally. Cephalomedullary devices used for hip fracture fixation often have proximal nail diameters greater than 15 mm, which can risk fracturing an intact femur in smaller patients. Consider using a recon nail device with a reduced proximal diameter for patients with smaller canals measuring 11 mm or less
- Template implants preoperatively. Know the expected diameter and length of the implant to ensure that the implant is available, and have a slightly smaller implant in the room and on standby, so that if rapid or excessive bleeding from the canal is encountered, the implant can be immediately inserted to provide tamponade. A reamer can be placed temporarily in the canal to provide tamponade until the implant is ready
- Consider using a canal lavage/irrigator during reaming, particularly if performing simultaneous nailing of more than one long bone
- Be mindful of the radius of curvatures of the bone and the implant. The most common complication of a radius mismatch is perforation of the nail anteriorly. To avoid this, a starting point positioned slightly anterior

on the greater trochanter will aim the distal end of the nail more posteriorly. Obtain a lateral radiograph distally during insertion to view the trajectory of the nail. Do not hesitate to downsize or shorten the implant if a breach of the anterior cortex is threatened distally

- Cement augmentation is not routinely recommended, and should be reserved selectively for locations in which the added cement may contribute to the stability of the fixation construct, such as the metadiaphyseal junctions

Distal Femur and Proximal Tibia

Similar to other periarticular sites, internal fixation devices with or without PMMA augmentation are appropriate when bone stock and histology are favorable, and when immediate weight-bearing is reasonable (Figure 9-13). Resection with prosthetic reconstruction should be considered for lesions with extensive involvement of the epiphysis (Figure 9-14). Close attention should be paid to the stability and function of the extensor mechanism. The rotating platform within these implant systems may permit excessive external rotation of the extremity immediately after surgery, so rehabilitation in a supportive brace should be strongly considered until full recovery of the extensor mechanism is observed.

Tibial Shaft and Fibula

Metastatic bone disease and myeloma of the tibia are much less common than lesions of the femur and humerus but are still best treated with intramedullary devices. The fibula, much like the clavicle, is an expendable bone that can be managed nonoperatively or resected en bloc.

Distal Tibia and Foot

Lesions of the distal tibia, tarsal, and metatarsal bones are uncommon, and prosthetic options in these locations are limited. These lesions are generally treated by curettage and cementation, with internal fixation devices as required. Arthrodesis can be considered in select cases, but these reconstructions require a prolonged period of protected weight-bearing until bony union, which is impaired after adjuvant radiotherapy. Lesions of the small bones of the foot and lesions that compromise the stability of the foot or ankle may be best treated with amputation.

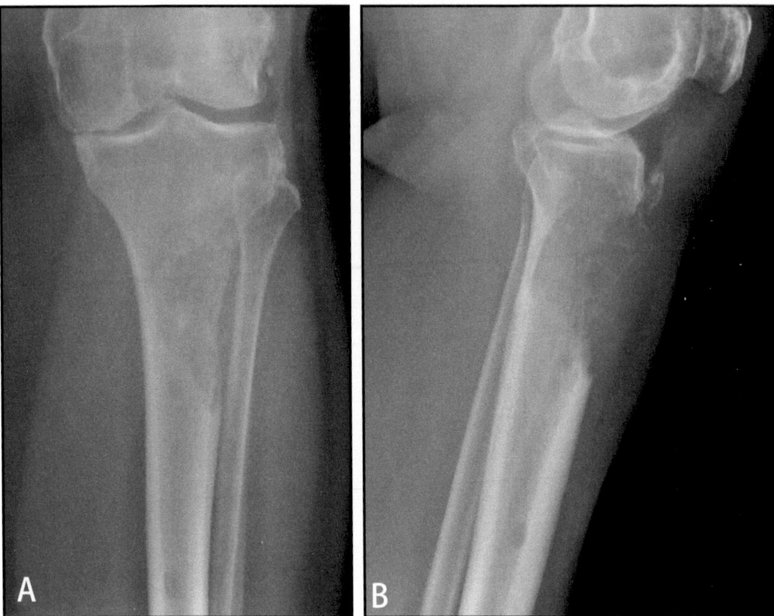

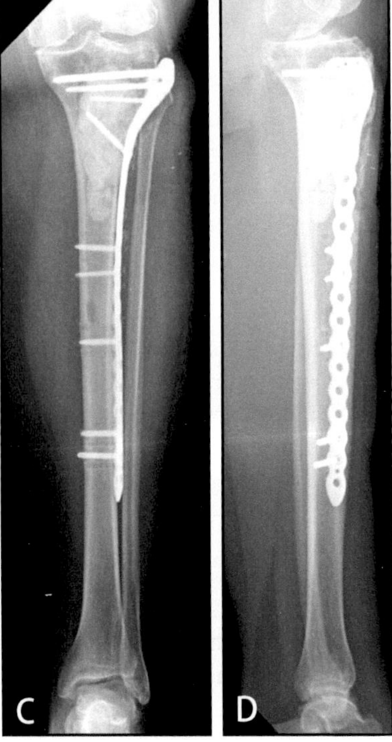

Figure 9-13. A 57-year-old woman presents with intense pain in the left knee with ambulation. (A) Anteroposterior and (B) lateral radiographs demonstrate an ill-defined destructive lesion of the medial proximal tibia, with a second radiolucent lesion in the shaft distally. Biopsy was consistent with metastatic breast cancer. (C and D) The patient underwent curettage resection with polymethyl methacrylate reconstruction and percutaneous open reduction internal fixation.

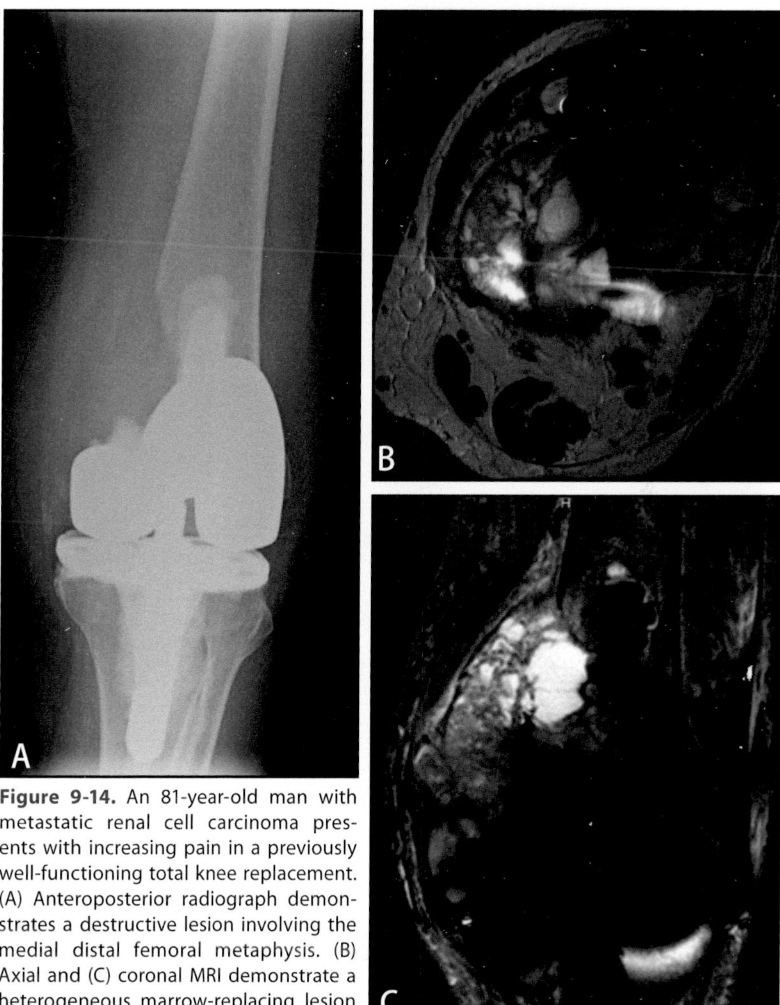

Figure 9-14. An 81-year-old man with metastatic renal cell carcinoma presents with increasing pain in a previously well-functioning total knee replacement. (A) Anteroposterior radiograph demonstrates a destructive lesion involving the medial distal femoral metaphysis. (B) Axial and (C) coronal MRI demonstrate a heterogeneous marrow-replacing lesion with extensive soft tissue involvement. Biopsy confirmed metastatic renal cell carcinoma.

Management of Pelvic and Spinal Disease

The spine and pelvis are the 2 most common sites of metastatic disease to the bone. With strong ligamentous structures providing more intrinsic support to the spine and pelvis, there is greater overall stability within the spine and pelvis, even when pathologic fractures occur. Lesions of

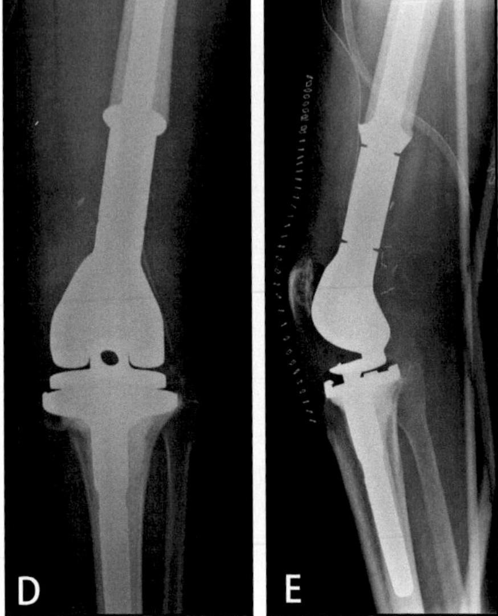

Figure 9-14 continued. (D and E) The patient underwent resection of the distal femur and endoprosthetic replacement.

non–weight-bearing areas of the pelvis are therefore treated with nonoperative modalities such as radiotherapy, thermal ablation, or percutaneous cement augmentation (cementoplasty). Non–weight-bearing areas of the pelvis can also be resected en bloc for difficult or refractory cases.

Management of juxta-acetabular lesions can be a complex undertaking, and treatment is determined by a combination of factors, including the extent of acetabular involvement, whether the joint can be salvaged, and the general condition of the patient. Nonoperative and percutaneous interventions are recommended in patients with limited life expectancy (Figure 9-15). For a resection with a complex reconstruction of the hip to be considered feasible, the patient must reasonably be expected to tolerate the extent of the surgery, demonstrate the motivation and functional capacity to participate in the rehabilitation necessary to return to full ambulation, and survive long enough to benefit from the procedure (Figure 9-16). Figure 9-17 depicts an algorithm for management of periacetabular disease.

Metastatic bone disease and myeloma of the spine involves in the thoracic spine in 70% of cases, followed by the lumbar (20%) and cervical spine (10%).[10] Spinal disease can present as incidental findings during staging of a new cancer diagnosis or with symptoms ranging from mild axial neck or back pain to vertebral collapse, neurological impairment, and paralysis. Radiotherapy is the mainstay of treatment for lesions that do not cause segmental instability, deformity, or neurological impairment. Patients with incomplete cord compression may be best managed with surgical

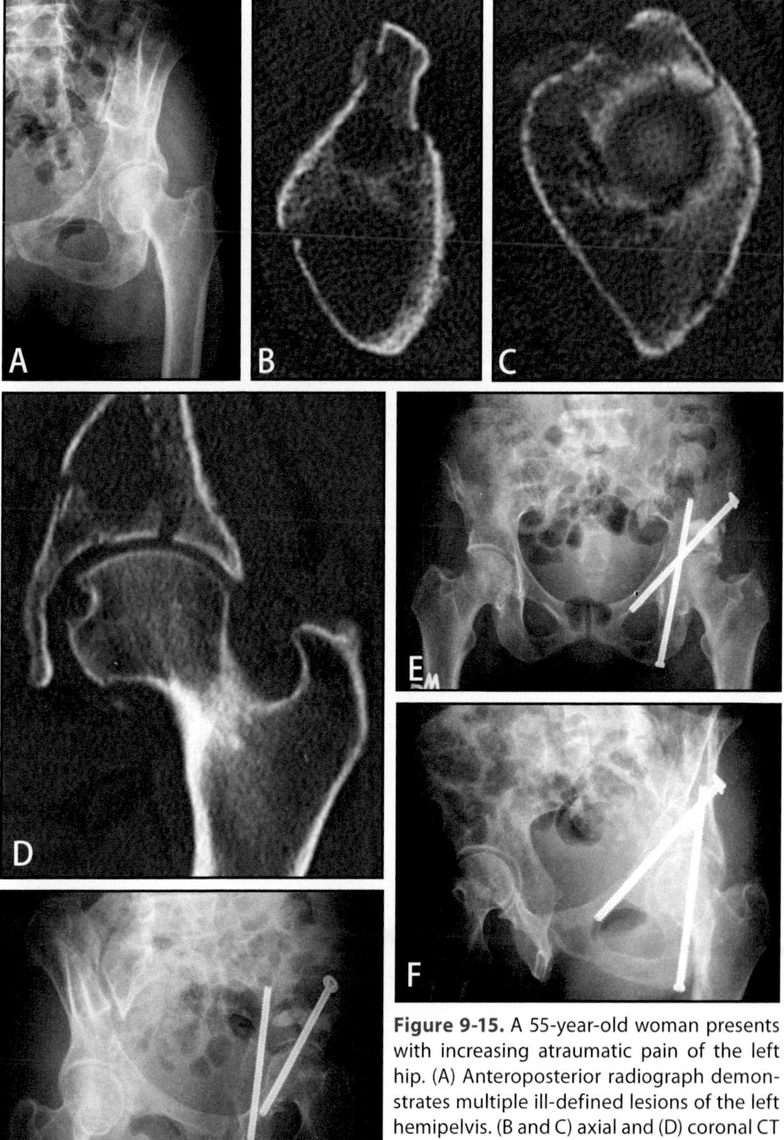

Figure 9-15. A 55-year-old woman presents with increasing atraumatic pain of the left hip. (A) Anteroposterior radiograph demonstrates multiple ill-defined lesions of the left hemipelvis. (B and C) axial and (D) coronal CT demonstrates a pathologic fracture of the left acetabulum through lucent lesions of the superior and posterior acetabulum. A biopsy confirmed metastatic triple-positive breast cancer. (E, F, and G) The fracture was treated with percutaneous screw fixation of the acetabular columns and cement augmentation.

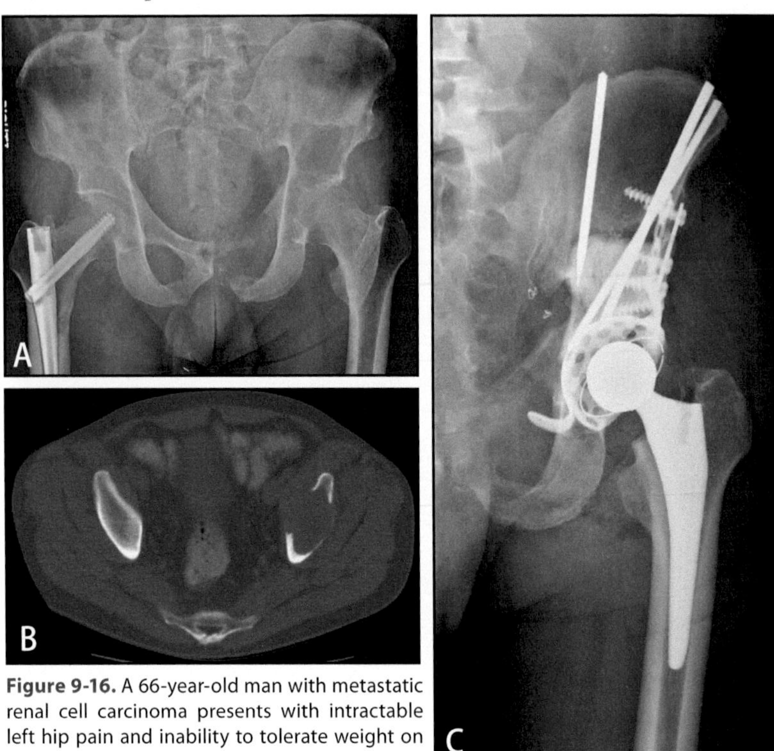

Figure 9-16. A 66-year-old man with metastatic renal cell carcinoma presents with intractable left hip pain and inability to tolerate weight on the right lower extremity. (A) Anteroposterior radiograph and (B) axial CT demonstrate a destructive, lytic lesion involving the superior acetabulum and medial obturator ring of the left hemipelvis. (C) The patient underwent resection of the acetabular lesion with internal fixation and total hip arthroplasty with cement and cage reconstruction.

decompression, with the caveat that surgical treatment of metastatic spine disease frequently requires addressing pathology that causes anterior cord compression at the same time as posterior hardware stabilization.[11] Similar to complex reconstruction of metastatic disease of the acetabulum, a combined anteroposterior treatment approach to spinal disease demands that patients be able to tolerate and recover from this aggressive intervention, generally a life expectancy greater than 3 months (Tables 9-3 and 9-4).

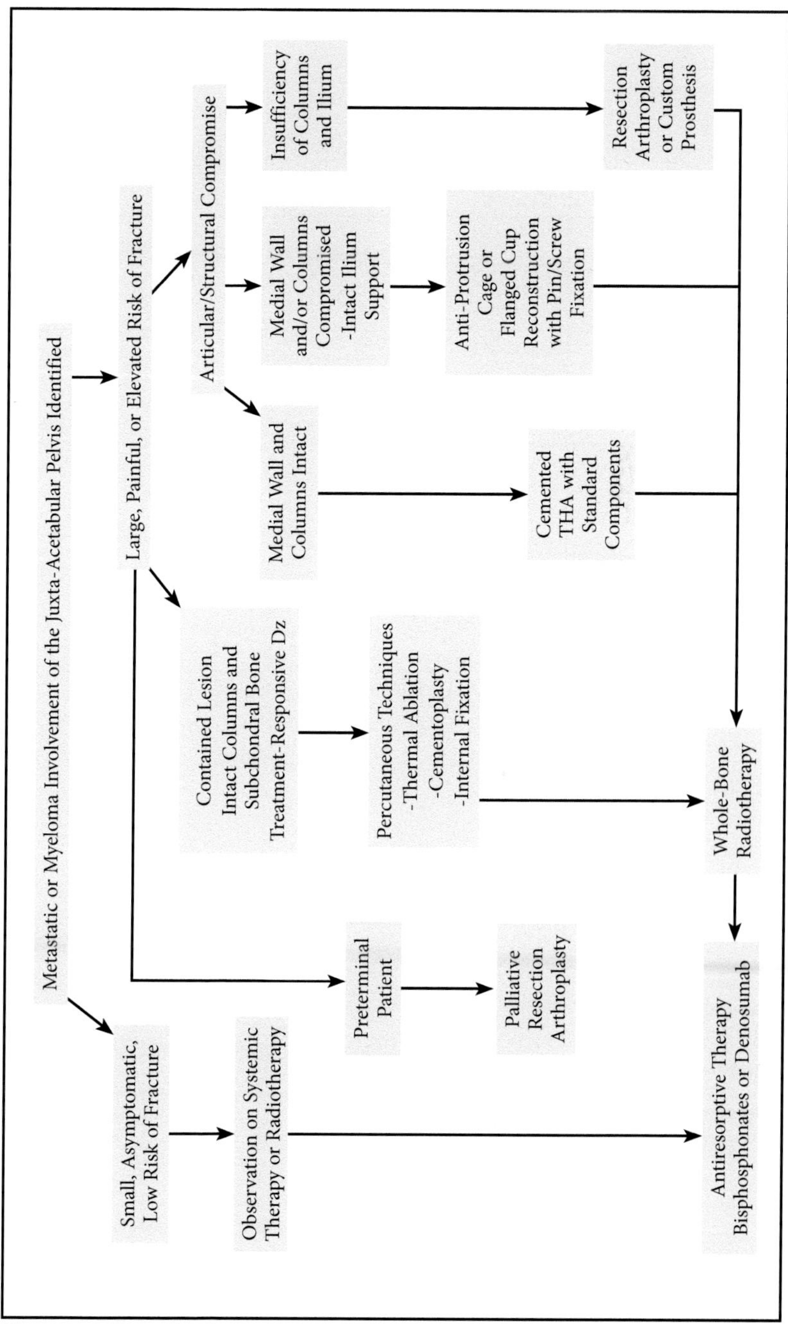

Figure 9-17. Algorithm for management of periacetabular disease.

Table 9-3

Tokuhashi Score for Prediction of Metastatic Spinal Disease Prognosis

CRITERIA	SCORE
General condition/ performance status	0 = Poor 1 = Moderate 2 = Good
Number of extraspinal bone mets	0 = >3 1 = 1 or 2 2 = 0
Number of vertebral mets	0 = >3 1 = 2 2 = 1
Mets to major internal organs	0 = Unremovable 1 = Removable 2 = None
Primary cancer site	0 = Lung, osteosarcoma, stomach, bladder, esophagus, pancreas 1 = Liver, gallbladder, unidentified 2 = Others 3 = Kidney, uterus 4 = Rectum 5 = Thyroid, prostate, breast, carcinoid
Cord palsy	0 = Complete (Frankel A: complete motor and sensory. Frankel B: complete motor, incomplete sensory) 1 = Incomplete (Frankel C: incomplete but useless motor. Frankel D: useful motor present) 2 = None (Frankel E: no neurological symptoms)
Score 0 to 8: survival <6 months Score 9 to 11: survival 6 to 12 months Score 12 to 15: survival >12 months	
Abbreviation: mets = metastases. (Adapted from Tokuhashi Y, Matsuzaki H, Oda H, Oshima M, Ryu J.[12])	

Table 9-4

Tomita Score for Surgical Strategy for Metastatic Bone Disease of the Spine

CRITERIA	SCORE
Primary tumor	1 = Slow growth (breast, prostate, etc) 2 = Moderate growth (kidney, uterus, etc) 4 = Rapid growth (lung, stomach, etc)
Visceral mets	0 = None 2 = Treatable 4 = Untreatable
Osseous mets	1 = Solitary or oligometastatic 2 = Multiple
Score 2 to 3: good long-term local control; wide or marginal excision Score 4 to 5: moderate local control; marginal or intralesional excision Score 6 to 7: short-term local control; palliative surgery Score 8 to 10: terminal; supportive care	

Abbreviation: mets = metastases. (Adapted from Tomita K, Kawahara N, Kobayashi T, Yoshida A, Murakami H, Akamaru T.[13])

Aftercare for Patients with Metastatic Bone Disease and Myeloma

Orthopaedic practitioners must consider themselves a member of a multidisciplinary cancer care team. After obtaining tissue for diagnosis and special studies, and after optimizing skeletal stability and function, a surgeon must coordinate with other specialists to ensure timely initiation of adjuvant therapies.

The surgeon should assist the patient in making appropriate arrangements for consultation with a radiation oncologist. Whole-bone radiotherapy should be delivered to the stabilized bone and other symptomatic lesions. This can be initiated immediately after incisional healing, typically 2 to 3 weeks. Single-fraction treatments of external-beam radiation of 8 Gy are reasonable for palliation in terminal patients, but risk local progression and construct failure long term.[14] Hyperfractionated regimens totaling an average of 30 Gy are standard, but radioresistant tumors such as renal cell carcinoma may require higher dosages or alternative methods of radiation delivery such as stereotactic body radiation therapy or proton beam therapy.

The surgeon should also ensure that the patient is initiated on antiresorptive therapy. This is most conveniently added to the treatments provided by the medical oncology specialist, but a primary care provider or endocrinologist is also appropriate. Bisphosphonate and denosumab therapy have been shown to interfere with osteoclast activity and halt the RANKL (receptor activator of nuclear factor kappa-B ligand) pathway responsible for tumor-mediated lysis of bone. This has been shown to reduce the rate of skeletal-related events; the development of additional symptomatic lesions requiring treatment.[15]

Take-Aways

1. A destructive bone lesion in a patient older than 40 years should be considered metastatic bone disease or myeloma until proven otherwise.
2. The peritrochanteric femur is a high-risk location for metastatic bone disease and myeloma, and painful lesions in this location warrant more aggressive intervention.
3. Careful preoperative planning of stabilization procedures can avoid preventable complications, including uncontrolled bleeding, iatrogenic fracture, and construct failure.
4. Management of metastatic bone disease and myeloma includes communication with radiation and medical oncology practitioners to coordinate adjuvant therapies that reduce the risk of construct failure and other skeletal-related events.

Commonly Tested Topics for Trainees

- A nuclear medicine bone scan may be negative in the setting of multiple myeloma or rapidly destructive malignancies. In these patients, staging should be pursued with skeletal survey.
- The work-up for a destructive bone lesion in an adult should include laboratory and imaging evaluation for myeloma and the most common carcinomas with known spread to bone (BLT-Kosher Pickle), and likely will require biopsy for tissue confirmation prior to any surgical treatments.
- Patients with spinal disease with an incomplete neurologic deficit, low overall burden of disease, and favorable life expectancy are more likely to benefit from aggressive surgical decompression.

- Postoperative whole-bone external-beam radiotherapy is necessary after stabilization of metastatic bone disease, which reduces subjective pain scores and decreases the risk of construct failure.

References

1. Rougraff BT, Kneisl JS, Simon MA. Skeletal metastases of unknown origin. A prospective study of a diagnostic strategy. *J Bone Joint Surg Am.* 1993;75(9):1276-1281. doi:10.2106/00004623-199309000-00003.
2. Piccioli A, Maccauro G, Spinelli MS, Biagini R, Rossi B. Bone metastases of unknown origin: epidemiology and principles of management. *J Orthop Traumatol.* 2015;16(2):81-86. doi: 10.1007/s10195-015-0344-0.
3. Saad F, Lipton A, Cook R, Chen YM, Smith M, Coleman R. Pathologic fractures correlate with reduced survival in patients with malignant bone disease. *Cancer.* 2007;110(8):1860-1867. doi:10.1002/cncr.22991.
4. Damron TA, Nazarian A, Entezari V, et al. CT-based structural rigidity analysis is more accurate than Mirels scoring for fracture prediction in metastatic femoral lesions. *Clin Orthop Relat Res.* 2016;474(3):643-651. doi:10.1007/s11999-015-4453-0.
5. Mirels H. Metastatic disease in long bones. A proposed scoring system for diagnosing impending pathologic fractures. *Clin Orthop Relat Res.* 1989;249:256-264.
6. Gainor BJ, Buchert PU. Fracture healing in metastatic bone disease. *Clin Orthop Relat Res.* 1983;178:297-302. doi:10.1097/00003086-198309000-00041.
7. Kurup AN, Callstrom MR. Image-Guided percutaneous ablation of bone and soft tissue tumors. *Semin Intervent Radiol.* 2010;27(3):276-284. doi:10.1055/s-0030-1261786.
8. Biermann JS, Holt GE, Lewis VO, Schwartz HS, Yaszemski MJ. Metastatic bone disease: diagnosis, evaluation, and treatment. *J Bone Joint Surg Am.* 2009;91(6):1518-1530.
9. Xing Z, Moon BS, Satcher RL, Lin PP, Lewis VO. A long femoral stem is not always required in hip arthroplasty for patients with proximal femur metastases. *Clin Orthop Relat Res.* 2013;471(5):1622-1627. doi:10.1007/s11999-013-2790-4.
10. Brihaye J, Ectors P, Lemort M, Van Houtte P. The management of spinal epidural metastases. *Adv Tech Stand Neurosurg.* 1988;16:121-176. doi: 10.1007/978-3-7091-6954-4_4.
11. Patchell RA, Tibbs PA, Regine WF, et al. Direct decompressive surgical resection in the treatment of spinal cord compression caused by metastatic cancer: a randomised trial. *Lancet.* 2005;3(4):288-295.
12. Tokuhashi Y, Matsuzaki H, Oda H, Oshima M, Ryu J. A revised scoring system for preoperative evaluation of metastatic spine tumor prognosis. *Spine (Phila Pa 1976).* 2005;30(19):2186-2191. doi:10.1097/01.brs.0000180401.06919.a5.
13. Tomita K, Kawahara N, Kobayashi T, Yoshida A, Murakami H, Akamaru T. Surgical strategy for spinal metastases. *Spine (Phila Pa 1976).* 2001;26(3):298-306. doi:10.1097/00007632-200102010-00016.
14. Townsend PW, Smalley SR, Cozad SC, Rosenthal HG, Hassanein RE. Role of postoperative radiation therapy after stabilization of fractures caused by metastatic disease. *Int J Rad Biol Phys.* 1995;31(1):43-49. doi:10.1016/0360-3016(94)E0310-G.
15. Quinn RH, Randall RL, Benevenia J, Berven SH, Raskin KA. Contemporary management of metastatic bone disease: tips and tools of the trade for general practitioners. *J Bone Joint Surg Am.* 2013;95(20):1887-1895. doi:10.2106/00004623-201310160-00011.

10

Bone Sarcomas in Adults, Chondrosarcoma, and Chondrogenic Tumor Syndromes

Overview

Destructive bone lesions in older adults warrant a thorough evaluation and work-up. Sarcomas of bone are vastly outnumbered by metastatic and myelomatous lesions, but should be identified promptly to provide life-saving and limb-sparing treatment. Improper management of bone sarcomas will preclude salvage of the extremity. We will discuss the clinical and radiologic features of the most common bone sarcomas in older adults, and present an algorithm for management of chondroid tumors.

Bone sarcomas in older adults present as painful, ill-defined, destructive lesions with imaging features that may overlap with metastatic bone disease and myeloma. Primary bone sarcomas in adults older than 40 years are much less common than metastatic and myeloma lesions. This can lead to false confidence in assuming that a destructive bone lesion in an older patient is metastatic bone disease or myeloma. The consequences of mismanagement of primary bone sarcomas include increased risk of disease recurrence, compromise of the affected bone and soft tissue, loss of limb, and adverse effects on prognosis. Recognition of the clinical and imaging features of adult bone sarcomas and adherence to the principles of biopsy and diagnosis can help the practitioner avoid these preventable adverse events.

Wallace, MT
Handbook of Musculoskeletal Tumors (pp 159-177).

Chondrosarcoma

Chondrosarcoma is the most common sarcoma of bone in adults older than 40 years. Unlike pediatric sarcomas of bone, the majority of chondrosarcomas are low-to-intermediate-grade tumors, characterized by slow, indolent progression over time. Patients generally report a long duration of aching pain, which is often mistaken for arthritis, tendinopathy, or other degenerative disease. Compared with inactive enchondromas, which are frequently identified incidentally, 81% of chondrosarcomas are painful, and only 19% are incidental findings.[1] Occasionally chondrosarcoma will present with pathologic fracture.

The majority of chondrosarcomas arise de novo, but a smaller number arise in pre-existing cartilage lesions, including osteochondromas, periosteal chondromas, or enchondromatosis. These are termed secondary chondrosarcomas, of which more than 95% are low-grade tumors. By contrast, primary chondrosarcomas exhibit a wide range of clinical behavior, ranging from lower-grade lesions with extremely favorable prognoses to high-grade tumors with a fulminant and ultimately fatal course. Table 10-1 summarizes the clinical spectrum of chondrosarcoma.[2,3]

The diagnosis of malignant cartilage tumors differs greatly from other bone and soft-tissue tumors. Histologically, the differentiation between lower and intermediate grades of cartilage tumors is extremely difficult, even for experienced bone pathologists. Even higher-grade aggressive chondrosarcomas will display marked tumor heterogeneity, with areas of relatively well-differentiated cartilage adjacent to higher-grade tumor, which can lead to significant sampling error with biopsy. The anatomic location of the lesion also can create misleading correlations between the clinical and radiologic appearance and the histopathology, because benign lesions of the small tubular bones of the hands and feet can appear more aggressive radiologically without any significant risk of local recurrence or metastatic spread. Lesions within the pelvis and spine can appear benign radiographically and histologically, but carry a significant risk of local recurrence and aggressive transformation with inadequate surgical margins.[4] For this reason, the diagnosis and grading of chondrosarcomas is often performed with clinical correlation and defining radiologic features (Figure 10-1).

Imaging Findings Suggestive of Chondrosarcoma

Computed Tomography (Best Study)

- Large lesions, greater than 5 cm to 10 cm
- Bony lysis[5]

- Endosteal scalloping more than two-thirds of cortical thickness
- Cortical disruption/defect
- Cortical/adaptive changes
  - Thickening
  - Expansion
  - Deformity
  - Periosteal reaction
- Changes in mineralization[6]
  - Faint or amorphous calcifications
  - Juxtaposed areas of variable mineralization
  - Lysis within previously mineralized areas
  - Erosion into stalk of exostosis

Magnetic Resonance Imaging

- Soft-tissue mass
- High T2-fluid (myxoid) content
- Discontinuous tumor, skip lesions
- Significantly thickened cartilage cap in an exostosis (>20 mm in younger patients, >10 mm in older individuals)
- Periosteal reaction
- Peritumoral edema

Technetium-99m Bone Scan

- Increased radiotracer uptake
- Discontinuous tumor or osseous metastatic diseas

Although histologic grading of cartilage tumors is difficult, certain findings can be confirmatory of malignant cartilage:

- Multinucleate cells
- Significant hypercellularity
- Multiple cells within lacunar spaces
- Entrapment/permeation of host bone
- High-Grade pleomorphism: round cell or spindle cell component

There is no effective chemotherapy or radiotherapy for chondrosarcoma, and surgical resection is the only recommended treatment. Intermediate and high-grade lesions warrant a wide resection with negative surgical margins (Figure 10-2). Premalignant and low-grade tumors without soft-tissue extension or aggressive features may be amenable to intralesional resection with

Table 10-1 Chondrosarcoma Variants and Prognosis[2,3]			
GRADE	**VARIANT**	**DEFINING FEATURES**	**LONG-TERM OUTCOME**
Premalignant	Chondrosarcoma in situ, also known as: • Grade 0 • Grade ½ • Enchondrosarcoma • Atypical enchondroma • Borderline	Subtle bony erosions without reactive or adaptive changes	Extremely favorable 0% metastatic risk
Low grade	Clear cell chondrosarcoma	Epiphyseal location	Extremely favorable 100% 5-year survival with appropriate margins
	Grade 1 intramedullary chondrosarcoma (60%)	Bony lysis without cytologic atypia, soft-tissue extension, or adaptive changes	Extremely favorable 0% metastatic risk 5% to 10% local recurrence
Intermediate grade	Grade 2 intramedullary chondrosarcoma (36%)	Aggressive features with soft-tissue mass and myxoid change	Favorable 11% metastatic risk 15% to 20% local recurrence
High grade	Grade 3 intramedullary chondrosarcoma	Rapid growth with sparse mineralization	Moderate 30% metastatic risk 33% local recurrence *Risk of metastasis correlates with local recurrence
	Mesenchymal chondrosarcoma	Aggressive growth with significant soft-tissue mass and round cell component	Poor 40% metastatic risk
Pleomorphic	Dedifferentiated chondrosarcoma	High-grade spindle cell tumor adjacent to lower-grade chondroid lesion	Very poor 0% to 20% 5-year survival

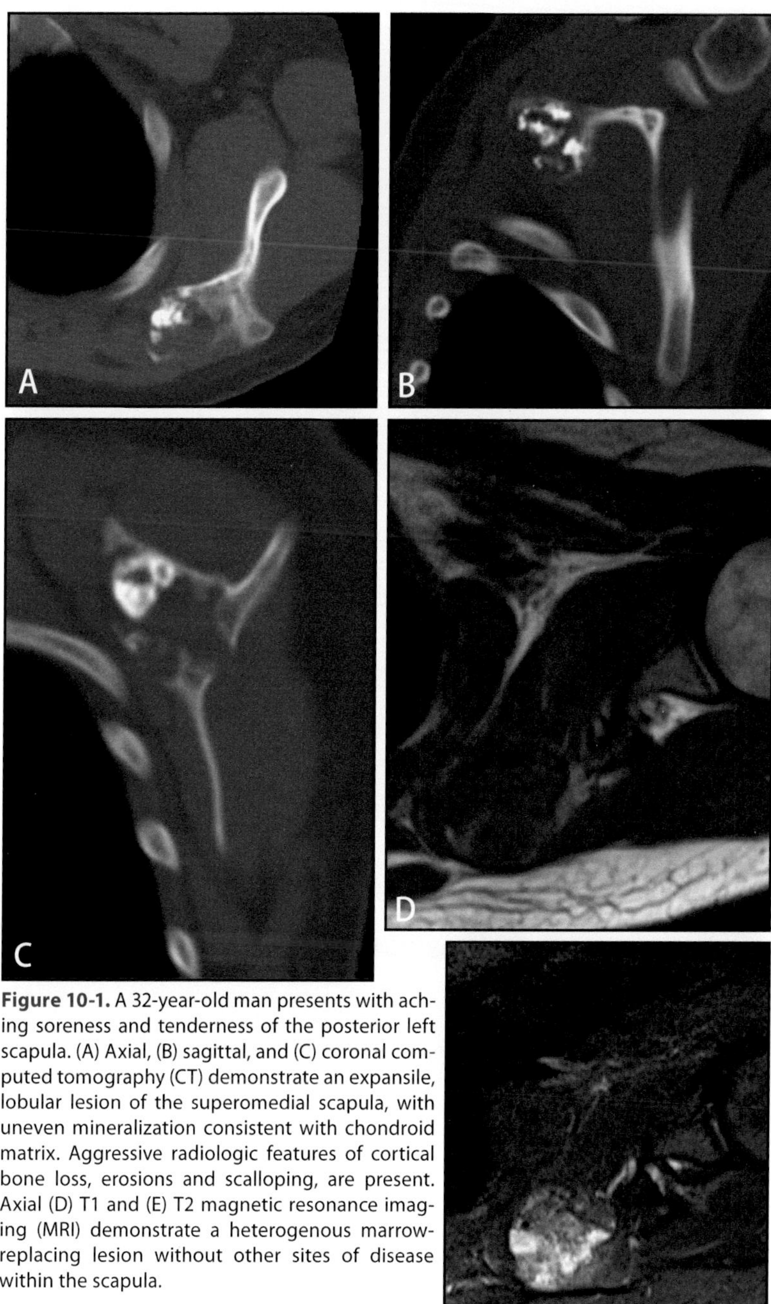

Figure 10-1. A 32-year-old man presents with aching soreness and tenderness of the posterior left scapula. (A) Axial, (B) sagittal, and (C) coronal computed tomography (CT) demonstrate an expansile, lobular lesion of the superomedial scapula, with uneven mineralization consistent with chondroid matrix. Aggressive radiologic features of cortical bone loss, erosions and scalloping, are present. Axial (D) T1 and (E) T2 magnetic resonance imaging (MRI) demonstrate a heterogenous marrow-replacing lesion without other sites of disease within the scapula.

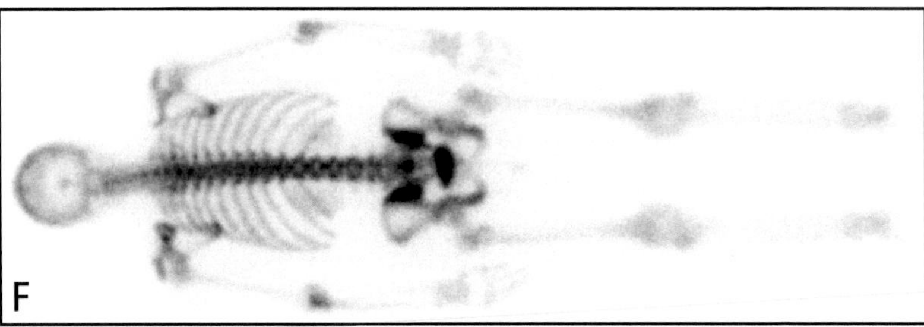

Figure 10-1 continued. Technetium-99m bone scintigraphy (F) demonstrates increased uptake in the superior scapula. Grade 2 chondrosarcoma was confirmed, and the patient was treated with subtotal scapulectomy.

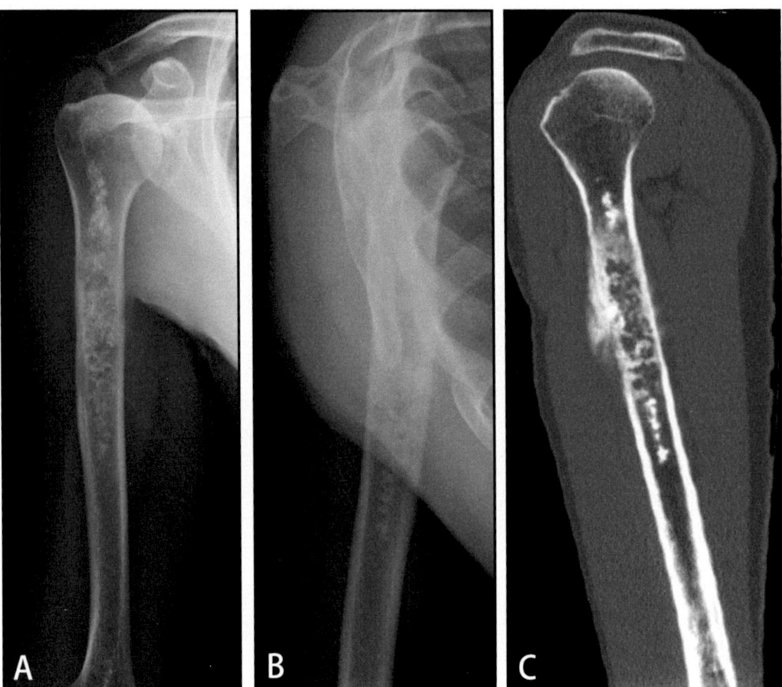

Figure 10-2. A 71-year-old man presents with vague right upper arm pain for several months. (A) Anteroposterior and (B) lateral radiographs demonstrate a mineralized chondroid lesion extending along the proximal half of the humeral diaphysis. The center of the lesion demonstrates some subtle areas of endosteal scalloping and lucencies within an otherwise well-mineralized lesion. (C) Coronal and (D and E) axial CT demonstrates cortical erosions and extension of the mineralized lesion into the surrounding soft tissue, highly suggestive for high-grade chondrosarcoma.

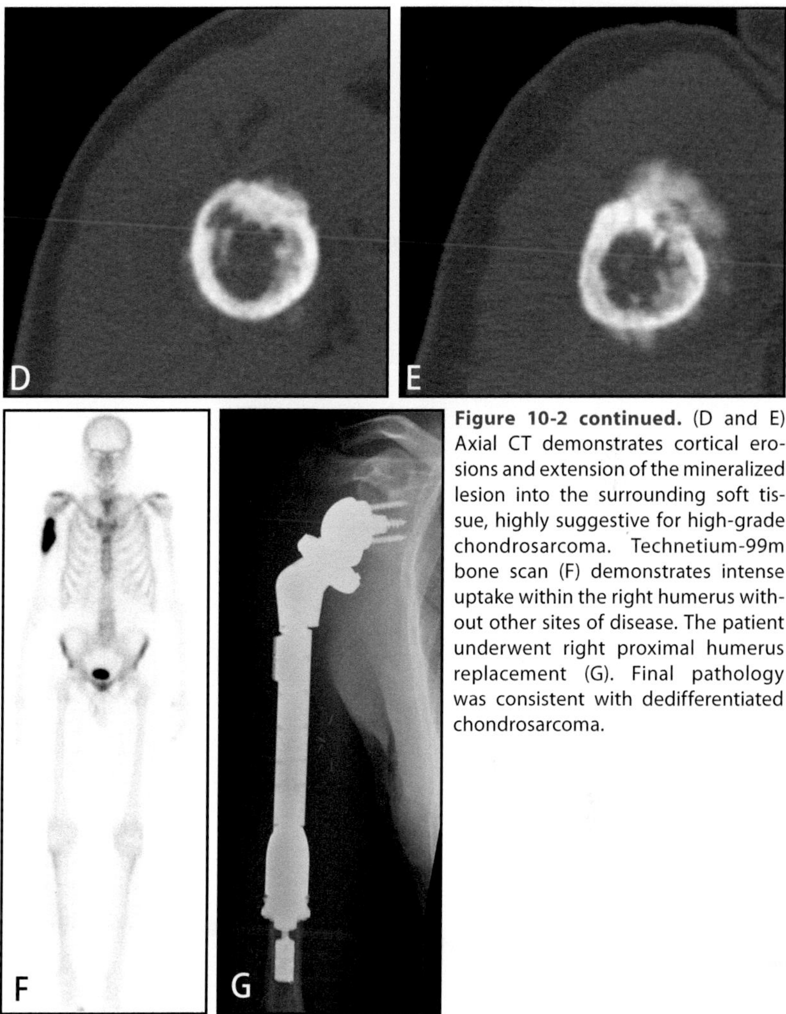

Figure 10-2 continued. (D and E) Axial CT demonstrates cortical erosions and extension of the mineralized lesion into the surrounding soft tissue, highly suggestive for high-grade chondrosarcoma. Technetium-99m bone scan (F) demonstrates intense uptake within the right humerus without other sites of disease. The patient underwent right proximal humerus replacement (G). Final pathology was consistent with dedifferentiated chondrosarcoma.

extended curettage, high-speed burring, and local adjuvant use[7] (Figure 10-3). As with all other sarcomas, this should be performed by experienced clinicians familiar with the assessment and natural history of these lesions. Figure 10-4 depicts an algorithm for the management of aggressive cartilage tumors.

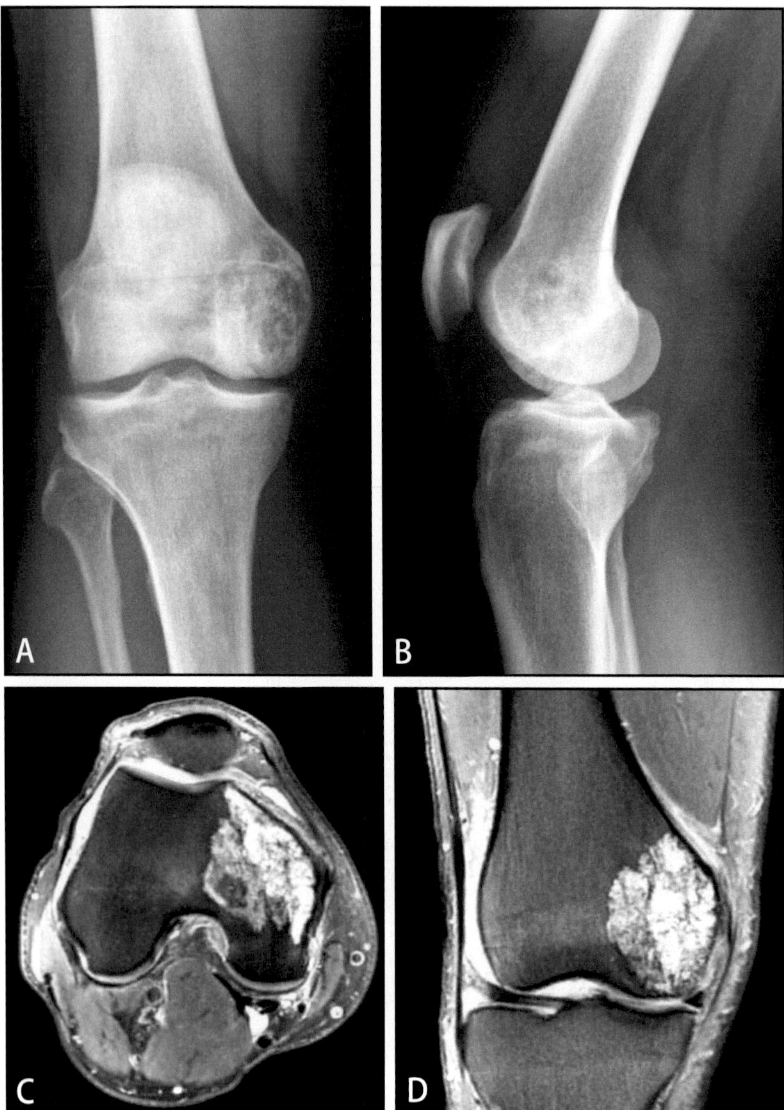

Figure 10-3. A 52-year-old man presents with long-standing achiness in the right knee for several years. (A) Anteroposterior and (B) lateral radiographs demonstrate a lesion within the right medial femoral condyle with lobular growth and mineralization consistent with chondroid matrix. Subtle cortical erosions are observed medially. (C) Axial and (D) coronal T2-weighted MRI demonstrates a well-defined marrow-replacing process with endosteal scalloping without soft-tissue extension.

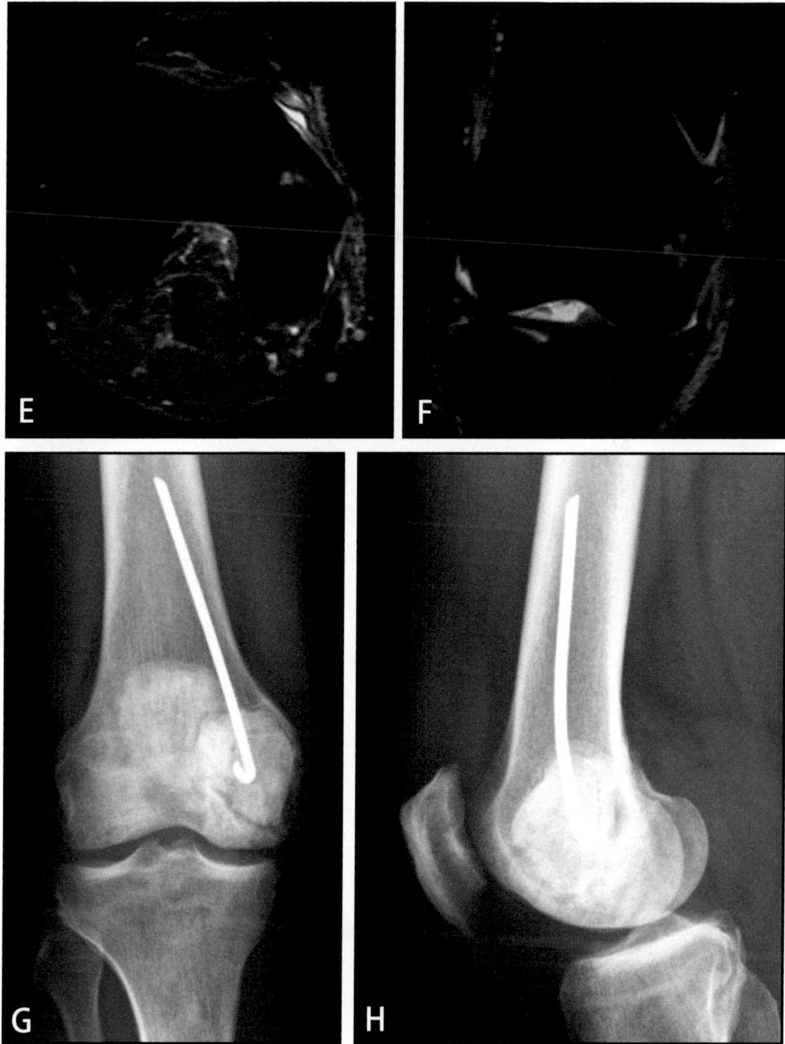

Figure 10-3 continued. (E and F) Comparison MRI from 12 years prior confirms interval growth. Biopsy confirmed grade I chondrosarcoma. (G and H) Extended curettage with cryotherapy, bone grafting of subchondral bone, and polymethyl methacrylate cementation was performed.

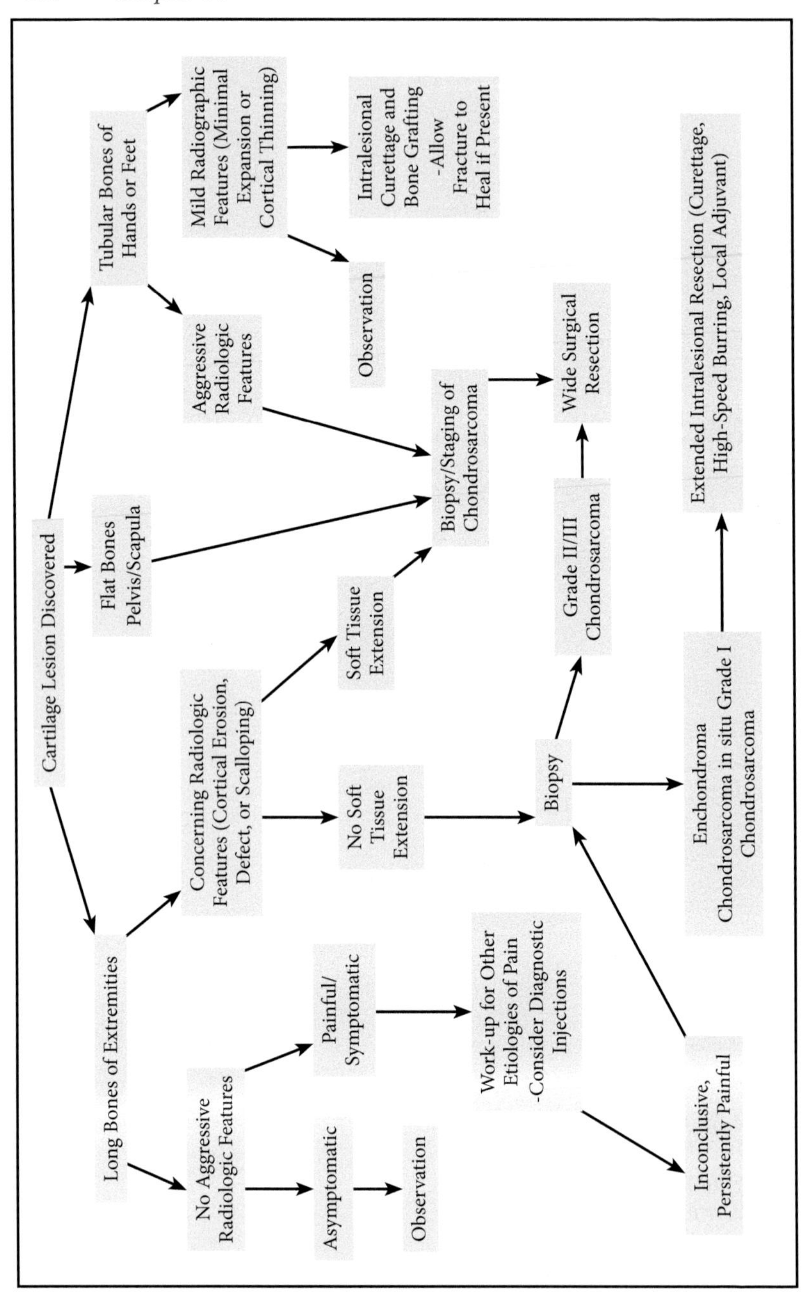

Figure 10-4. Algorithm for management of aggressive cartilage tumors.

Osteochondroma and Multiple Hereditary Exostosis

Osteochondroma, also known as exostosis, is a non-neoplastic developmental anomaly in which an ectopic focus of growth plate cartilage projects away from growing areas of the immature skeleton. They can occur in any skeletal location, but are most common in the metaphysis of long bones, where they typically grow away from the adjacent physis. The estimated incidence of osteochondromas in the general population is approximately 0.5% to 1%, and 15% of those patients will present with multiple exostoses.[8]

Most exostoses are asymptomatic, discovered incidentally or as a palpable bony bump. Osteochondromas can be definitively diagnosed when the exostosis demonstrates continuous cortical and medullary flow into the normal bone. Lesions can be expected to mirror physeal growth, and will demonstrate continued growth until skeletal maturity. Osteochondromas that grow after skeletal maturity are worrisome, and these and any painful lesions should be investigated.

Etiologies of Painful Osteochondromas

- Soft-tissue irritation, overlying bursitis
- Mechanical impingement of joints or adjacent bones
- Entrapment or tethering of nerves or blood vessels
- Growth arrest, angular deformity
- Fracture of stalk (Figure 10-5)
- Spinal cord compression
- Encroachment of intrapelvic structures
- Malignant degeneration (less than 1% of solitary osteochondromas)

Multiple hereditary exostosis (MHE) is an autosomal dominant disorder that affects 1 or 2 individuals per 100,000 (Figure 10-6). Mutations in the *EXT1* and *EXT2* genes account for the majority of cases, and a smaller number of cases are attributed to *EXT3* mutations. *EXT1* is associated with a greater severity of disease, and possibly a higher risk of malignant transformation, which is estimated to occur in 5% to 10% of MHE patients.[9]

Asymptomatic osteochondromas can be observed until skeletal maturity. Patients with MHE should be monitored long-term for changes in osteochondromas. This should include physical examination of osteochondromas that can be easily palpated and measured, and periodic radiographic monitoring for lesions of the hips and pelvis that cannot be easily palpated. Resection of symptomatic osteochondromas should include the entirety of the cartilage

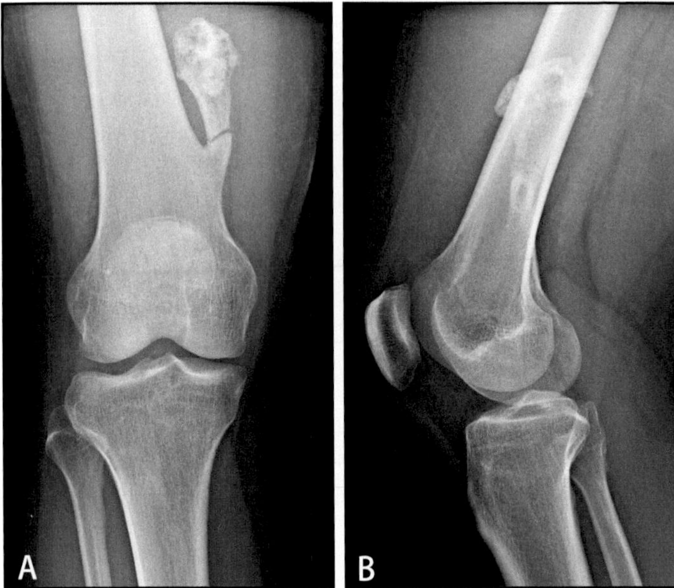

Figure 10-5. A 17-year-old boy presents with right distal thigh pain after a collision during a basketball game. (A) Anteroposterior and (B) lateral radiographs demonstrate a pedunculated, well-defined osteochondroma with a transverse fracture through the base of the stalk of the lesion. The patient was managed with observation.

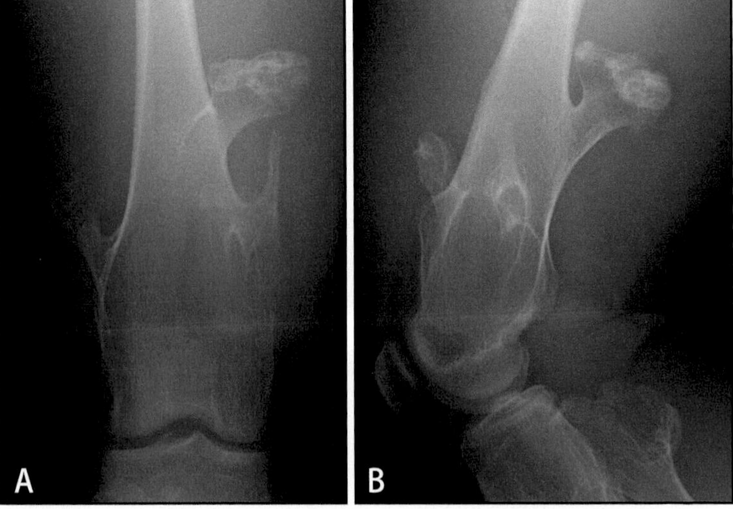

Figure 10-6. A 16-year-old boy with a history of multiple bony prominences presents with catching and pain in the back of the right knee. (A) Anteroposterior and (B) lateral radiographs demonstrate several pedunculated and sessile exostoses about the distal femur, proximal tibia, and proximal fibula. This is characteristic of multiple hereditary exostosis.

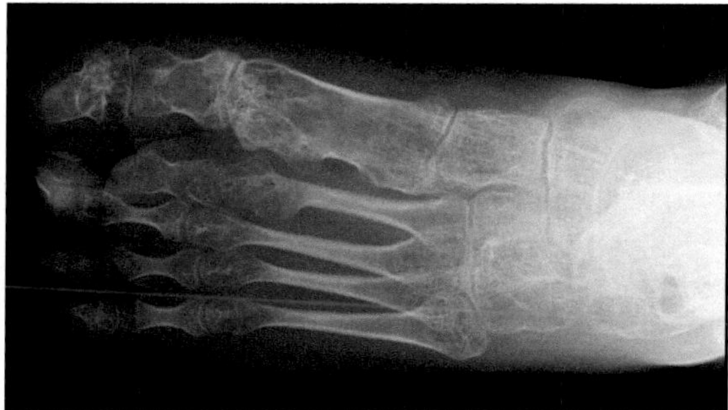

Figure 10-7. Anteroposterior radiograph of the right foot in a patient with Ollier's disease, demonstrating diffuse cartilaginous lesions within multiple bones.

cap and perichondral ring when feasible because the risk of recurrence is high in skeletally immature patients with incomplete resection. Patients with MHE frequently require deformity correction with osteotomy, lengthening, or guided growth procedures about the forearm, knee, and ankle, and should be performed only by experienced practitioners.

Ollier's Disease and Maffucci Syndrome

Ollier's disease and Maffucci syndrome are related disorders caused by a somatic mutation in the *IDH1* or *IDH2* genes, which causes multiple, diffuse enchondromatosis of the affected areas (Figure 10-7). Deformities, shortening of the extremities, and pathologic fractures are common. Maffucci syndrome is further characterized by hemangiomas and lymphangiomas of the skin, soft tissue, and viscera, with an elevated risk of malignant transformation (Table 10-2).

Other Adult Bone Sarcomas

Undifferentiated pleomorphic sarcoma, formerly referred to as malignant fibrous histiocytoma of bone, is a spindle cell malignancy of bone in patients older than 40 years. They are predominantly painful, lytic, and often radiographically indistinguishable from metastatic bone disease. Histologic features include pleomorphic spindle cells in a storiform arrangement without discernable malignant osteoid. Treatment is similar to pediatric osteosarcoma, with chemotherapy and wide surgical resection (Figure 10-8). Similar to conventional osteosarcoma, 5-year survival rates correlate to chemotherapy response, and average around 60% for patients with isolated disease.[11]

Table 10-2

Risk of Secondary Chondrosarcoma in Chondrogenic Disorders

DISORDER	CLINICAL FEATURES	RISK OF MALIGNANCY
Solitary osteochondroma	Sessile or pedunculated, surface-based lesion confluent with medullary canal	Less than 1%
Multiple hereditary exostosis	Multiple osteochondromas, short stature, extremity deformities	5% to 10%
Ollier's disease	Enchondromatosis, asymmetric dwarfism, extremity deformities	20% to 40%
Maffucci syndrome	Enchondromatosis, hemangiomatosis	50% or greater

Adapted from Verdegaal SH, Bovée JV, Pansuriya TC, et al.[10]

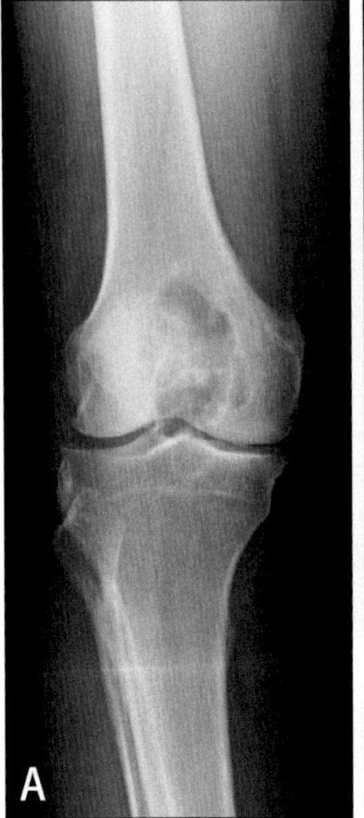

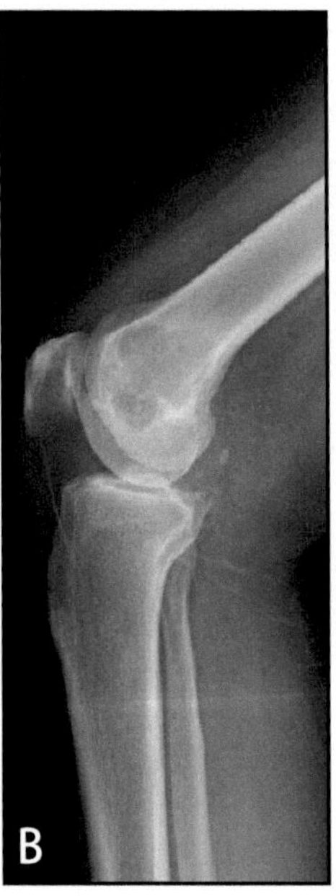

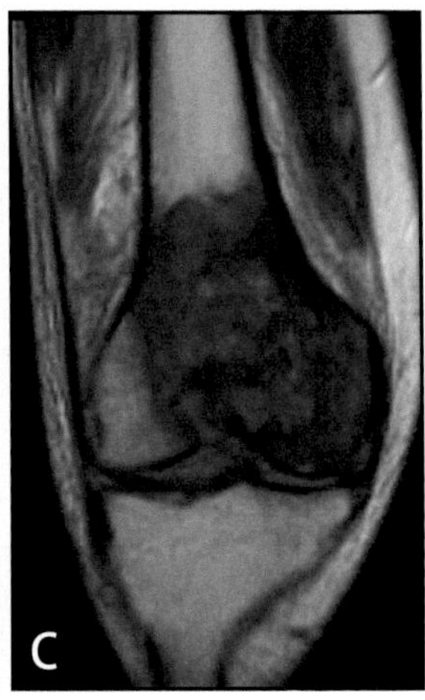

Figure 10-8. A 68-year-old man presents with worsening right knee pain. (A) Anteroposterior and (B) lateral radiographs demonstrate a destructive lesion of the right distal femur with extension to the surface of the trochlea. (C) Coronal T1-weighted MRI, and coronal and axial T2-weighted MRI obtained after an ill-advised arthroscopic biopsy demonstrate a marrow-replacing process with perilesional edema within the distal femur and contamination/growth within the joint synovium.

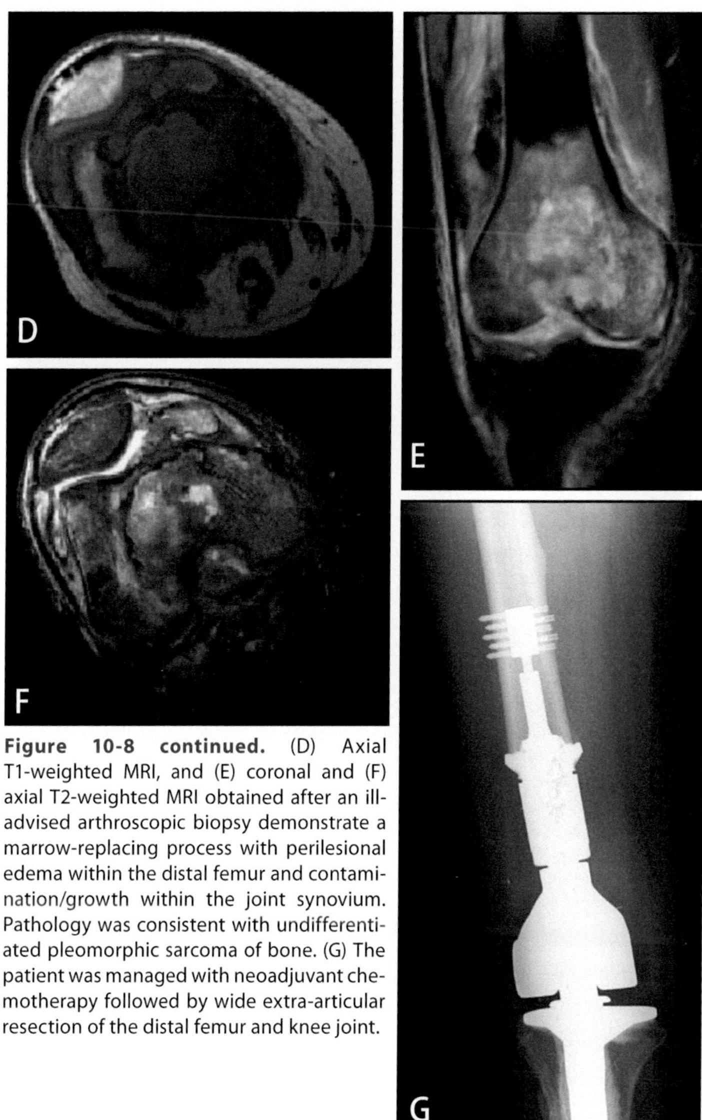

Figure 10-8 continued. (D) Axial T1-weighted MRI, and (E) coronal and (F) axial T2-weighted MRI obtained after an ill-advised arthroscopic biopsy demonstrate a marrow-replacing process with perilesional edema within the distal femur and contamination/growth within the joint synovium. Pathology was consistent with undifferentiated pleomorphic sarcoma of bone. (G) The patient was managed with neoadjuvant chemotherapy followed by wide extra-articular resection of the distal femur and knee joint.

Fibrosarcoma is a spindle cell malignancy of older adults, often identified secondary to irradiation and other disorders of bone. The grade of lesion is variable, and correlates directly with prognosis. Histologic features include spindle cells in bands with changing orientation, giving a "herringbone"

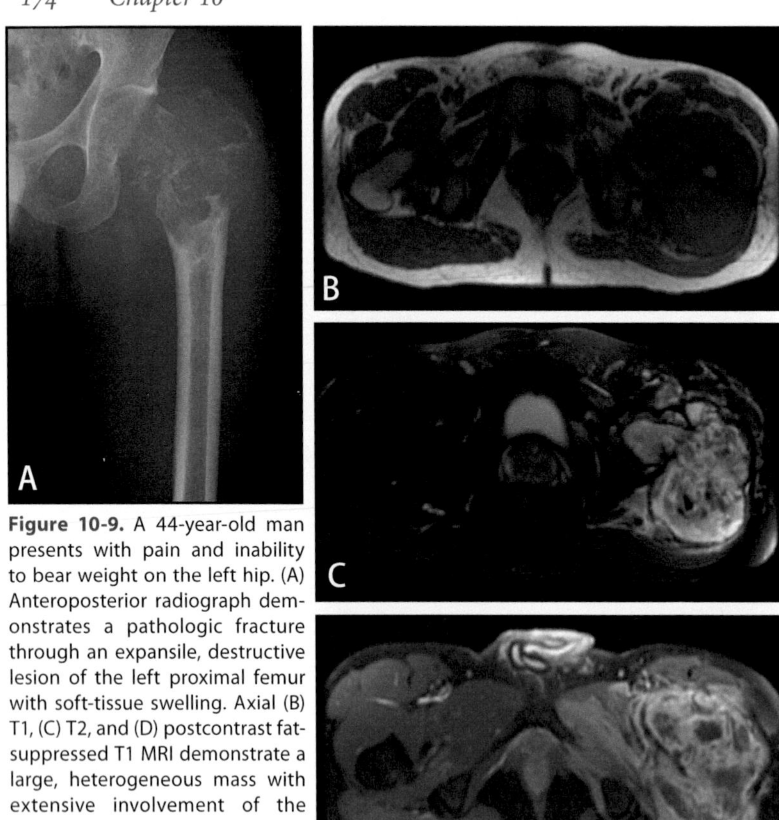

Figure 10-9. A 44-year-old man presents with pain and inability to bear weight on the left hip. (A) Anteroposterior radiograph demonstrates a pathologic fracture through an expansile, destructive lesion of the left proximal femur with soft-tissue swelling. Axial (B) T1, (C) T2, and (D) postcontrast fat-suppressed T1 MRI demonstrate a large, heterogeneous mass with extensive involvement of the bone and surrounding soft tissue, with areas of solid and rim post-contrast enhancement.

pattern to the tumor with variable degrees of collagen and myxoid background. Low-grade lesions are treated with wide surgical resection only. High-grade tumors are managed similarly to undifferentiated pleomorphic sarcoma as previously described.

Angiosarcoma is an extremely aggressive high-grade malignancy of vasogenic tissue. Multifocal disease within the extremity with proximal migration from a primary site is common, and urgent amputation may be necessary to achieve an adequate surgical margin (Figure 10-9).

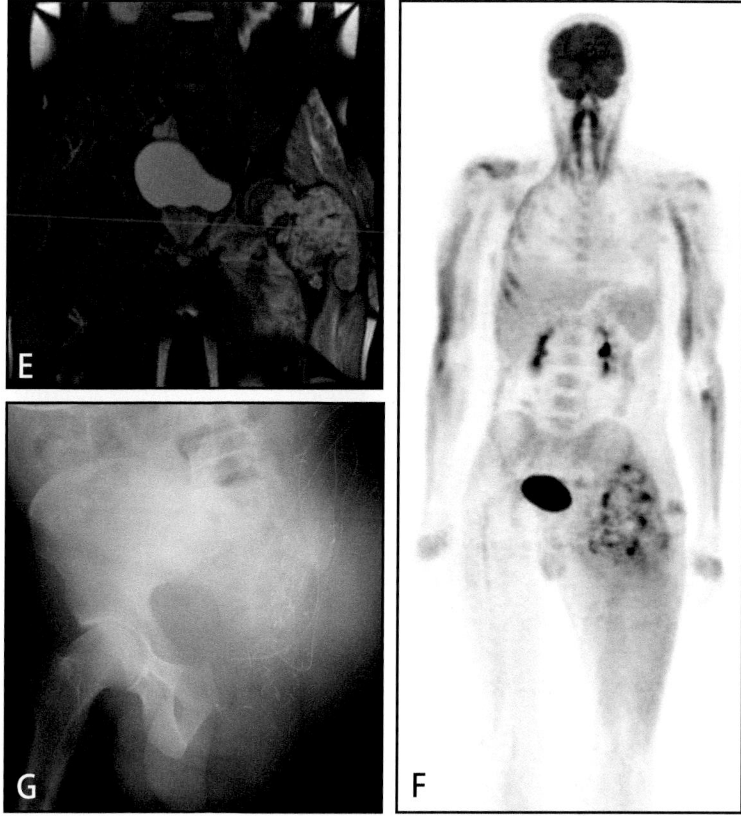

Figure 10-9 continued. (E) Coronal T2 MRI demonstrates extensive peritumoral edema within the surrounding musculatures. (F) Positron emission tomography-CT demonstrates fluorodeoxyglucose activity within the left hip. (G) The patient was managed with external hemipelvectomy.

Adamantinoma is a very rare, low-to-intermediate-grade bone sarcoma with an overwhelming predilection for the anterior cortex of the tibial diaphysis. The majority of cases occur in the third and fourth decade of life, and metastases occur in 30% of patients. Histologic analysis demonstrates a characteristic biphasic appearance of epithelial islands in a spindle cell osteofibrous background.[12] No effective chemotherapy or radiotherapy is established, and treatment consists of wide surgical resection.

Take-Aways

1. Chondrosarcoma is the most common bone sarcoma in older adult patients. The diagnosis is often suggested radiographically, and fine-cut CT is the imaging study of choice for evaluation.
2. Osteochondromas are common lesions of cartilage with a low risk of malignant degeneration. Pain in the area of an osteochondroma should be thoroughly evaluated, but is more commonly attributed to mechanical effects on adjacent structures.
3. Undifferentiated pleomorphic sarcoma and fibrosarcoma of bone have a similar radiologic appearance to metastatic bone disease, but are managed with chemotherapy and surgical resection similar to primary osteosarcoma.

Commonly Tested Topics for Trainees

- Chondrosarcoma is a radioresistant and chemoresistant disease. The mainstay of treatment remains surgical resection. Low-grade lesions without soft-tissue extension can be managed with extended intralesional resection. Intermediate and high-grade tumors require wide surgical resection.
- Secondary chondrosarcomas are typically lower-grade lesions. The risk of chondrosarcoma development is low for solitary osteochondroma and multiple hereditary exostosis, and significant with Ollier's disease and Maffucci syndrome.
- Enchondromatosis with soft-tissue phleboliths is characteristic of Maffucci syndrome.
- Adamantinoma is an intermediate-grade sarcoma with a classically tibial diaphyseal location and biphasic histologic appearance. Treatment is wide surgical resection.

References

1. Pritchard DJ, Lunke RJ, Taylor WF, Dahlin DC, Medley BE: Chondrosarcoma: a clinicopathologic and statistical analysis. *Cancer.* 1980;45(1):149-157. doi:10.1002/1097-0142(19800101)45:1<149::aid-cncr2820450125>3.0.co;2-a.
2. Andreou D, Ruppin S, Fehlberg S, Pink D, Werner M, Tunn PU. Survival and prognostic factors in chondrosarcoma: results in 115 patients with long-term follow-up. *Acta Orthop.* 2011;82(6):749-755. doi:10.3109/17453674.2011.636668.

3. Grimer RJ, Gosheger G, Taminiau A, et al. Dedifferentiated chondrosarcoma: prognostic factors and outcome from a European group. *Eur J Cancer.* 2007;43(14):2060-2065. doi:10.1016/j.ejca.2007.06.016.
4. Tsuchiya H, Ueda Y, Morishita H, et al. Borderline chondrosarcoma of long and flat bones. *J Cancer Res Clin Oncol.* 1993;119(6):363-368. doi:10.1007/BF01208847.
5. Murphey MD, Andrews CL, Flemming DJ, Temple HT, Smith WS, Smirniotopoulos JG. From the archives of the AFIP. Primary tumors of the spine: radiologic pathologic correlation. *Radiographics.* 1996;16(5):1131-1158. doi:10.1148/radiographics.16.5.8888395.
6. Rosenthal DI, Schiller AL, Mankin HJ. Chondrosarcoma: correlation of radiological and histological grade. *Radiology.* 1984;150(1):21-26. doi:10.1148/radiology.150.1.6689763.
7. Meftah M, Schult P, Henshaw RM. Long-term results of intralesional curettage and cryosurgery for treatment of low-grade chondrosarcoma. *J Bone Joint Surg Am.* 2013;95(15):1358-1364. doi:10.2106/JBJS.L.00442.
8. Gaumer GR, Weinberg DS, Collier CD, Getty PJ, Liu RW. An osteological study on the prevalence of osteochondromas. *Iowa Orthop J.* 2017;37:147-150.
9. Porter DE, Lonie L, Fraser M, et al. Severity of disease and risk of malignant change in hereditary multiple exostoses. A genotype-phenotype study. *J Bone Joint Surg Br.* 2004;86(7):1041-1046. doi:10.1302/0301-620X.86B7.14815.
10. Verdegaal SH, Bovée JV, Pansuriya TC, et al. Incidence, predictive factors, and prognosis of chondrosarcoma in patients with Ollier disease and Maffucci syndrome: an international multicenter study of 161 patients. *Oncologist.* 2011;16(12):1771-1779. doi:10.1634/theoncologist.2011-0200.
11. Jeon DG, Song WS, Kong CB, Kim JR, Lee SY. MFH of bone and osteosarcoma show similar survival and chemosensitivity. *Clin Orthop Relat Res.* 2011;469(2):584-590. doi:10.1007/s11999-010-1428-z.
12. Most MJ, Sim FH, Inwards CY. Osteofibrous dysplasia and adamantinoma. *J Am Acad Orthop Surg.* 2010;18(6):358-366.

Section **IV**

Soft-Tissue Tumors

11

Benign Soft-Tissue Tumors

Overview

Due to their ubiquity, soft-tissue lumps and bumps are something every clinician will encounter on a frequent basis. Most of these lesions will represent benign or non-neoplastic diagnoses, but each should be diligently investigated to avoid delaying the diagnosis of or mismanagement of a more aggressive entity. We will discuss the most common benign soft-tissue tumors that present to clinical attention, how to accurately identify them clinically and radiologically, and discuss basic treatments for these lesions.

The ratio of benign to malignant soft-tissue masses is unknown, but the overwhelming majority of soft-tissue lumps and bumps are benign. Many of these disorders can be managed with little more than observation, but doing so demands a high level of confidence in the diagnosis. There is considerable overlap between the radiologic findings of benign and malignant soft-tissue neoplasms, so lesions that cannot be definitively diagnosed between clinical and radiologic evaluations require biopsy. For lesions that meet surgical indications, a marginal resection is usually appropriate. Patients should be counseled that even benign soft-tissue tumors can recur, but this does not suggest an elevated risk of malignant transformation.

Wallace, MT
Handbook of Musculoskeletal Tumors (pp 181-193).

Lipomatous Tumors

Benign lipomatous masses are the most common soft-tissue neoplasms encountered in clinical practice, though the true incidence is unknown. Subcutaneous lipomas can be identified by their soft, rubbery, and freely mobile texture on physical examination. Deeper lesions are often substantially larger, but can be definitively identified by their characteristic fat signal on all magnetic resonance imaging (MRI) sequences (Figure 11-1). These determinate imaging findings and the high rates of sampling error observed with needle biopsy of well-differentiated fatty lesions generally render confirmation by biopsy unnecessary.[1]

Lipomas are characterized by an indolent clinical course, exhibiting an initial growth phase followed by slow to no growth over an extended period of time. Lipomas may appear to enlarge with weight gain, or may become more prominent with weight loss, but the risk of continued growth is low. As a result, most lipomas can be safely observed, either by clinical measurement or MR imaging for deeper lesions. Marginal resection is appropriate for growing lesions, symptomatic lesions, or lesions that patients find functionally unacceptable.

Atypical lipomatous tumor (ALT), historically referred to as well-differentiated liposarcoma, is a more active lesion of well-differentiated fat. ALTs tend to occur in deeper tissues, and are more infiltrative and demonstrate progressive growth over time. Radiologic and histological findings are similar to benign lipomas, but areas of fibrous stranding are common (Figure 11-2). The diagnosis is confirmed by the presence of ring and giant marker chromosomes with amplification of *HMGA2* and *MDM2* genes, which demonstrate 100% sensitivity and specificity.[2] ALTs with intrapelvic or retroperitoneal extension have a more aggressive clinical course, and the term "well-differentiated liposarcoma may be more appropriate for these tumors. For extremity ALTs, marginal excision is acceptable, although rates of local recurrence approach 10% to 15%, and recurrence after re-excision exceeds 50%. The risk of malignant dedifferentiation is estimated at approximately 4%.[3]

Benign lipomatous tumors can include areas of necrosis, calcification, ossification, or internal areas of chondroid, angiomatous, spindle cell, or smooth muscle differentiation. Hibernomas, for example, are peculiar lipomas of brown fat. These lesions often show atypical zones on MRI and often require biopsy. Once confirmed, marginal excision is recommended.

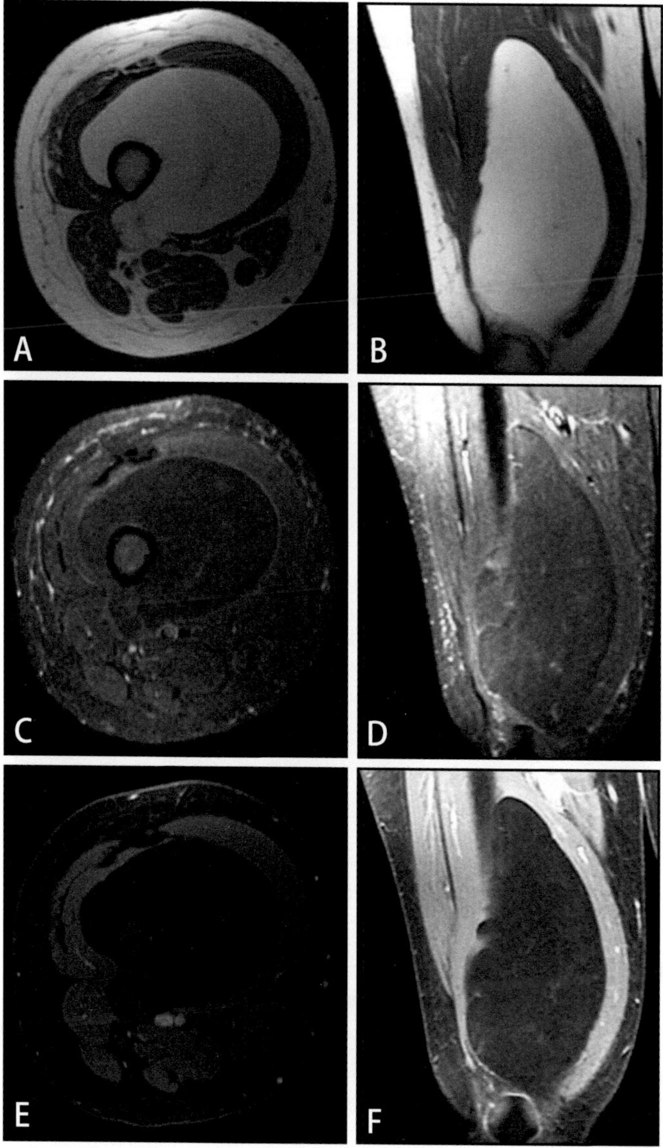

Figure 11-1. A 42-year-old woman presents with long-standing painless swelling of the right thigh, to the point that it interferes with clothing wear. T1 (A) axial and (B) coronal MRI sequences demonstrate a large homogenous mass within the quadriceps compartment. This mass is isointense to subcutaneous fat, with similar homogenous fat suppression on T2 (C) axial and (D) coronal sequences. (E) Axial and (F) coronal T1 fat-suppressed postcontrast imaging do not demonstrate areas of internal enhancement, confirming the diagnosis of a benign lipomatous soft-tissue tumor. Marginal excision was performed, and final pathology was consistent with intramuscular lipoma.

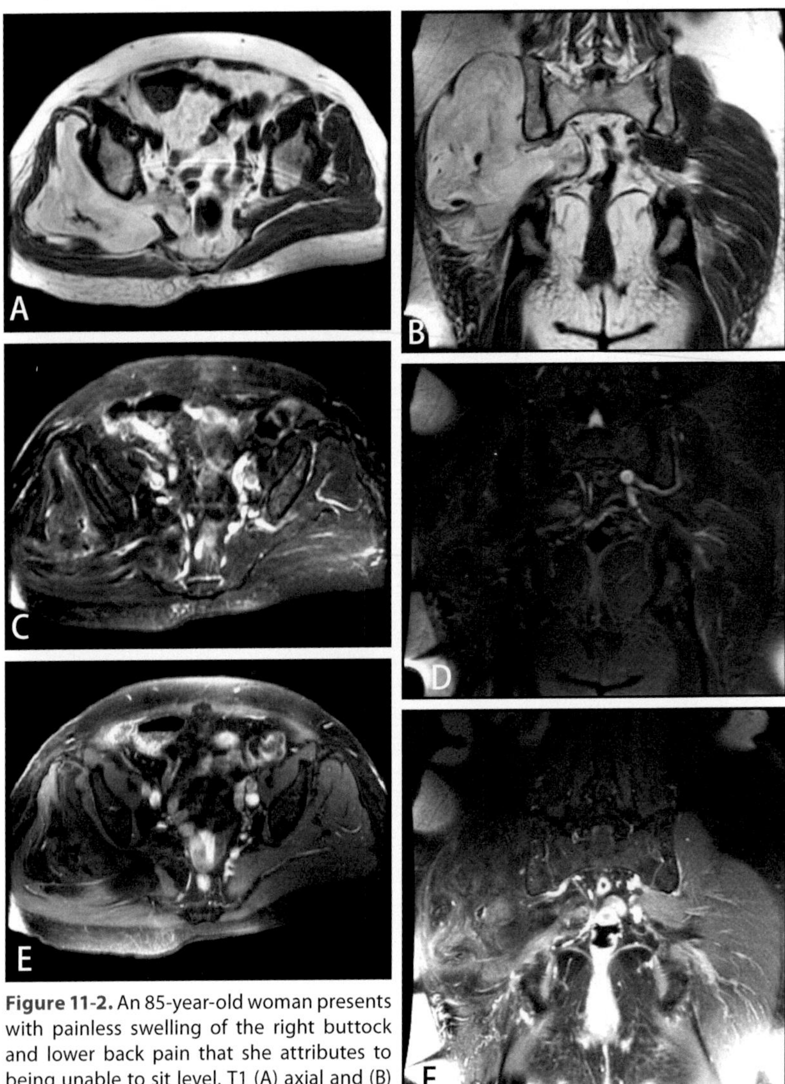

Figure 11-2. An 85-year-old woman presents with painless swelling of the right buttock and lower back pain that she attributes to being unable to sit level. T1 (A) axial and (B) coronal MRI demonstrate a large, hyperintense, lobulated mass within the gluteus minimus and medius musculature, with extension through the sciatic notch. T2 (C) axial and (D) coronal sequences demonstrate suppression of the mass with signal intensity similar to subcutaneous fat, and subtle linear areas of increased signal. T1 fat-suppressed postcontrast (E) axial and (F) coronal sequences do not demonstrate areas of significant or nodular enhancement, but subtle areas of linear enhancement. Marginal excision was performed, and final pathology demonstrated atypical lipomatous tumor with fibrous bands and *MDM2* amplification.

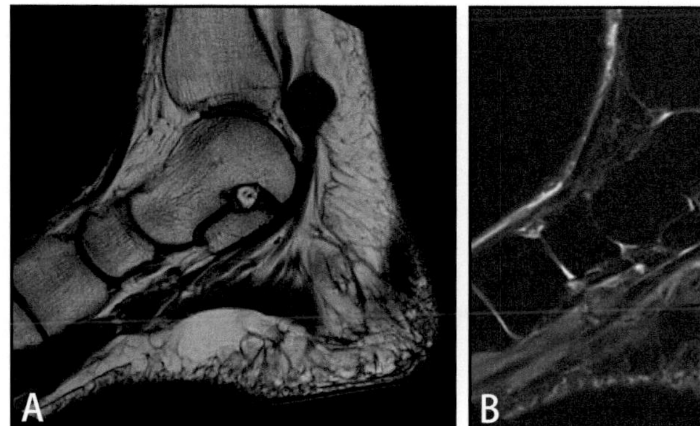

Figure 11-3. A 57-year-old woman presents with a tender nodule over the posteromedial aspect of the right ankle. Examination demonstrated a mobile mass with tender radiation of pain into the medial and plantar foot with palpation. Sagittal (A) T1 and (B) T2 MRI demonstrate a well-defined, fusiform mass adjacent to the posterior tibial tendon, with low T1 and bright T2 signal. There is a characteristic "tail sign" at the distal extent of the lesion, consistent with a peripheral nerve sheath tumor. Biopsy confirmed the diagnosis of schwannoma, and the patient was treated with marginal resection.

Nerve Sheath Tumors

Peripheral nerve sheath tumors are the second most common soft-tissue neoplasms encountered clinically. Peripheral nerve sheath tumors most commonly occur in young adults, and may develop as solitary lesions or multifocal syndromes such as neurofibromatosis or schwannomatosis. These tumors may be asymptomatic, but are frequently painful, and may cause radiating pain when present in major extremity nerves. Lesions that develop in major extremity nerves are often mobile side to side, but restricted in the proximal-to-distal direction (Figure 11-3).

Marginal excision is typically curative. Schwannomas, or neurilemomas, occur on the surface of the nerve fascicles, and are easier to resect than neurofibromas, which tend to invest more within nerve fibers. Plexiform neurofibromas are associated with type 1 neurofibromatosis (NF1), which is characterized by multiple cutaneous neurofibromas, café-au-lait macules, axillary or inguinal freckling, Lisch nodules in the iris or optic glioma, long-bone pseudarthrosis, or scoliosis. The risk of malignant peripheral nerve sheath tumor (MPNST) in NF1 patients is 10% to 13%, and 50% of MPNSTs occur in NF1 patients.[4,5] MPNSTs are radiologically indistinguishable from benign peripheral nerve sheath tumors, so biopsy is necessary for confirmation. In the setting of NF1, a positron emission tomography-computed

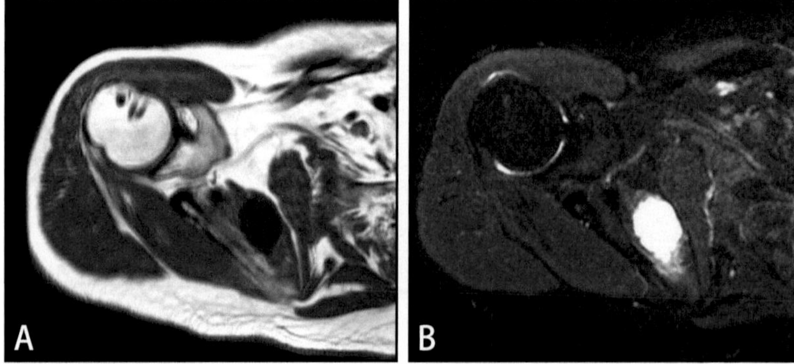

Figure 11-4. A 53-year-old man presents with an incidental finding during evaluation for chronic rotator cuff insufficiency. (A) T1 and (B) T2 MRI sequences demonstrate a well-defined lesion within the subscapularis muscle, hypointense to surrounding muscle on T1 and brightly hyperintense on T2. Biopsy confirmed a diagnosis of benign intramuscular myxoma, and the patient underwent marginal resection.

tomography can be used to compare uptake values between multiple lesions, and identify fluorodeoxyglucose-avid lesions for biopsy.

Myxoid, Fibrous, and Vascular Lesions

Intramuscular myxomas are painless tumors of mesenchymal cells and abundant extracellular myxoid material. These lesions are generally non-tender, intramuscular, and deep to compartment fascia. As with other cellular tumors, these lesions demonstrate low signal intensity on T1-weighted MRI, and very high signal intensity on T2-weighted MRI, so the imaging findings can be nonspecific. A biopsy is therefore required to differentiate benign myxoma from more aggressive myxoid-producing malignancies. Myxoid material has a loose, gelatinous consistency on biopsy, similar to runny mucus. Mazabraud syndrome consists of multiple myxomas with polyostotic fibrous dysplasia. Once confirmed, treatment consists of marginal excision (Figure 11-4).

Fibromatosis

Extra-abdominal desmoid tumors are aggressively proliferating fibroblastic lesions that most commonly develop in areas of confluent fascial planes such as the posterior shoulder, hip, knee, and elbow or forearm of younger adults. These lesions are composed of very dense collagen, and are very firm on evaluation. The general consistency of fibromatosis is that of a firm rubber

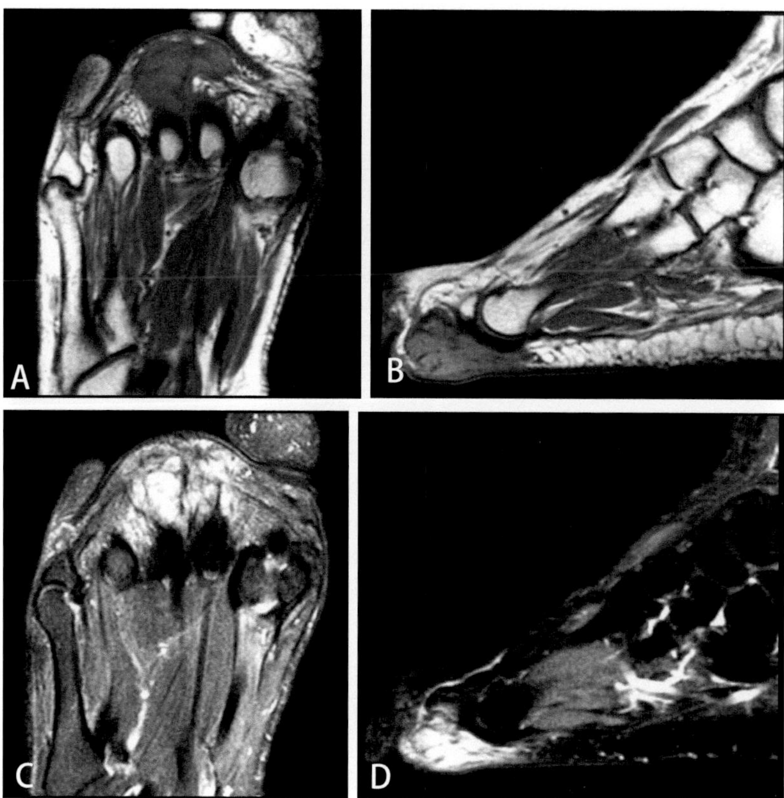

Figure 11-5. A 57-year-old man presents with painless, firm masses over bilateral plantar feet. T1 (A) axial and (B) sagittal and T2 (C) axial and (D) sagittal MRI of the right foot.

ball with attempted needle biopsy. Most are asymptomatic, but may present with locoregional pain and contracture of the nearby joint. The clinician must be aware of the association between extra-abdominal desmoids tumors and Gardner syndrome/familial adenomatous polyposis, and these patients should be referred for screening colonoscopy. There is also an association between fibromatoses of the palmar fascia (Dupuytren disease), plantar fascia (Ledderhose syndrome), and penile fascia (Peyronie disease), so discovery of fibromatosis in one location should prompt screening of other at-risk locations (Figure 11-5).

The natural history of fibromatosis is often unpredictable; lesions may demonstrate persistent growth, stabilization after a period of initial growth, or occasionally, spontaneous regression. Despite their locally aggressive features, the risk of distant spread and mortality is negligible. There is no

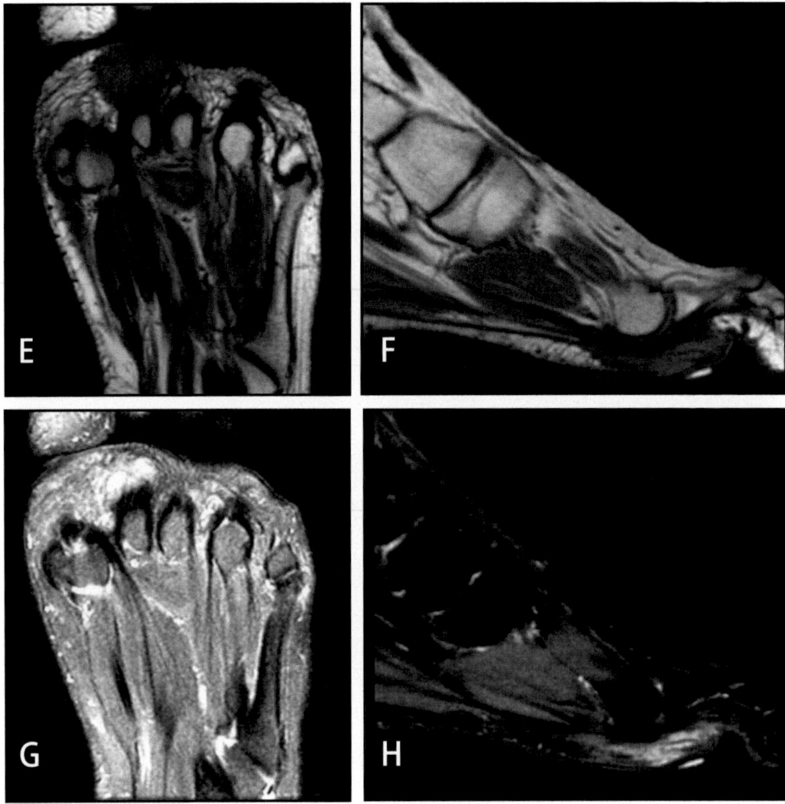

Figure 11-5 continued. T1 (E) axial and (F) sagittal and T2 (G) axial and (H) sagittal MRI of the left foot demonstrate infiltrative T1-hypointense, T2-hyperintense masses of the plantar forefeet bilaterally. The margins of the tumors are indistinct and spread broadly over the distal extent of the plantar fasciae. Streaks of hypointense signal on T1 and T2 sequences are consistent with dense collagen tissue. Biopsy confirmed plantar fibromatoses.

broad consensus as to the management of extra-abdominal desmoid tumors. Wide resections with negative margins are associated with high rates of local recurrence up to 50%, so the treatment of extra-abdominal desmoids has evolved recently to focus on nonoperative modalities such as observation, nonsteroidal anti-inflammatory drugs, antihormonal agents, and low-dose chemotherapy.[6] Surgery with adjuvant radiotherapy may be considered in severe cases, but significant post-treatment morbidity should be anticipated. Treatment should therefore be performed by experienced practitioners, preferably within a multidisciplinary team that includes radiation and medical oncology colleagues for multimodal treatment. When in doubt, it is always safest to avoid operative intervention, particularly for asymptomatic tumors.

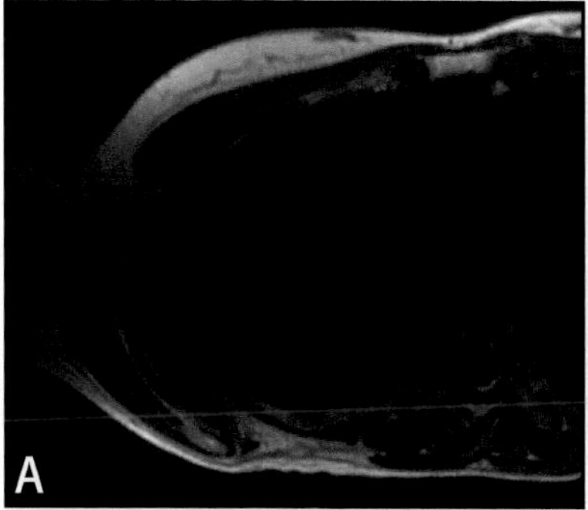

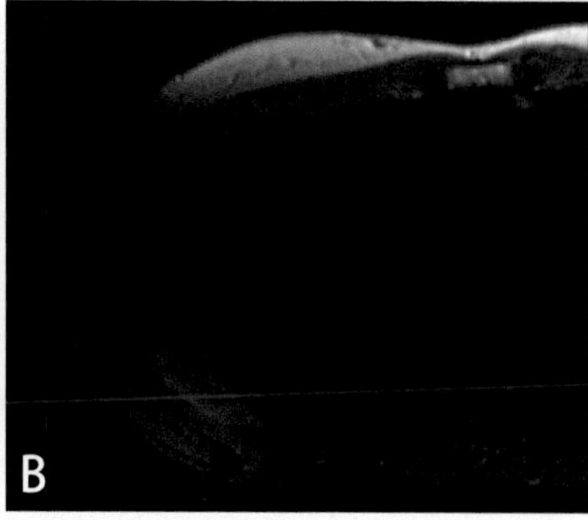

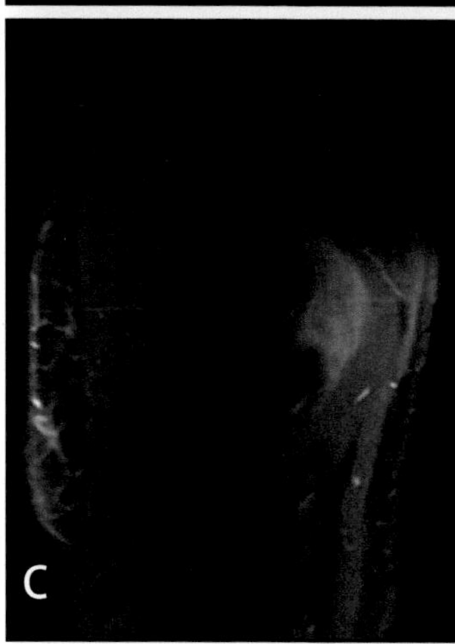

Figure 11-6. A 57-year-old woman with a history of competitive swimming presents with painful snapping of the right scapula. T1 (A) axial, T1 (B) postcontrast axial and (C) sagittal MRI demonstrates a broad-based lesion between the inferior left scapula and the posterolateral chest wall with solid postcontrast enhancement. Biopsy confirmed a diagnosis of elastofibroma, and the patient was treated with marginal excision.

Padded shoe inserts with cutouts for plantar fibromatoses are a helpful first-line intervention for Ledderhose disease, and collagenase injections have demonstrated efficacy in the treatment of Dupuytren disease.

Elastofibromas

Elastofibromas are lesions of collagen and elastin fibers that mimic fibromatoses, but are classically located between the chest wall of the seventh and eighth ribs and the inferior angle of the scapula. They typically present with a painless snapping of the scapula in older patients with repetitive overhead activity, and often occur bilaterally. Observation and symptomatic treatment are appropriate, but for painful lesions and those that significantly impair shoulder function, marginal excision is generally curative (Figure 11-6).

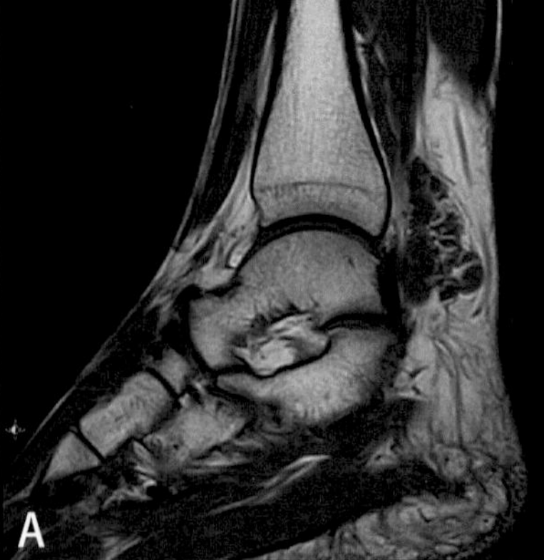

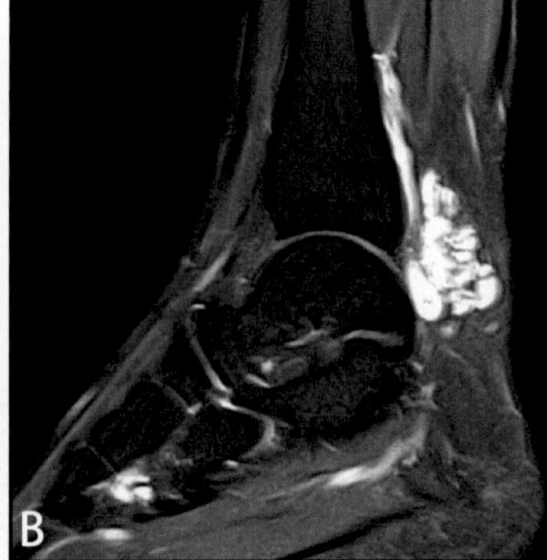

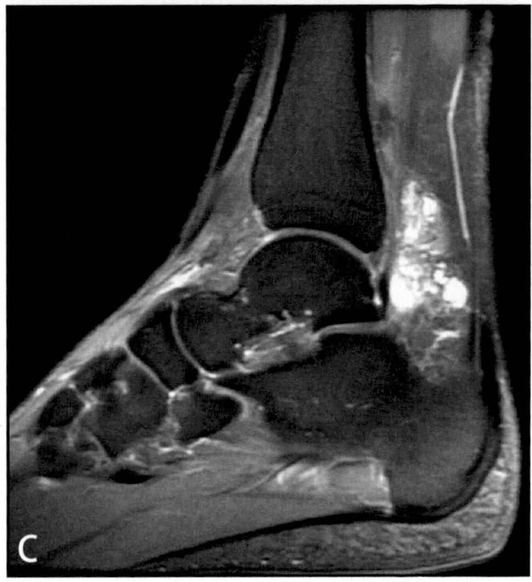

Figure 11-7. A 25-year-old male presents with vague discomfort in the posterior right ankle. Sagittal (A) T1, (B) T2, and T1 (C) postcontrast MRI demonstrate a lobular mass with streaks of T1-hyperintense fat separating T2-hyperintense fluid-filled zones with postcontrast enhancement, consistent with soft-tissue hemangioma.

Hemangioma

Low-flow venous and capillary malformations and high-flow arteriovenous malformations, are non-neoplastic proliferations of blood vessels that can occur in any tissue, including bone, viscera, or soft tissues. Most are asymptomatic, incidental findings that require little more than observation, but some can present with acute episodes of painful thrombophlebitis, uncomfortable engorgement with activity or temperature, or acute bleeding episodes when located within the joint synovium. Symptomatic lesions can be managed with percutaneous sclerotherapy, embolization, surgical resection, or any combination of the 3 (Figure 11-7). The tendency for neovascularization within these lesions is associated with notable rates of recurrence, which patients must be aware of prior to surgical resection.[7]

The majority of soft-tissue tumors present with indeterminate findings, and these require tissue biopsy for diagnosis. Some defining imaging features can help identify those masses that can be definitively diagnosed without a biopsy, or provide a reasonable clinical suspicion of the diagnosis prior to biopsy. Table 11-1 illustrates common soft-tissue masses with characteristic imaging findings.

Take-Aways

1. Benign fatty tumors (lipoma and ALT) can be definitively identified on MRI. Marginal excision is appropriate.
2. Peripheral nerve sheath tumors can be identified by their characteristic clinical and imaging findings, but in the setting of multifocal disease, cannot be distinguished from MPNST without a biopsy.
3. Extra-abdominal desmoids are associated with aggressive growth patterns and high rates of local recurrence after resection. Nonoperative management is recommended when feasible.

Commonly Tested Topics for Trainees

- In the setting of benign lipomatous tumors, fluorescent in situ hybridization for *MDM2* is sensitive and specific for ALT.
- Identification of a plexiform neurofibroma should prompt evaluation for NF1, which is associated with a 10% to 13% risk of malignancy.
- Extra-abdominal desmoids should be investigated for associated Gardner syndrome.

Table 11-1

Characteristic Imaging Features of Common Soft-Tissue Masses

DIAGNOSIS	CLINICAL FINDINGS	PLAIN RADIOGRAPHY	MRI
Lipoma	Rubbery Mobile	Radiolucent shadow within soft tissue	Homogenous, bright T1-fat signal Isointense to subcutaneous fat on all sequences
Atypical lipomatous tumor	Deep, rubbery, and compressible	Radiolucent shadow within soft tissue	Homogenous, bright T1-fat signal Isointense to subcutaneous fat on all sequences Fibrous stranding
Peripheral nerve sheath tumors (schwannoma and neurofibroma)	Painful, tender Mobile side to side, but tethered proximal to distal Tinel's sign Sharp distributional pain with needle biopsy	None	Bright T2 signal Fusiform shape Target sign "Tail" sign: fluid within distended epineurium Plexiform tumor diagnostic of NF1
Intramuscular myxoma	Nonspecific Gelatinous, "snot-like" material on biopsy	None	Intensely bright T2 signal Hypointense on T1, darker than surrounding skeletal muscle
Fibromatosis	Dense/firm to palpation Association with Gardner syndrome	None	Irregular, infiltrative borders Low on T1, bright on T2
Vascular malformation/ hemangioma	Boggy, ill-defined Fluctuations in size Atraumatic hemarthrosis	Phleboliths (calcified thrombi)	Serpiginous vascular channels of bright T2 signal separated by streaks of T1-bright fat signal Significant postcontrast enhancement

Abbreviations: MRI, magnetic resonance imaging; NF1, neurofibromatosis 1.

References

1. Gaskin CM, Helms CA. Lipomas, lipoma variants, and well-differentiated liposarcomas (atypical lipomas): results of MRI evaluations of 126 consecutive fatty masses. *AJR Am J Roentgen.* 2004;182(3):733-739. doi:10.2214/ajr.182.3.1820733.
2. Mandahl N, Bartuma H, Magnusson L, Isaksson M, Macchia G, Mertens F. HMGA2 and MDM2 expression in lipomatous tumors with partial, low-level amplification of sequences from the long arm of chromosome 12. *Cancer Genet.* 2001;204(10):550-556. doi:10.1016/j.cancergen.2011.09.005.
3. Mavrogenis AF, Lesensky J, Romagnoli C, Alberghini M, Letson GD, Ruggieri P. Atypical lipomatous tumors/well-differentiated liposarcomas: clinical outcomes of 67 patients. *Orthopedics.* 2011;34(12):893-898. doi:10.3928/01477447-20111021-11.
4. Evans DG, Baser ME, McGaughran J, Sharif S, Howard E, Moran A. Malignant peripheral nerve sheath tumours in neurofibromatosis 1. *J Med Genet.* 2002;39(5):311-314. doi:10.1136/jmg.39.5.311.
5. Farid M, Demicco EG, Garcia R, et al. Malignant peripheral nerve sheath tumors. *Oncologist.* 2014;19(2):193-201. doi:10.1634/theoncologist.2013-0328.
6. Murphey MD, Ruble CM, Tyszko SM, Zbojniewicz AM, Potter BK, Miettinen M. From the archives of the AFIP: musculoskeletal fibromatoses: radiologic-pathologic correlation. *Radiographics.* 2009;29(7):2143-2173. doi:10.1148/rg.297095138.
7. Tang P, Hornicek FJ, Gebhardt MC, Cates J, Mankin HJ. Surgical treatment of hemangiomas of soft tissue. *Clin Orthop Relat Res.* 2002;399:205-210. doi:10.1097/00003086-200206000-00025.

12

Soft-Tissue Sarcomas

Overview

Malignant soft-tissue tumors are uncommon cancers that arise from mesenchymal tissue. Although substantially less common than benign soft-tissue masses, soft-tissue sarcomas (STS) are among the most common musculoskeletal lesions to be misdiagnosed and mismanaged. The work-up, biopsy, and diagnosis of soft-tissue lesions have been discussed previously. We will present the most common STS based on patient age and anatomic location, and review the treatment of STS. As with all other primary musculoskeletal malignancies, the management of STS should be performed by experienced practitioners, and prompt referral is recommended.

Approximately 9000 new cases of STS are diagnosed each year in the United States, for an estimated incidence of 3.5 cases per 100,000 individuals annually.[1] Owing to their relative rarity compared with benign soft-tissue tumors, the diagnosis is not often considered by the unwary practitioner, and errors in diagnosis and management are common. Delays in diagnosis, misdiagnosis, and improper surgery leading to otherwise-preventable limb loss are potential outcomes when the proper methods of work-up and biopsy are not observed.

STS are a heterogeneous group of more than 50 different histological subtypes, with a wide range of growth behaviors, metastatic potential, and responsiveness to adjunctive treatments. Symptomatology may vary, but STS most commonly present as painless, enlarging, and well defined on imaging.

Wallace, MT
Handbook of Musculoskeletal Tumors (pp 195-210).

More than half occur in extremity locations, and 70% are deep to fascia. More than 80% occur in patients older than 15 years, but many sarcoma subtypes display a predilection for certain ages.[2]

Common Soft-Tissue Sarcoma Subtypes Based on Age

Childhood (Younger Than 15 Years)

- Rhabdomyosarcoma (embryonal; most common STS of childhood)
- Infantile fibrosarcoma

Adolescent and Young Adult (16 to 39 Years)

- Synovial sarcoma (most common STS of young adults; most common STS of the foot)
- Rhabdomyosarcoma (alveolar)
- Clear cell sarcoma
- Epithelioid sarcoma (most common STS of the hand)
- Primitive neuroectodermal tumor/extraskeletal Ewing sarcoma
- Extraskeletal osteosarcoma
- Alveolar soft part sarcoma

Adult (40 to 60 Years)

- Undifferentiated pleomorphic sarcoma (UPS; most common STS of adults)
- Rhabdomyosarcoma (pleomorphic)
- Liposarcoma (myxoid and round cell)
- Malignant peripheral nerve sheath tumor
- Extraskeletal chondrosarcoma
- Kaposi sarcoma

Older Adult (Older Than 60 Years)

- Liposarcoma (dedifferentiated and pleomorphic; most common STS of older adults)
- Leiomyosarcoma
- Fibrosarcoma

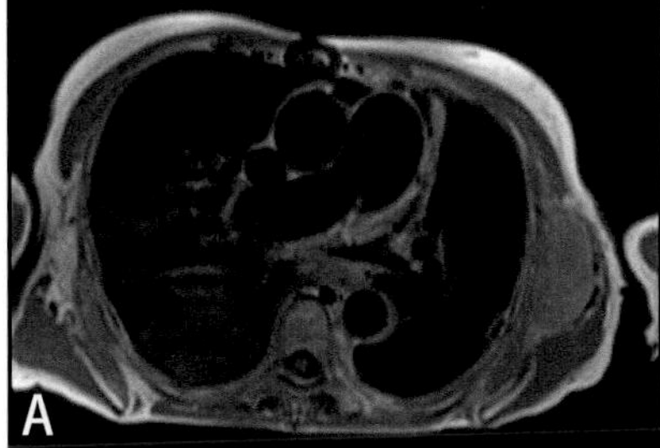

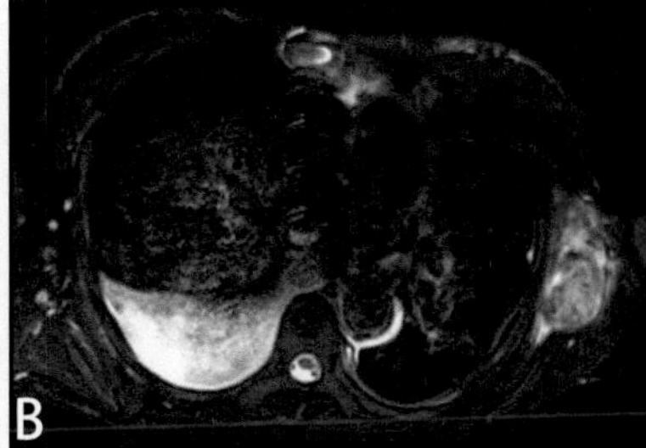

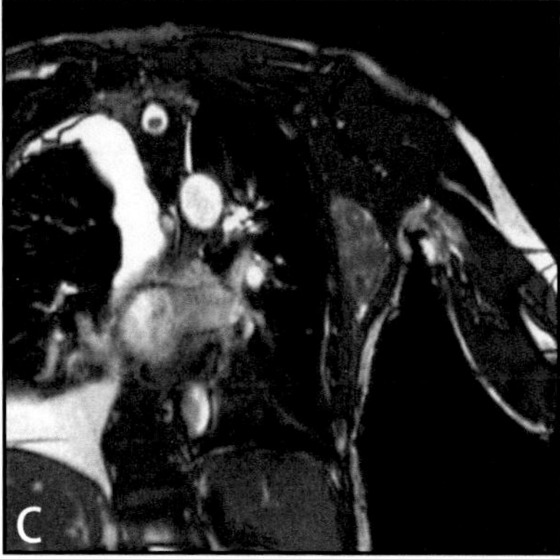

Figure 12-1. An 81-year-old woman with a history of left breast cancer treated with mastectomy and radiation 15 years prior to presentation now presents with a painless swelling in the left axilla. Axial (A) T1, (B) T2, and (C) coronal T2 MRI demonstrate a heterogeneous mass within the left latissimus abutting the chest wall. A biopsy confirmed fibrosarcoma, a histologically distinct diagnosis from previous breast carcinoma, consistent with postradiation sarcoma.

- Angiosarcoma
- Myxofibrosarcoma

Very few specific risk factors have been associated with STS; most tumors develop spontaneously. Sarcomas have been reported to occur in burns, fracture sites, and areas of surgery, but trauma is not a consistently validated risk factor, and may be a source of misdiagnosis. Kaposi sarcoma has a known relationship with HIV and immunosuppression, but other infectious, environmental, and chemical exposures classically correlated with other malignancies are not consistently observed in STS. Radiation exposure is a verifiable risk factor, and soft-tissue tumors in areas of prior radiation treatment should be evaluated as potential postradiation STS (Figure 12-1). Familial cancer syndromes known to be associated with STS include neurofibromatosis 1 (malignant peripheral nerve sheath tumor), Li-Fraumeni syndrome (rhabdomyosarcoma, osteosarcoma, leiomyosarcoma, liposarcoma, and UPS), and retinoblastoma (leiomyosarcoma, fibrosarcoma, and rhabdomyosarcoma).[3]

Most STS disseminate by hematogenous spread and deposit in the lungs via the pulmonary circuit. Staging of most STS with locoregional magnetic resonance imaging (MRI) and computed tomography of the chest is generally adequate. However, some select subtypes demonstrate patterns of spread that warrant additional staging as discussed in Chapter 2 (Figure 12-2).

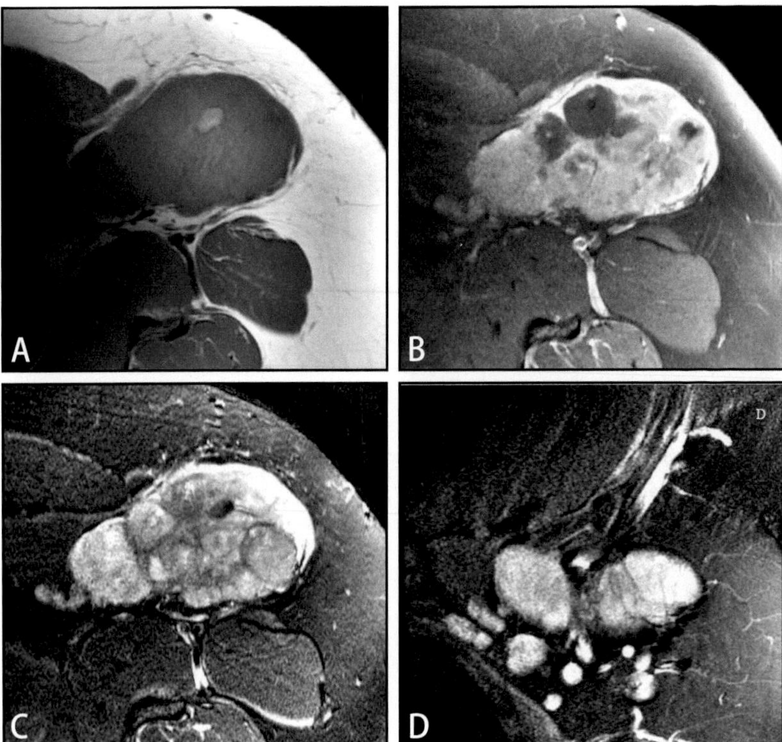

Figure 12-2. A 43-year-old man presents with a painless lump in the left axilla. Axial MRI demonstrates a well-defined, heterogeneous lesion that is hypointense on (A) T1, and (B) internal enhancement with gadolinium. Axial MRI demonstrates a well-defined, heterogeneous lesion that is (C) hyperintense signal on T2-weighted sequences with (D) extensive regional lymphadenopathy. Biopsy demonstrated pleomorphic rhabdomyosarcoma. The patient was managed with systemic therapy, preoperative radiotherapy, and wide surgical resection.

Soft-Tissue Sarcomas That Demonstrate Lymphatic Spread

(Mnemonic RACES or ESARC)

Rhabdomyosarcoma
Angiosarcoma
Clear cell sarcoma
Epithelioid sarcoma
Synovial sarcoma

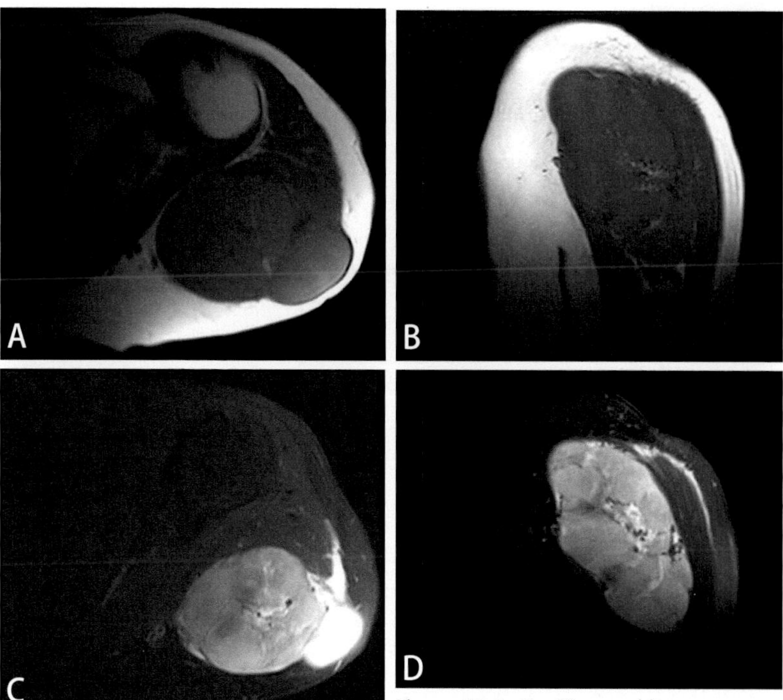

Figure 12-3. An 80-year-old woman presents with painless swelling of the left posterior shoulder. MRI demonstrates a well-defined mass within the posterior deltoid that is hypointense on (A) axial and (B) coronal T1, and hyperintense on (C) axial and (D) coronal T2. A biopsy confirmed the diagnosis of undifferentiated pleomorphic sarcoma, and the patient was managed with wide surgical resection and adjuvant radiotherapy.

Undifferentiated Pleomorphic Sarcoma

UPS, formerly known as malignant fibrous histiocytoma, is the most common STS, and the most common STS of adults. UPS is composed of high-grade, pleomorphic spindle cells without apparent tissue differentiation. The majority of UPS occur in subfascial locations within the extremities, and management consists of wide surgical resection with adjuvant radiotherapy. Chemosensitivity is unpredictable in UPS but is often considered in healthy patients with lesions that are high grade, subfascial, and larger than 5 cm in diameter (Figure 12-3).

Table 12-1

Management of Liposarcoma Subtypes

SUBTYPE	DIAGNOSTIC FEATURES	TREATMENT
Well-Differentiated	Low-grade Retroperitoneal location *MDM2* amplification	Marginal to conservatively wide surgical resection
Myxoid	Subfascial location Bright T2 signal t(12;16) translocation, TLS-CHOP	Preoperative radiotherapy (exquisitely radiosensitive) Wide surgical resection Consider systemic therapy for high-risk patients
Round cell	High grade Round cell component >5%	Preoperative radiotherapy Wide surgical resection Systemic therapy
Dedifferentiated	High-grade cellular component juxtaposed to well-differentiated tumor	Wide surgical resection Adjuvant radiotherapy Consider systemic therapy
Pleomorphic	Aggressively high grade High rate of malignant spread	Wide surgical resection Adjuvant radiotherapy and systemic therapy Palliation

Liposarcomas

Liposarcomas are malignancies of fatty tissue and represent the second most common STS. Five distinct subtypes exist, and the amount of internal fat signal present can be variable. Liposarcomas are known for atypical patterns of spread, and screening of the retroperitoneum and/or skeleton should be performed. Table 12-1 summarizes the management considerations of the subtypes of liposarcoma (Figure 12-4).

Synovial Sarcoma

Synovial sarcoma is the most common STS of young adults, and the most common STS of the foot. The clinical presentation can range from rapid

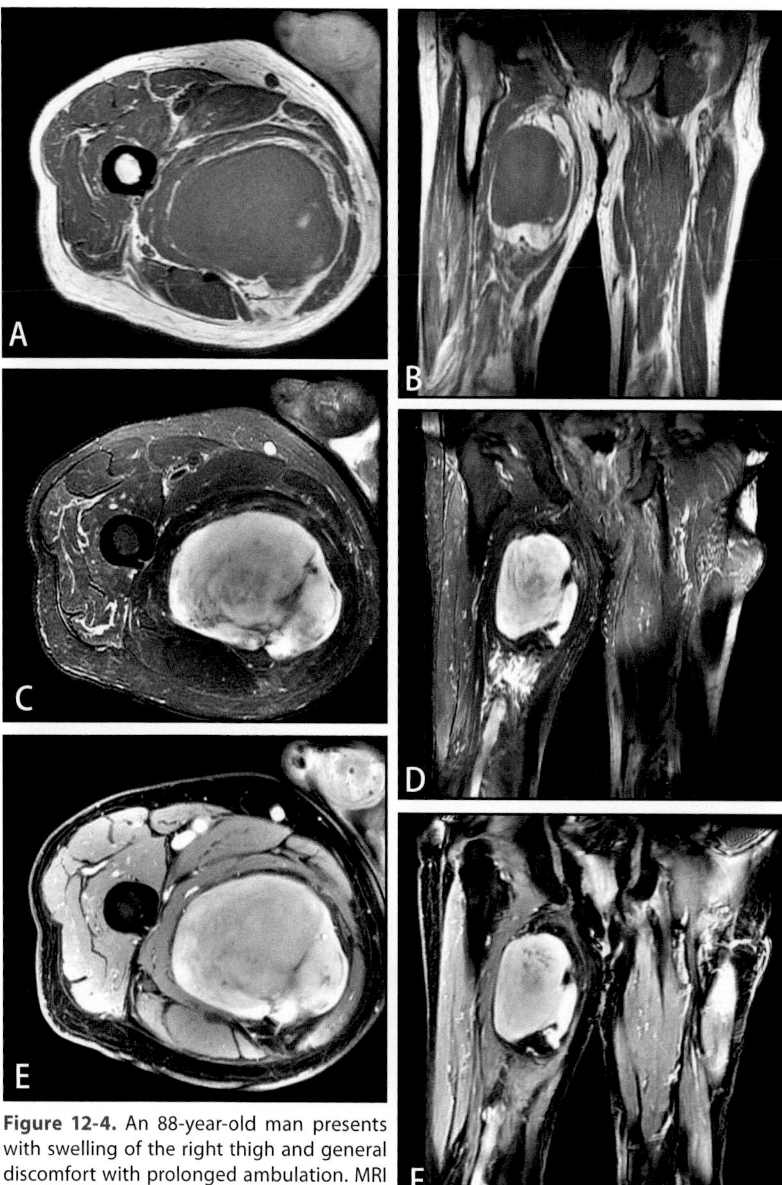

Figure 12-4. An 88-year-old man presents with swelling of the right thigh and general discomfort with prolonged ambulation. MRI demonstrates a well-defined lesion that is (A and B) hypointense on T1, (C and D) hyperintense on T2, (E and F) with internal enhancement on fat-suppressed postcontrast sequences. This lesion is located within a larger area of well-differentiated fatty tumor, hyperintense on T1 and isointense to subcutaneous fat on all imaging sequences. A biopsy was consistent with dedifferentiated liposarcoma. The patient was managed with wide surgical resection and adjuvant radiotherapy.

aggressive growth to a slower, more indolent progression. Synovial sarcomas are identified by their monophasic or biphasic histology, and by a characteristic t(X;18) translocation associated with an *SYT-SSX* gene rearrangement. Up to 30% of synovial sarcomas will exhibit lace-like dystrophic calcifications of the soft tissue, which can be identified radiologically.[4] Synovial sarcomas are high-grade tumors with an elevated risk of metastatic spread. Owing to the younger average patient age and the demonstrated chemosensitivity of synovial sarcoma, these tumors are managed with an aggressive regimen, including wide surgical resection, adjuvant radiotherapy, and systemic chemotherapy.

Rhabdomyosarcoma

Rhabdomyosarcoma is the most common soft-tissue tumor of children. The embryonal subtype, which generally occurs in young children, is the most common form and carries a more favorable prognosis than the alveolar form, which occurs in teenagers and young adults. The diagnosis of alveolar rhabdomyosarcoma is often facilitated by identification of gene fusions involving *PAX* and *FOX* genes. A smaller subset of rhabdomyosarcomas occurs in adults. These pleomorphic rhabdomyosarcomas demonstrate very poor differentiation and are very aggressive clinically (Figure 12-5). Treatment of rhabdomyosarcoma is multimodal, with systemic chemotherapy, wide surgical resection, and possible radiotherapy.

Epithelioid Sarcoma

Epithelioid sarcoma is the most common soft-tissue tumor of the hand. These tumors classically present as small nodular growths that may mimic granulomas or palmar fibromas. Proximal migration to myofascial sites, tendons, and lymph nodes are typical and require lymph node evaluation and imaging of the entire extremity for staging. Treatment of epithelioid sarcoma consists of wide surgical resection and adjuvant radiotherapy.

Surgical Treatment

STS are not curable by chemotherapy or radiotherapy alone and remain primarily a surgical disease. This demands meticulous surgical technique that should be performed by experienced practitioners only. Wide surgical resection with negative margins remains the mainstay of treatment of STS.

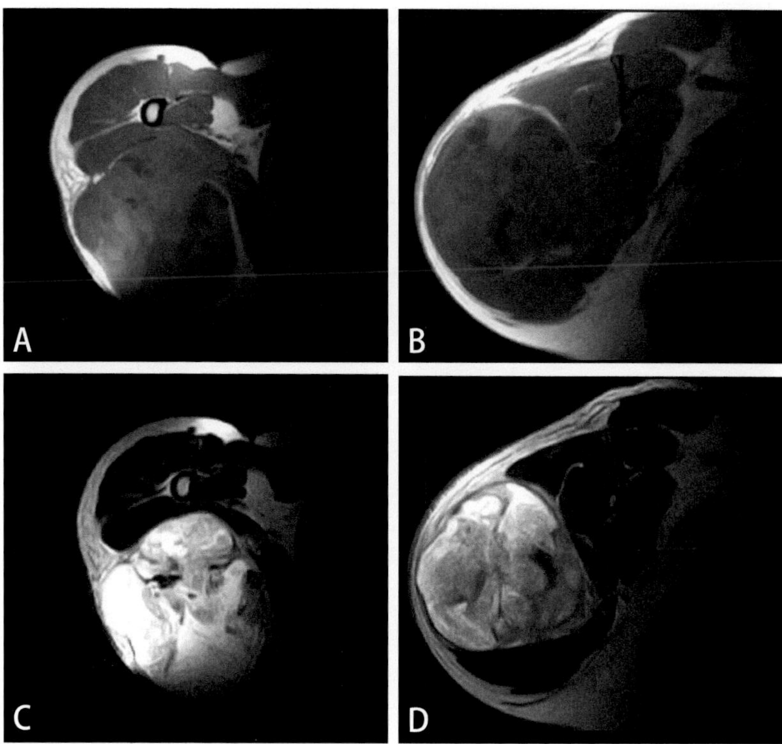

Figure 12-5. A 43-year-old man presents with painless swelling over the right posterior shoulder. MRI demonstrates a heterogeneous mass within the right posterior deltoid, with low and intermediate signal on T1 (A) axial and (B) coronal sequences, and high signal on (C) axial and (D) sagittal T2 sequences. A biopsy confirmed pleomorphic rhabdomyosarcoma. The patient was treated with wide surgical resection, adjuvant radiotherapy and chemotherapy.

This is defined as complete excision of the tumor with a surrounding cuff of normal tissue (Figure 12-6). In sarcoma surgery, the thickness of this cuff of normal tissue is undefined; lesions that abut neurovascular structures and fascial boundaries may be resected with a thinner margin of intact fascia, epineurium, or vascular sheath.

STS generally grow centrifugally, displacing structures outward and growing with respect for fascial and anatomic boundaries. This facilitates limb salvage for 90% of STS patients, when a wide margin can be achieved without sacrifice of critical structures. Vessels that require resection can be reconstructed with vascular grafts. Lesions that abut bone may require sacrifice (stripping) of the periosteum, and lesions that penetrate the periosteum will require sacrifice of the involved bone and subsequent reconstruction. Even

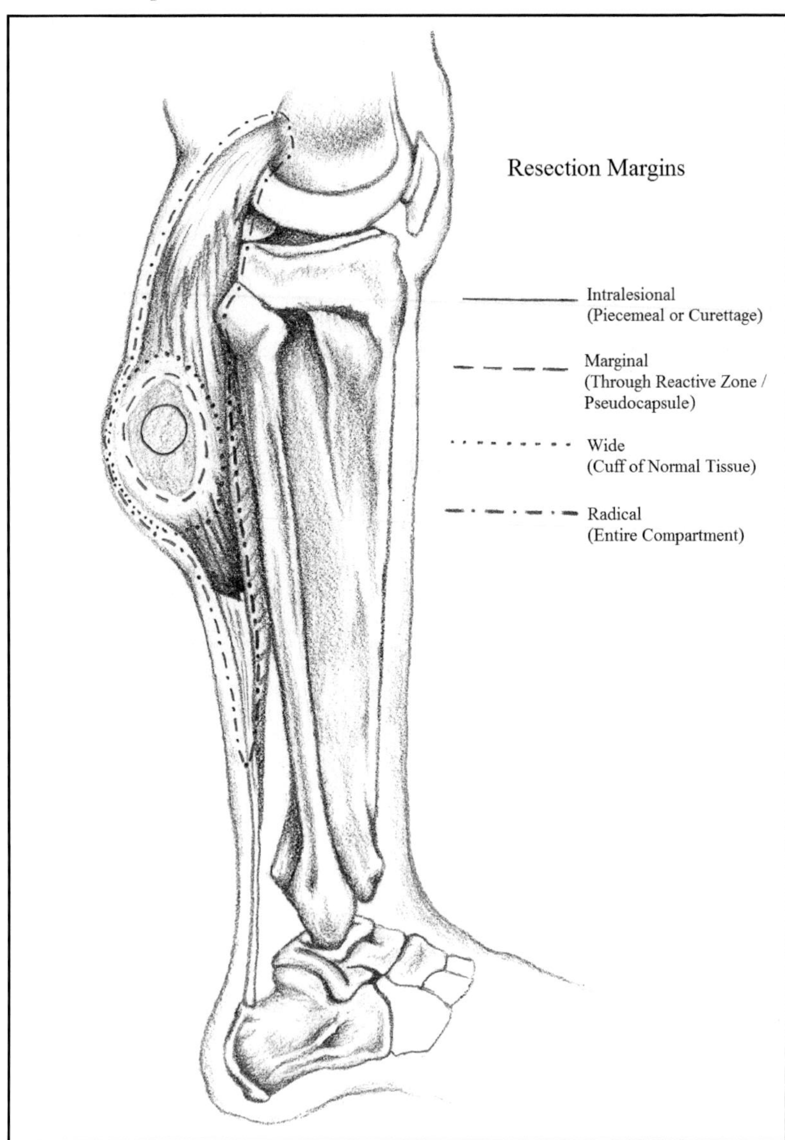

Figure 12-6. Diagram of surgical resection margins.

the loss of 1 major peripheral nerve can be expected to result in a functional extremity, but sacrifice of 2 or more nerves is an indication for limb ablation. Other indications for amputation include fungating tumors, extensively infiltrating lesions that involve multiple compartments, or a postresection defect without acceptable reconstructive options.

Radiotherapy

For low-grade STS, wide surgical resection is often the only treatment required, as rates of local recurrence are less than 10%. Local recurrence rates of intermediate-to-high-grade STS, however, are approximately 20% to 30% without adjuvant treatment. Radiotherapy is generally added for higher-grade tumors to reduce any microscopic tumor around the primary lesion. This has been observed to reduce the risk of locally recurrent disease to less than 10%.[5] Many different methods of radiation delivery exist, but STS consistently require radiation dosages between 50 Gy and 70 Gy, delivered in a hyperfractionated protocol over a 4 to 6 week period. Radiation can be delivered either preresection or postresection, and the decision may be made on a case-by-case basis or based on institutional preferences. Table 12-2 illustrates the risks and benefits of radiotherapy delivered in the preoperative and postoperative settings. Myxoid liposarcomas and round cell tumors display significant radiosensitivity and are best approached with preoperative radiotherapy (Figure 12-7).

It is important to note that the addition of radiation as an adjuvant treatment is not a substitute for inadequate surgery. The risk of local recurrence remains unacceptably high with an intralesional or marginal resection margin, so radiotherapy cannot be relied on to mitigate a positive surgical margin. Grossly and microscopically positive margins require re-resection until negative margins are obtained.

Radiotherapy in excess of 30 Gy is associated with depletion of osteoblast and osteoclast cell populations within bone. This impaired remodeling potential contributes to an elevated risk of postradiation insufficiency fracture. Female sex, advanced age, higher radiation dose, and sacrifice of more than 10 cm of periosteum at the time of resection contribute to a greater risk of fracture, and prophylactic stabilization should be considered in these patients.[7]

Chemotherapy and Prognosis

Refinements in surgical and radiation techniques have helped optimize rates of local recurrence, but rates of 5-year survival have remained unchanged for the past several decades. The prognosis for STS is determined principally by the biological aggressiveness of the lesion, reflected in the histologic grade

Table 12-2

Comparison of Preoperative and Postoperative Radiotherapy

	PREOPERATIVE XRT	POSTOPERATIVE XRT
DOSAGE	50 Gy to 60 Gy, with option for postoperative boost	60 Gy to 70 Gy
TIMING	Surgery performed 3.5 to 5 weeks after completion of XRT to allow for recovery of tissue	Radiation performed 3 to 4 weeks after surgery to allow for wound healing
RADIATION FIELD	Smaller: several cm around known mass	Larger: several cm around entire surgical field; marked intraoperatively with surgical clips
TUMOR RESPONSE	Facilitation of resection • Volumetric reduction variable • Maturation of tumor capsule	N/A
WOUND HEALING	Impaired: 35% wound complication rate	Normal: 17% wound complication rate
LONG-TERM LOCAL TOXICITY • *Fibrosis* • *Lymphedema* • *Contracture*	Reduced	Elevated
LOCAL RECURRENCE	No difference	No difference
OVERALL SURVIVAL	No difference	No difference

Abbreviations: N/A, not applicable; XRT, x-ray radiation therapy. (Adapted from O'Sullivan B, Davis AM, Turcotte R, et al.[6])

of the tumor. Low-grade lesions have an excellent long-term prognosis, with 5-year survival rates greater than 95%. This compares favorably to the 70% to 80% survival rates for intermediate-grade tumors, and the 50% to 60% survival rates for high-grade malignancies. Pleomorphic variants of STS carry a poor prognosis, with 5-year survival rates between 10% and 30%.

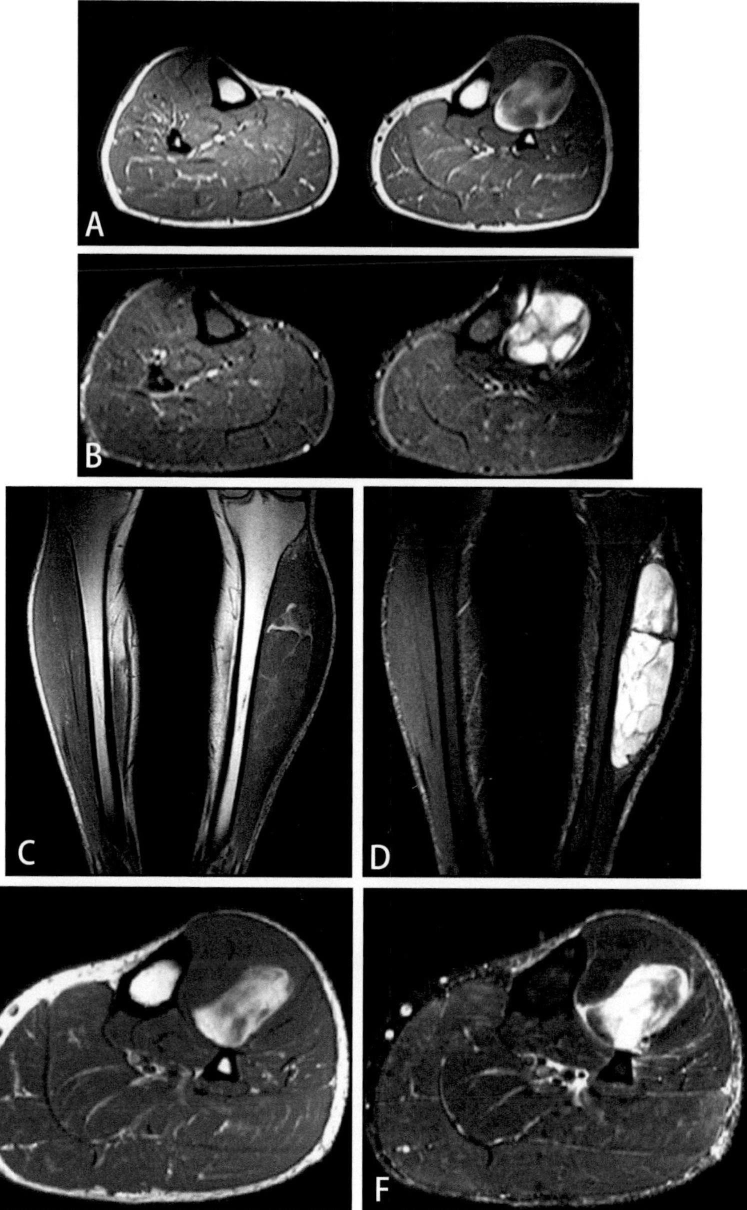

Figure 12-7. A 59-year-old man presents with vague swelling of the left lower leg. MRI demonstrates a well-defined mass within the anterior compartment of the left lower leg that is largely hypointense on (A and C) T1, and (B and D) hyperintense on T2, with streaks of internal fat signal consistent with a lipogenic tumor. Biopsy confirmed a diagnosis of myxoid liposarcoma. Axial (E) T1 and (F) T2 MRI after preoperative radiotherapy demonstrates a volumetric reduction in tumor size.

Table 12-3

Sensitivity of Sarcoma Subtypes to Chemotherapy

CHEMOSENSITIVE	UNKNOWN SENSITIVITY	CHEMORESISTANT
Embryonal and alveolar rhabdomyosarcomas	Undifferentiated pleomorphic sarcoma	Clear cell sarcoma
PNET/extraskeletal Ewing	Myxofibrosarcoma	Alveolar soft part sarcoma
Synovial sarcoma	Pleomorphic rhabdomyosarcoma	Extraskeletal chondrosarcoma
Myxoid and round cell liposarcomas	Pleomorphic liposarcoma	Dedifferentiated chondrosarcoma
	Epithelioid sarcoma	
	Leiomyosarcoma	
	Malignant peripheral nerve sheath tumor	
	Angiosarcoma	

Abbreviation: PNET, primitive neuroectodermal tumor.

To improve historical rates of survival, there is a clear need to establish effective regimens of systemic therapy. However, the heterogeneity of sarcoma subtypes, variable sensitivities to chemotherapy, and wide range of patient ages that affect the ability of individuals to receive and tolerate systemic treatments render statistical validation of chemotherapy for STS extremely difficult. Large-scale studies have not shown consistent efficacy of systemic therapy for STS, and even suggest an increased risk of end-organ injury that may confer a negative survival benefit.[8] Currently, chemotherapy is considered on a case-by-case basis for large, deep, and high-grade tumors in patients physiologically capable of tolerating an aggressive regimen (Figure 12-8). Table 12-3 depicts the relative sensitivity of sarcoma subtypes to conventional chemotherapy.

Take-Aways

1. Soft-tissue tumors that are painless, deep to fascia, and larger than 5 cm should be investigated as potential STS until definitively proven otherwise.
2. Low-grade STS are managed with wide surgical resection only, with excellent rates of long-term survival.

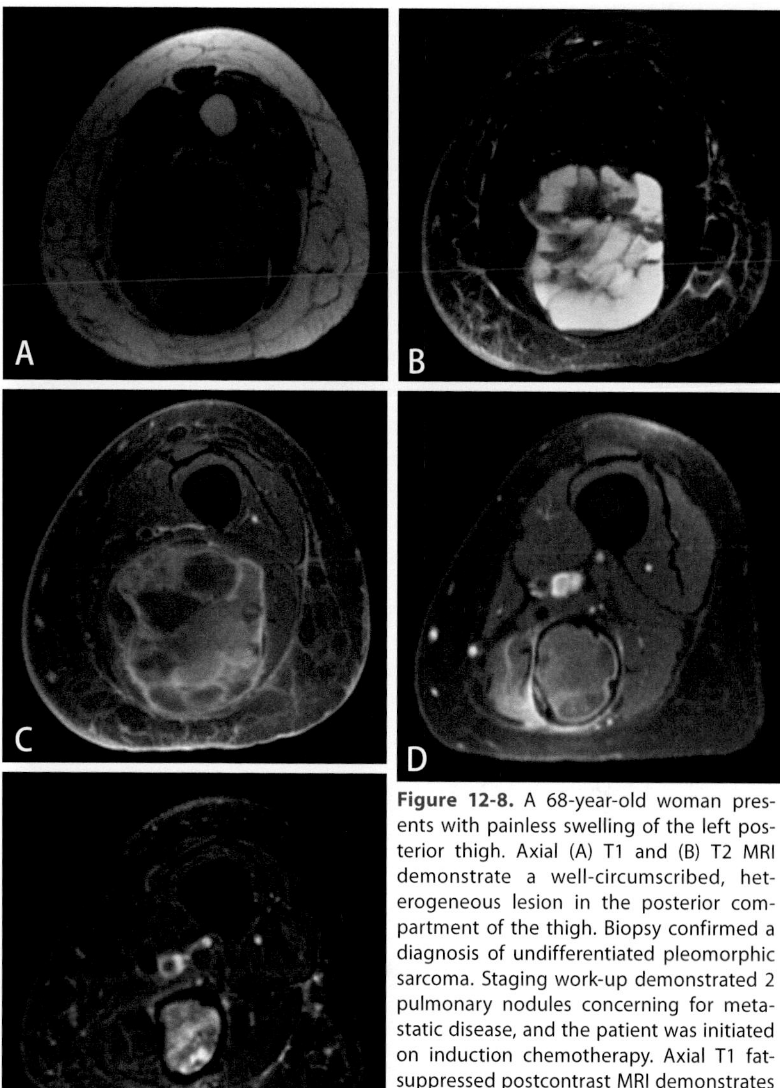

Figure 12-8. A 68-year-old woman presents with painless swelling of the left posterior thigh. Axial (A) T1 and (B) T2 MRI demonstrate a well-circumscribed, heterogeneous lesion in the posterior compartment of the thigh. Biopsy confirmed a diagnosis of undifferentiated pleomorphic sarcoma. Staging work-up demonstrated 2 pulmonary nodules concerning for metastatic disease, and the patient was initiated on induction chemotherapy. Axial T1 fat-suppressed postcontrast MRI demonstrates volumetric reduction of the tumor from (C) baseline presentation, (D) the conclusion of 6 cycles of chemotherapy, (E) followed by preoperative radiotherapy.

3. High-grade STS are managed with wide surgical resection and adjuvant radiotherapy. Chemotherapy may be considered in select patients.

Commonly Tested Topics for Trainees

- Rhabdomyosarcoma, angiosarcoma, clear cell sarcoma, epithelioid sarcoma, and synovial sarcoma (RACES) are tumors with known propensity for lymphangitic spread and should be investigated with lymph node screening.
- Synovial sarcoma is the most common STS in adults, characterized by biphasic histology, soft-tissue calcifications, and a characteristic t(X;18) translocation.
- Compared with postoperative radiotherapy, preoperative radiotherapy is associated with less local toxicity, but higher rates of wound complication, and identical oncologic outcomes.

References

1. American Cancer Society. *Cancer Treatment & Survivorship Facts & Figures 2016-2017*. Atlanta: American Cancer Society; 2016.
2. Mastrangelo G, Coindre JM, Ducimetière F, et al. Incidence of soft tissue sarcoma and beyond: a population-based prospective study in 3 European regions. *Cancer.* 2012;118(21)5339-5348. doi:10.1002/cncr.27555.
3. Ognjanovic S, Olivier M, Bergemann TL, Hainaut P. Sarcomas in TP53 germline mutation carriers: a review of the IARC TP53 database. *Cancer.* 2012;118(5):1387-1396. doi:10.1002/cncr.26390.
4. Murphey MD, Gibson MS, Jennings BT, Crespo-Rodríguez AM, Fanburg-Smith J, Gajewski DA. From the archives of the AFIP: imaging of synovial sarcoma with radiologic-pathologic correlation. *Radiographics.* 2006;26(5):1543-1565. doi:10.1148/rg.265065084.
5. Albertsmeier M, Rauch A, Roeder F, et al. External beam radiation therapy for resectable soft tissue sarcoma: a systematic review and meta-analysis. *Ann Surg Oncol.* 2018;25(3):754-767. doi:10.1245/s10434-017-6081-2.
6. O'Sullivan B, Davis AM, Turcotte R, et al. Preoperative versus postoperative radiotherapy in soft-tissue sarcoma of the limbs: a randomised trial. *Lancet.* 2002;359(9325):2235-2241. doi:10.1016/S0140-6736(02)09292-9.
7. Gortzak Y, Lockwood GA, Mahendra A, et al. Prediction of pathologic fracture risk of the femur after combined modality treatment of soft tissue sarcoma of the thigh. *Cancer.* 2010;116(6):1553-1559. doi:10.1002/cncr.24949.
8. Adjuvant chemotherapy for localised resectable soft-tissue sarcoma of adults: meta-analysis of individual data. Sarcoma Meta-analysis Collaboration. *Lancet.* 1997;350(9092):1647-1654. doi:10.1016/S0140-6736(97)08165-8.

Section V

Anatomic-Specific Considerations

13

Intra-Articular Lesions

Overview

Intra-articular lesions are commonly discovered after a prolonged period of treatment for presumed degenerative joint disease or other soft-tissue injury. Once identified, synovial lesions require the same diligence in evaluation as other tumors, but this can be performed safely by an awareness of the presenting clinical and imaging findings of the most common synovitic processes. We will discuss the most common lesions arising from the joint, how to identify these disorders, and discuss recommendations for treatment.

The majority of intra-articular growths are benign and non-neoplastic processes. These lesions typically present with a long, indolent course of recurrent joint effusions, vague joint pains, and occasionally symptoms of mechanical impingement such as restricted motion, locking, or giving way of the joint. Synovial-based lesions can manifest in localized, discrete nodules, or with diffuse involvement of the joint. Extra-articular involvement is occasionally observed, and does not imply malignant transformation. True intra-articular malignancies are exceedingly rare, but care should be taken that the lesion is diagnosed definitively prior to any invasive intervention. Indeterminate lesions should be referred to oncologic specialists to avoid contamination of the joint, which would require extra-articular resections that can be quite morbid.

The diagnosis of intra-articular lesions is typically determined radiologically. Magnetic resonance imaging (MRI) findings of proliferation of the joint

Wallace, MT
Handbook of Musculoskeletal Tumors (pp 213-222).

lining, effusion, and bony erosions on both sides of a joint are characteristic markers of a synovitic process. Radiographs are frequently useful because patterns of mineralization can be diagnostic of hemangioma, synovial chondromatosis, calcific tendinitis, and pseudogout.

The natural history of most synovial lesions when left untreated is progressive growth, loss of joint cartilage, and erosions of the bone. Treatment is generally medical management combined with radical synovectomy for control of symptoms and reduced tumor burden, but recurrence rates are high.

Pigmented Villonodular Synovitis/ Tenosynovial Giant Cell Tumor

As its name suggests, pigmented villonodular synovitis, or PVNS, is a nodular proliferation of synovium characterized by macrophages, histiocytes, and giant cells thought to be more reactive than neoplastic in etiology. There are often variable amounts of hemorrhage and iron-rich hemosiderin, which pigments the tissue a tan to deep brown color. The majority of cases are the diffuse-type disease, with extensive involvement of the anterior and posterior joint spaces, and extra-articular and intraosseous extension seen in advanced cases. A smaller subset of patients presents with localized nodular disease. This disease can also present in association with tendon sheaths in the soft tissues, particularly the hands and feet. These are often termed "giant cell tumor of tendon sheath," and are managed with marginal resection.

PVNS is most commonly observed in younger to middle-aged adults, and presents with achy joint pains, mechanical complaints, and recurrent blood-tinged effusions. PVNS is typically monoarticular, and the knee joint is the most common joint involved by PVNS. MRI will reveal typical findings of nodular synovium with areas of dark signal (dropout) both on T1 and T2 because of the hemosiderin deposits. Plain radiographs will be negative for intralesional calcifications, confirming the diagnosis and distinguishing PVNS from synovial chondromatosis (Figure 13-1).

Treatment for PVNS consists of surgical resection via radical synovectomy. Localized disease is generally curable with resection. For diffuse disease, this may require 2 separate approaches to the joint. Open as well as arthroscopic approaches have been employed with success, using each technique alone or for combined anterior and posterior approaches, but the risk of recurrence is greater with arthroscopic synovectomy.[1] Patients with advanced erosive or degenerative changes may be candidates for joint arthroplasty with wide synovectomy. Unfortunately, diffuse-type PVNS is associated with significant rates of local recurrence, between 20% and 30%.[2] Adjuvant treatments to

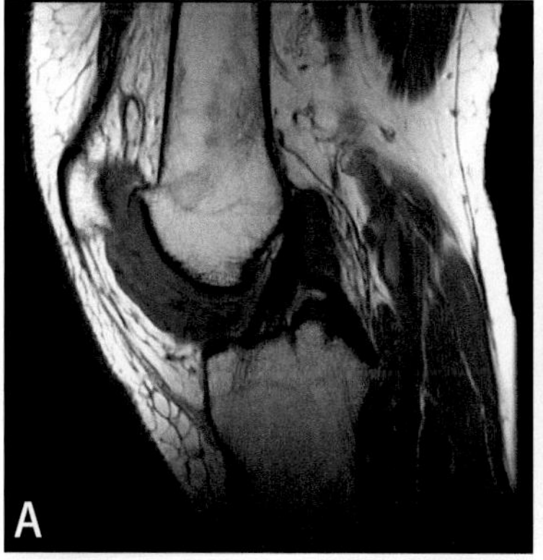

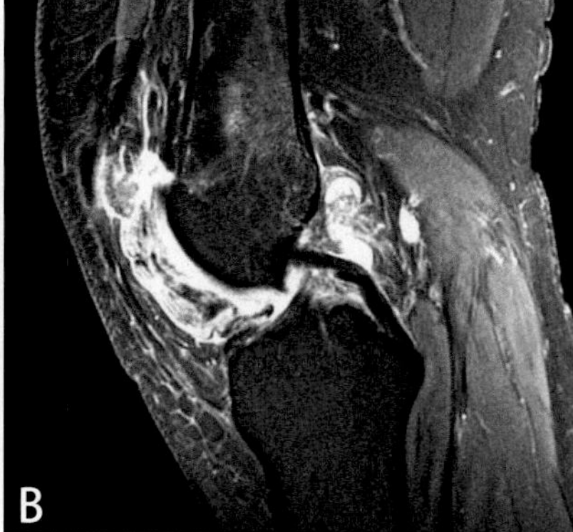

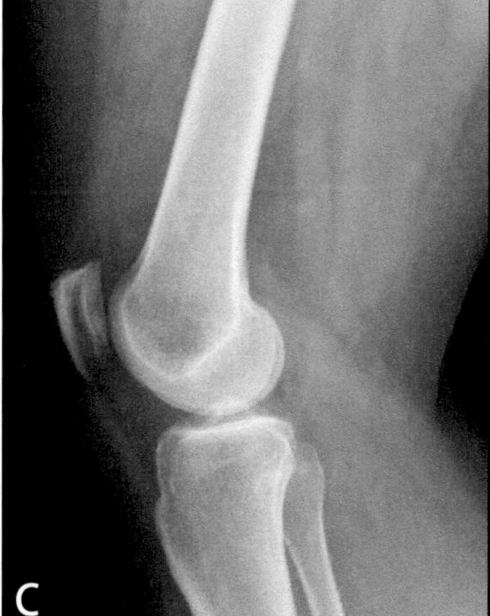

Figure 13-1. A 45-year-old woman presents with episodes of swelling and pain in the right knee. Sagittal (A) T1 and (B) T2 MRI demonstrate a heterogeneous, intra-articular proliferation in the anterior and posterior knee joint that is hypointense on T1 and hyperintense on T2, with areas of dark signal dropout on both sequences. (C) Lateral radiograph demonstrates effusion of the joint and intra-articular soft-tissue densities without mineralization, consistent with pigmented villonodular synovitis.

reduce this risk are being explored, ranging from external beam radiotherapy, intra-articular injections of radioisotope yttrium 90, to systemic treatments with tyrosine kinase and other multitarget inhibitors.

Synovial Chondromatosis

Synovial chondromatosis is a non-neoplastic cartilaginous metaplasia of the joint synovium, producing lobules of cartilage that can either break away to form small, loose bodies within the joint, or accumulate into larger nodules or plaques. Mechanical symptoms are common, either from loose body impingement or from mechanical blocking leading to restricted, painful range of motion.

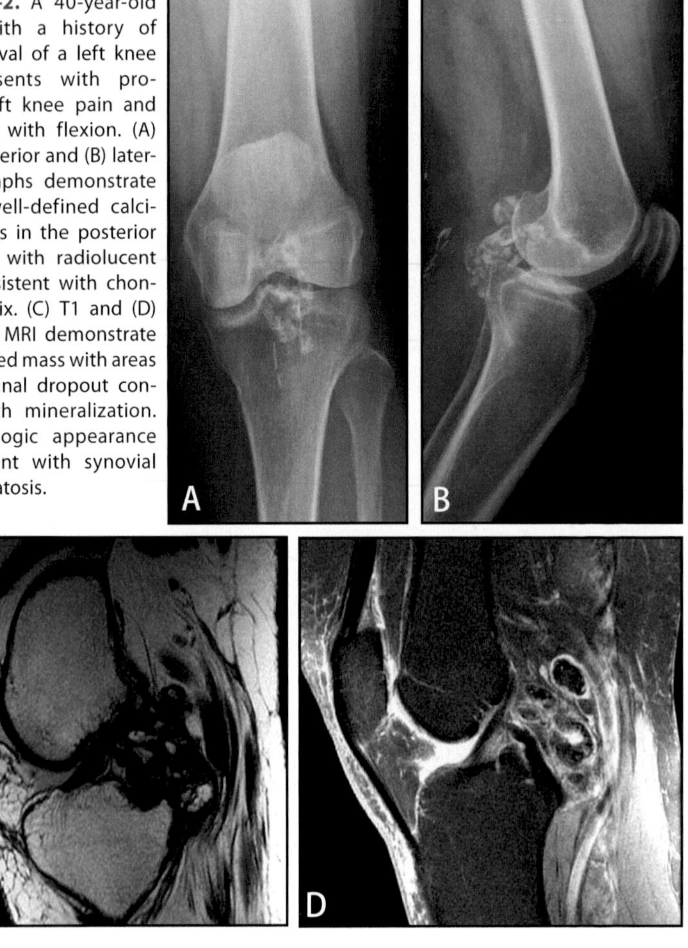

Figure 13-2. A 40-year-old woman with a history of prior removal of a left knee mass presents with progressive left knee pain and discomfort with flexion. (A) Anteroposterior and (B) lateral radiographs demonstrate multiple well-defined calcified lobules in the posterior knee joint with radiolucent zones consistent with chondroid matrix. (C) T1 and (D) T2 sagittal MRI demonstrate the lobulated mass with areas of dark signal dropout consistent with mineralization. The radiologic appearance is consistent with synovial chondromatosis.

Synovial chondromatosis can be definitively identified on appropriate imaging demonstrating lobules of intra-articular chondroid synovium with rim-like calcifications. MRI will demonstrate chondroid material that is low to intermediate on T1 and bright on T2, with areas of signal dropout due to calcification (Figure 13-2). Once identified, treatment of synovial chondromatosis is surgical, with removal of loose bodies and resection of involved synovium. Recurrences are common.

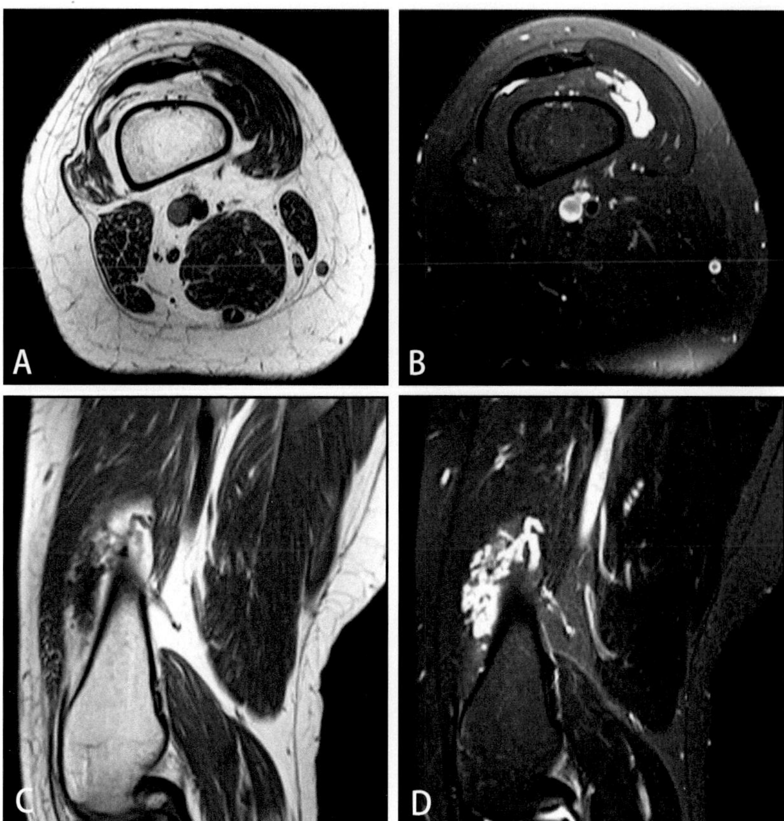

Figure 13-3. A 29-year-old man presents with a history of 3 episodes of painful, spontaneous, atraumatic hemarthrosis of the right knee. (A) Axial T1 and (B) T2 MRI demonstrate a lobular mass within the synovium of the knee joint. Sagittal (C) T1 and (D) T2 sequences demonstrate interspersed areas of fat separating fluid-bright areas connected to an apparent feeder vessel, diagnostic of synovial hemangioma.

Other Synovial Lesions

Synovial Hemangioma of the Joint

Synovial hemangiomas of the joint often present with recurrent spontaneous hemarthroses, occurring when vessels become caught and torn during normal joint motion. They can be diagnosed on MRI by characteristic streaks of fat-separating lobular vascular channels (Figure 13-3). As with vascular malformations in other locations, these lesions may be amenable to sclerotherapy or embolization, but intra-articular lesions may be best managed with resection/synovectomy.

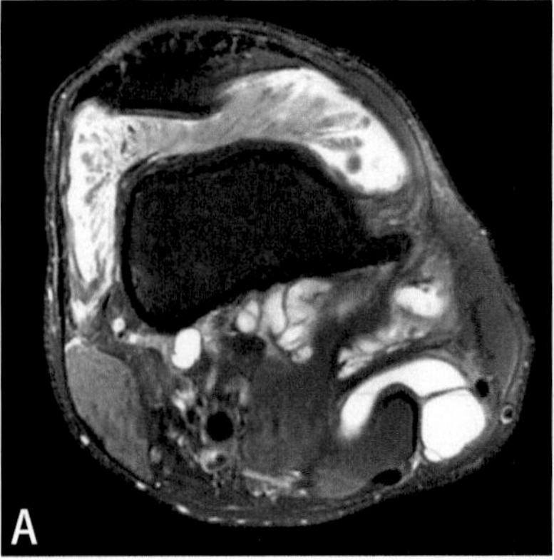

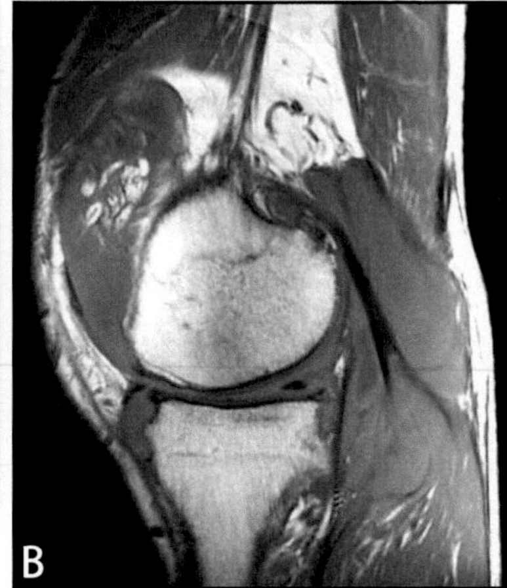

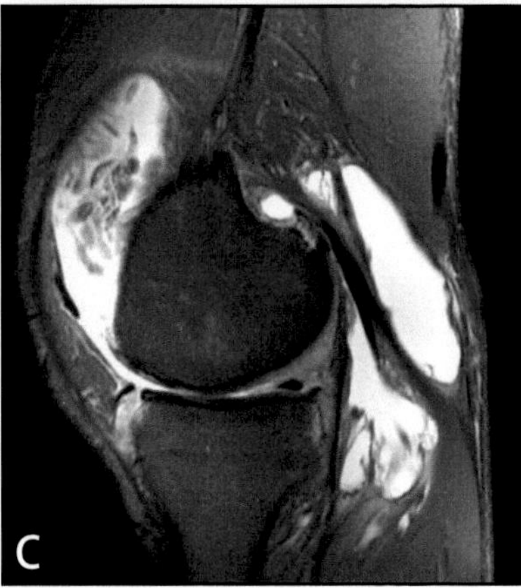

Figure 13-4. A 57-year-old man presents with painful, episodic swelling in bilateral knees. (A) Axial T2, and sagittal (B) T1 and (C) T2 MRI demonstrates a proliferative synovial process with characteristic hyperintense fat signal on T1, consistent with lipoma arborescens.

Lipoma Arborescens

Lipoma arborescens is a fatty proliferation of the synovium characterized by effusion and swelling of the joint, with characteristic villous structures containing well-differentiated fat (Figure 13-4). This disease may occur in bilateral joints, and symptomatic management with radical synovectomy is recommended.[3]

Chronic Inflammatory and Infectious Disorders of the Joint

Table 13-1 discusses the clinical and imaging presentations of the most common inflammatory joint diseases. In general, when loss of joint cartilage

TABLE 13-1

CLINICAL AND RADIOLOGICAL FEATURES OF CHRONIC SYNOVITIS

DISORDER	CLINICAL FEATURES	RADIOLOGIC APPEARANCE
Rheumatoid arthritis	Multiple joint involvement Small joints of hands/feet Upper cervical spine disease Morning stiffness Rheumatoid nodules Serum rheumatoid factor	Osteopenia Periarticular erosions Narrowing and collapse of joint space without osteophyte formation Subluxation or contracture of joints Pannus with pitting erosions of joint
Crystal deposition disorder • Gout • Pseudogout	Spontaneous, recurring episodes of painful effusions Periarticular tophi Birefringent crystals in joint fluid on polarized microscopy	Periarticular erosions Patellar lesions Chondrocalcinosis (pseudogout)
Chronic septic arthritis	Subclinical infectious symptoms Atypical pathologens Tuberculosis Fungus	Chronic lytic/sclerotic changes Patchy destruction of bone on both sides of joint Subluxation of joint
Neuropathic arthropathy	Central or peripheral neuropathy leading to cumulative repetitive microtrauma Diabetes mellitus Syringomyelia Myelomeningocele Tabes dorsalis (EtOH or syphilis)	Destruction and dissolution of the joint and bone Instability and migration of joint Smoothed, atrophic bone ends Cervical syrinx is the most common etiology for neuropathic arthropathy of the upper extremities

Abbreviation: EtOH, ethyl alcohol.

by infection and inflammation is not accompanied by hypertrophy of the bone with stabilizing osteophytes (Figure 13-5), the process will result in instability, migration, and resorption of the joint (Figure 13-6).

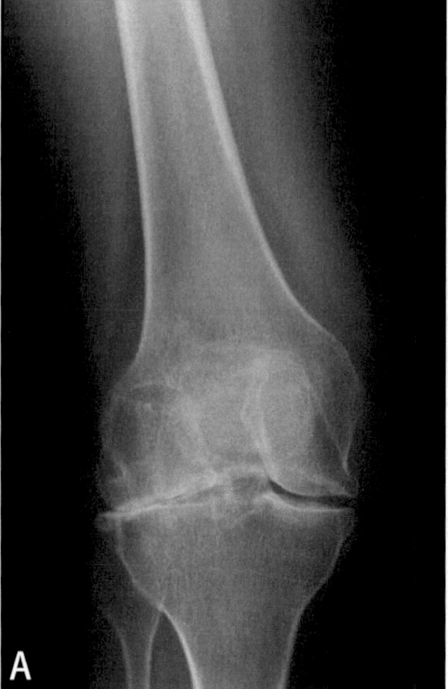

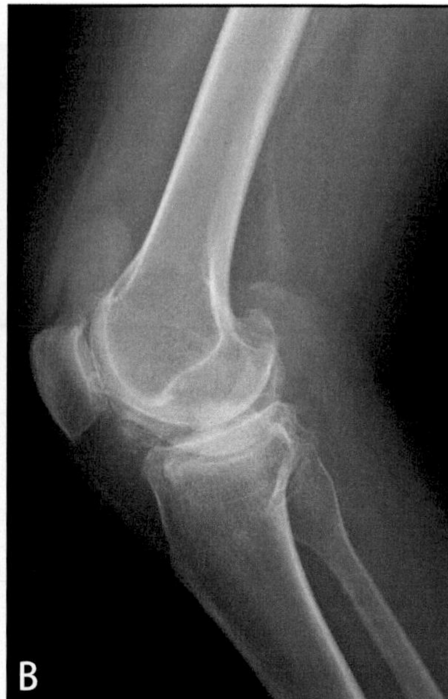

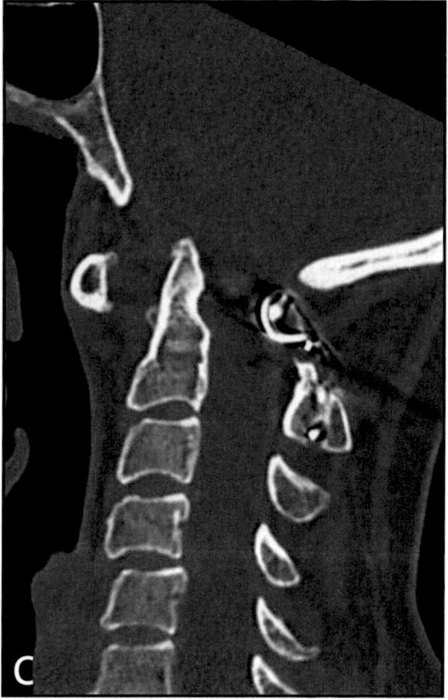

Figure 13-5. A 45-year-old woman with a long-standing history of rheumatoid arthritis presents with painful swelling and contracture of the right knee. (A) Anteroposterior and (B) lateral radiographs demonstrate loss of joint space and flattening/effacement of the lateral femoral condyle and tibial plateau. There is prominent synovitis evidenced by the periarticular soft-tissue densities within the suprapatellar, anterior, and posterior joint spaces. Reactive osteophyte formation is modest, consistent with inflammatory joint disease. (C) Diligent screening of the upper cervical spine was performed with sagittal computed tomography to demonstrate atlantoaxial instability and basilar invagination.

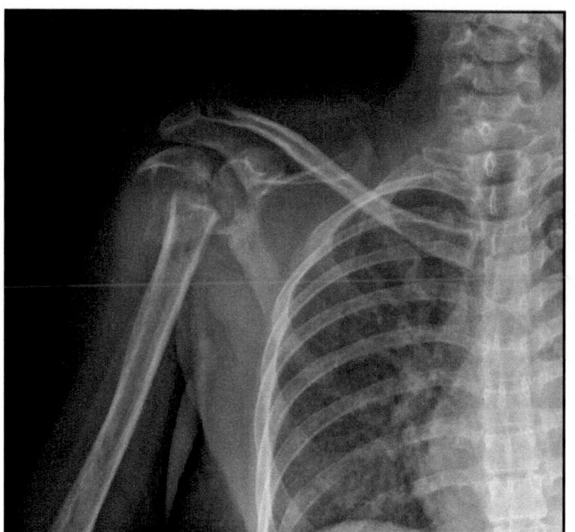

Figure 13-6. A 32-year-old woman with a history of substance abuse-related anoxic brain injury presents with bilateral foot contractures and painless weakness of the right shoulder without a history of trauma. Anteroposterior radiograph demonstrates fragmentation and resorption of the right proximal humerus with smoothened edges consistent with Charcot arthropathy.

Take-Aways

1. Intra-articular lesions are most commonly benign, and many can be definitively characterized on imaging evaluation. However, if unsure about the diagnosis or treatment of an intra-articular lesion, it is appropriate to refer to a musculoskeletal tumor specialist; contamination of a joint from an ill-conceived intra-articular approach can result in devastating consequences for the patient.
2. PVNS is the most common intra-articular mass. The diffuse type is associated with high rates of local recurrence, and is typically managed aggressively by radical synovectomy.
3. Synovial chondromatosis presents with mechanical interference of normal joint function due to chondroid metaplasia of the synovium. This is managed by removal of loose bodies and resection of involved synovium.

Commonly Tested Topics for Trainees

- PVNS and synovial chondromatosis both are characterized on MRI by nodules of synovial growth with dark areas of signal dropout on T1- and T2-weighted sequences. This is due to hemosiderin deposition in PVNS, which is typically radiolucent, and chondroid calcification in synovial chondromatosis, which is typically radiopaque.
- Recurrence rates of PVNS and synovial chondromatosis after arthroscopic synovectomy are high. Arthroscopy should be considered for limited or nodular-type disease, or as a part of combined modality approaches to resection when multiple open joint exposures carry a significant risk for postoperative stiffness, instability, or osteonecrosis.

References

1. De Ponti A, Sansone V, Malcherè M. Result of arthroscopic treatment of pigmented villonodular synovitis of the knee. *Arthroscopy.* 2003;19(6):602-607. doi:10.1016/S0749-8063(03)00127-0.
2. Flandry FC, Hughston JC, Jacobson KE, Barrack RL, McCann SB, Kurtz DM. Surgical management of diffuse pigmented villonodular synovitis of the knee. *Clin Orthop Relat Res.* 1994;300:183-192.
3. Kloen P, Keel SB, Chandler HP, Geiger RH, Zarins B, Rosenberg AE. Lipoma arborescens of the knee. *J Bone Joint Surg Br.* 1998;80(2):298-301.

14

Spine Tumors

Overview

The spine is the most common location for the development of metastatic bone disease, but is also a frequent location of common benign and malignant primary tumors of bone. We have reviewed most of the common lesions of the spine in prior discussions. We will consider vertebral body hemangioma, the most commonly identified spinal lesion, as well as chordoma, a primary malignancy of bone unique to the spine.

The most common spine tumors and their management have been covered in previous chapters. The unique anatomy of the spine presents complex challenges for management. Achieving an adequate oncologic outcome must often be balanced with protecting the mechanical stability of the spine and with consideration for protecting critical neural elements.

Benign active bone tumors are often adequately managed by intralesional resection. Unlike other skeletal sites, extension of the resection margin by aggressive burring and local adjuvant use in the spine is generally not recommended because of the close proximity of neural structures. For this reason, rates of local recurrence are often higher for lesions of the spine, and en bloc resection should be considered for locally active lesions when feasible.[1]

Treatment of malignant tumors of the spine must take into account the natural history of the primary diagnosis and expected responsiveness to treatments, as well as the functional status and life expectancy of the patient. Tumors with known radiosensitivity such as lymphoma, Ewing sarcoma,

Wallace, MT
Handbook of Musculoskeletal Tumors (pp 223-229).

and myeloma can be managed safely and noninvasively with radiation and systemic treatment. Tumors that demand resection of segments of the vertebra or en bloc spondylectomy of one or several spinal segments will require complex reconstruction, which should be performed only when the patient can be expected to survive, rehabilitate from, and achieve a lasting clinical and oncologic benefit from such an aggressive procedure. Metastatic bone disease to the spine, as discussed in Chapter 9, is managed with a more palliative approach. Percutaneous techniques and radiotherapy are mainstays of treatment, and surgery is considered for cases of intractable pain, deformity, spinal instability, or compression of the spinal cord and neural elements.

Vertebral Body Hemangioma

Hemangiomas are the most common benign and incidental findings of the spine, estimated to occur in slightly more than 10% of all individuals.[2] The overwhelming majority of vertebral hemangiomas are asymptomatic, but lesions can present with pain due to pathologic fracture, cord or nerve root compression, or spontaneous bleeding episodes.

Vertebral hemangiomas can be definitively identified radiologically. Vertical striations, known as "corduroy cloth" or "jail cell bars," combined with magnetic resonance imaging (MRI) findings of hyperintense signal on T1- (fat) and T2 (fluid)-weighted sequences are considered diagnostic (Figure 14-1). Identification of multiple hemangiomas should raise suspicion for specific syndromes such as Cobb, McCune-Albright, Maffucci, and Klippel-Trénaunay-Weber syndromes.

Most vertebral hemangiomas are managed with observation. Percutaneous injection of ethanol or cement and embolization may be considered for symptomatic lesions. Fractured or bleeding lesions that cause deformity or neural compression may require surgical decompression and stabilization.

Chordoma

Notochordal tumors are unique lesions of the spine that develop from rests of primitive notochordal tissue in the midline of the axial spine. Benign notochordal cell tumors and malignant chordoma both demonstrate a similar anatomic distribution, with one-third of lesions occurring in the sacrococcygeal region, one-third in the base of the skull, and one-third scattered within the mobile spine.[3]

Chordomas are slow-growing, low- to intermediate-grade malignancies that occur most commonly in middle-aged adults. They arise from the

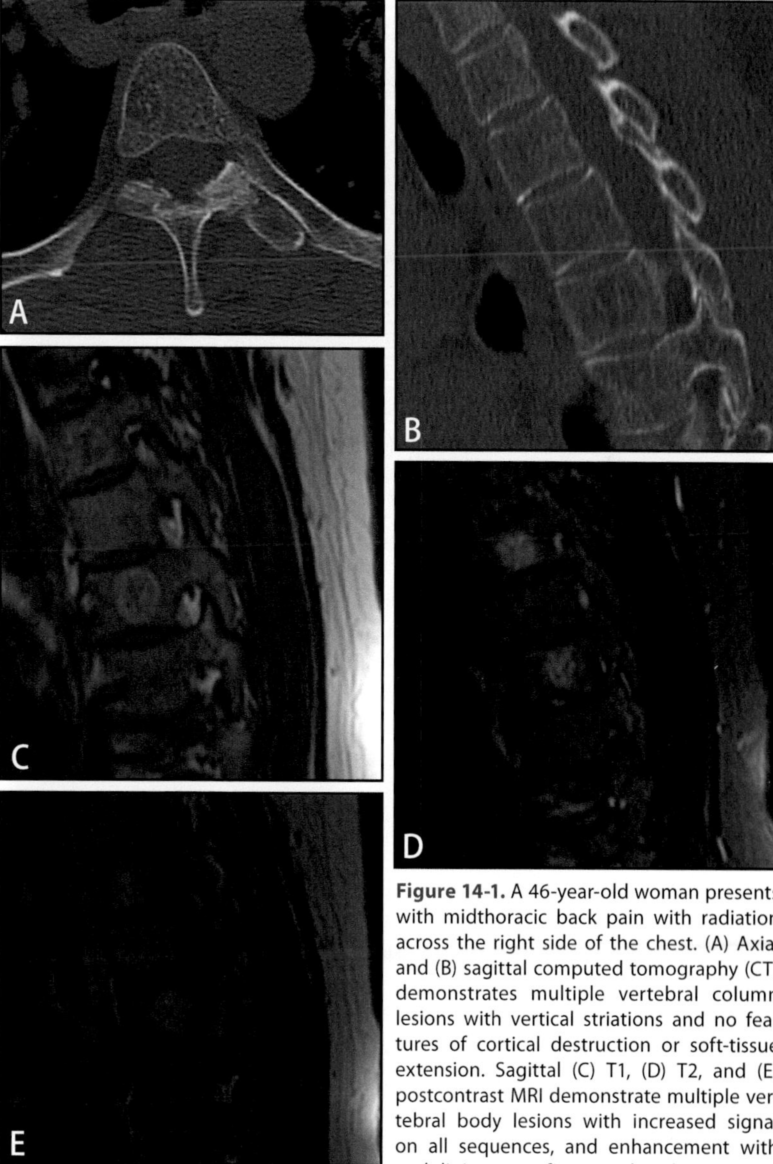

Figure 14-1. A 46-year-old woman presents with midthoracic back pain with radiation across the right side of the chest. (A) Axial and (B) sagittal computed tomography (CT) demonstrates multiple vertebral column lesions with vertical striations and no features of cortical destruction or soft-tissue extension. Sagittal (C) T1, (D) T2, and (E) postcontrast MRI demonstrate multiple vertebral body lesions with increased signal on all sequences, and enhancement with gadolinium, confirming the diagnosis of hemangioma. A midthoracic paracentral disc herniation was identified as the etiology of the patient's discomfort.

midline of the axial skeleton and tend to expand outside of the bone anteriorly, causing nonspecific pain that is often dismissed or ignored as degenerative spine disease. Frequently, an initial imaging work-up for lower back pain will miss a sacrococcygeal chordoma when the imaging does not extend through the tip of the coccyx. Chordomas can grow impressively large before their mass effect is discovered compressing adjacent vital structures such as major vessels, esophagus, trachea, cranial and lumbosacral nerve roots, bowel, and bladder.

Radiographs are often subtle to normal in appearance, and CT and MRI are generally required for diagnosis. CT often reveals destruction of the bone with midline soft-tissue extension, and mineralization within the soft-tissue components of the lesion. MRI will show characteristic growth from the midline of the spine into the anterior soft tissues, with heterogeneous low T1 and high T2 signal and enhancement with gadolinium contrast (Figure 14-2). Bone scintigraphy may be cold and is not helpful for distinguishing benign from malignant notochordal tumors. Chordomas are often delayed in diagnosis when imaging of the spine fails to extend through the sacrococcygeal region.

Chordoma is chemoresistant and relatively radioresistant at conventional dose gradients. The mainstay of treatment for chordoma is wide surgical resection with negative margins, which can result in significant postresection deficits. Lower-extremity strength, bowel, bladder, and sexual function are universally impaired with total sacrectomy. Preservation of S3 unilaterally or bilaterally can preserve bowel and bladder function in one-third to one-half of chordoma patients.[4] Patients must be counseled preoperatively about these long-term deficits. Lower sacrococcygeal resections from S3 to the coccyx can be safely performed from a posterior-only approach. Resections cephalad to the S2 foramina can be expected to result in significant bowel and bladder dysfunction, and a staged approach with anterior exposure and diverting colostomy, followed by completion of the resection posteriorly, should be considered. Sacrectomy resections that extend into S1 risk spinopelvic discontinuity and insufficiency fractures through the residual sacrum, and spinopelvic stabilization and reconstruction should be considered in these cases.

In spite of aggressive surgical treatment, local recurrence rates remain high with sacral chordoma, averaging 50% over 10 years. Local recurrences are inversely correlated with overall survival, which averages 60% and 35% at 5 and 10 years, respectively, with a median survival of slightly more than 6 years.[5] Late metastases are common, and the risk of disease progression exists decades after initial treatment. Radiotherapy has been employed to mitigate this risk, but conventional external beam therapy is limited by the relatively radioresistant nature of chordoma, as well as the limited dosage tolerated by adjacent pelvic, enteric, and other critical structures about the

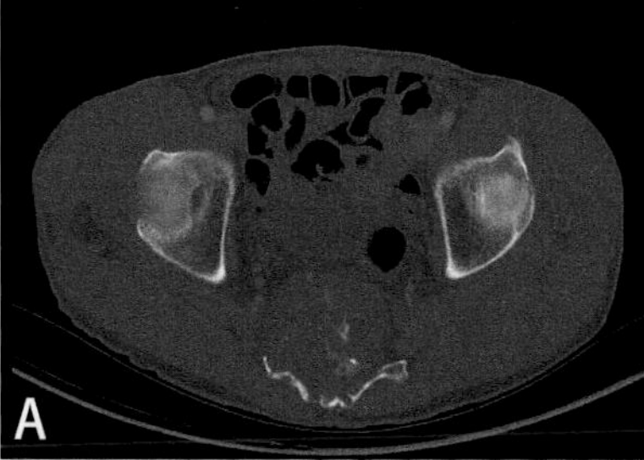

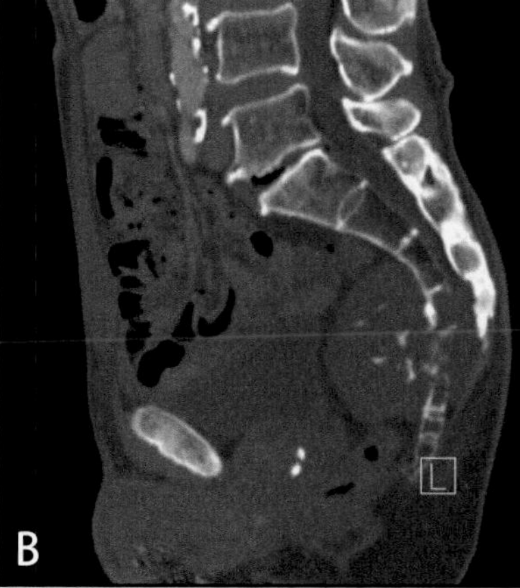

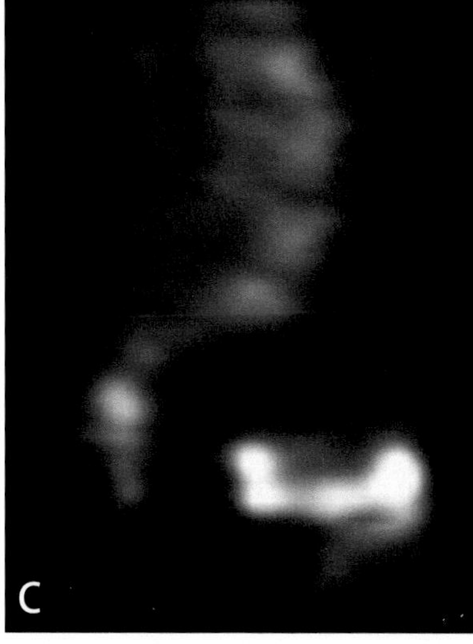

Figure 14-2. A 62-year-old man presents with rectal pain and constipation. (A) Axial and (B) sagittal CT demonstrates a midline, destructive lesion of the inferior sacrum with anterior soft-tissue extension and associated mineralization. (C) Technetium-99m bone scintigraphy demonstrates modest uptake in the distal sacrum. Axial (D) T1, (E) T2, post-contrast (F) T1, and sagittal.

spine and pelvis. Recently, more advanced techniques of radiation delivery such as stereotactic and intensity-modulated radiation therapy and hadron (proton or neutron) beam therapy are able to deliver higher cumulative doses of radiation to the tumor while sparing surrounding tissues. This has shown improvements in rates of local control in small series.[6]

Take-Aways

1. Benign tumors of the spine are generally managed with intralesional resection. For more active tumors such as osteoblastoma and giant cell tumor of bone, en bloc resection is recommended when feasible.
2. Chordomas are slow-growing malignancies of the midline spine with poor sensitivity to chemotherapy and radiotherapy. Wide surgical resection is the mainstay of treatment, and long-term outcomes are poor.

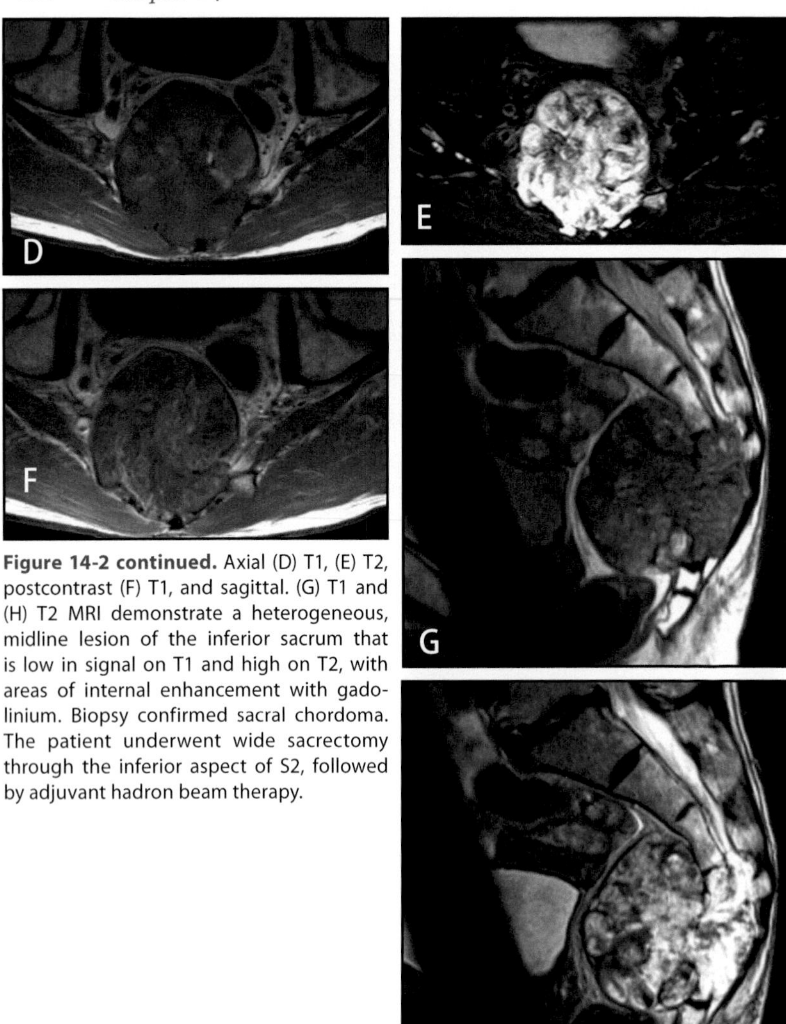

Figure 14-2 continued. Axial (D) T1, (E) T2, postcontrast (F) T1, and sagittal. (G) T1 and (H) T2 MRI demonstrate a heterogeneous, midline lesion of the inferior sacrum that is low in signal on T1 and high on T2, with areas of internal enhancement with gadolinium. Biopsy confirmed sacral chordoma. The patient underwent wide sacrectomy through the inferior aspect of S2, followed by adjuvant hadron beam therapy.

Commonly Tested Topics for Trainees

- Vertebral hemangiomas are common incidental findings in the spine, and can be definitively characterized on CT and MRI. Treatment is generally nonoperative.

- Chordoma recurrences after wide resection are common and are associated with increased risk of metastatic spread and mortality.
- Chordoma is associated with the highest rate of local recurrence of all malignant primary bone tumors.
- The morbidity after sacral resection is determined by the highest level of required nerve root sacrifice. S3 is the nerve root critical to preservation of at least partial bowel and bladder function.

References

1. Berry M, Mankin H, Gebhardt M, Rosenberg A, Hornicek F. Osteoblastoma: a 30-year study of 99 cases. *J Surg Oncol.* 2008;98(3):179-183. doi:10.1002/jso.21105.
2. Pastushyn AI, Slin'ko EI, Mirzoyeva GM. Vertebral hemangiomas: diagnosis, management, natural history and clinicopathological correlates in 86 patients. *Surg Neurol.* 1998;50(6):535-547. doi:10.1016/S0090-3019(98)00007-X.
3. McMaster ML, Goldstein AM, Bromley CM, Ishibe N, Parry DM. Chordoma: incidence and survival patterns in the United States, 1973-1995. *Cancer Causes Control.* 2001;12(1):1-11. doi:10.1023/A:1008947301735.
4. Todd LT, Yaszemski MJ, Currier BL, Fuchs B, Kim CW, Sim FH. Bowel and bladder function after major sacral resection. *Clin Orthop Relat Res.* 2002;397:36-39. doi:10.1097/00003086-200204000-00006.
5. Fuchs B, Dickey ID, Yaszemski MJ, Inwards CY, Sim FH. Operative management of sacral chordoma. *J Bone Joint Surg Am.* 2005;87(10):2211-2216. doi:10.2106/JBJS.D.02693.
6. Park L, Delaney TF, Liebsch NJ, et al. Sacral chordomas: impact of high-dose proton/photon-beam radiation therapy combined with or without surgery for primary versus recurrent tumor. *Int J Radiat Oncol Biol Phys.* 2006;65(5):1514-1521. doi:10.1016/j.ijrobp.2006.02.059.

15

Tumors of the Hands and Feet

Overview

The hands and feet experience a higher-than-expected burden of bone and soft-tissue tumors relative to their cumulative body mass. The clinical presentations and radiologic appearances of benign and malignant processes can be very similar, and errors in diagnosis and management are common when oncologic principles are not strictly observed. We will discuss the unique anatomic considerations for tumors of the hands and feet, and review lesions with a predilection for the hands and feet that have not been covered in prior chapters.

The hands and feet are characterized by complex anatomic orientations of multiple compact structures. Small compartments in close proximity are separated by thinner bony cortices and fascial boundaries. This allows for easier penetration of tumors into and out of bones and across anatomic barriers into adjacent structures. This accounts for the tendency of benign lesions to display radiographically aggressive patterns of growth not seen for identical lesions elsewhere in the body (Figure 15-1). Malignant tumors are likewise able to invade multiple adjacent compartments, and these masses often present earlier in the course of disease, as smaller lesions are more likely to become visible and interfere with function. As a result, benign tumors, malignant tumors, synovial lesions, and reactive lesions can all present with similar clinical and radiographic findings. For tumors of the hands and feet, size and appearance are no longer predictive of malignant potential, which

Wallace, MT
Handbook of Musculoskeletal Tumors (pp 231-240).

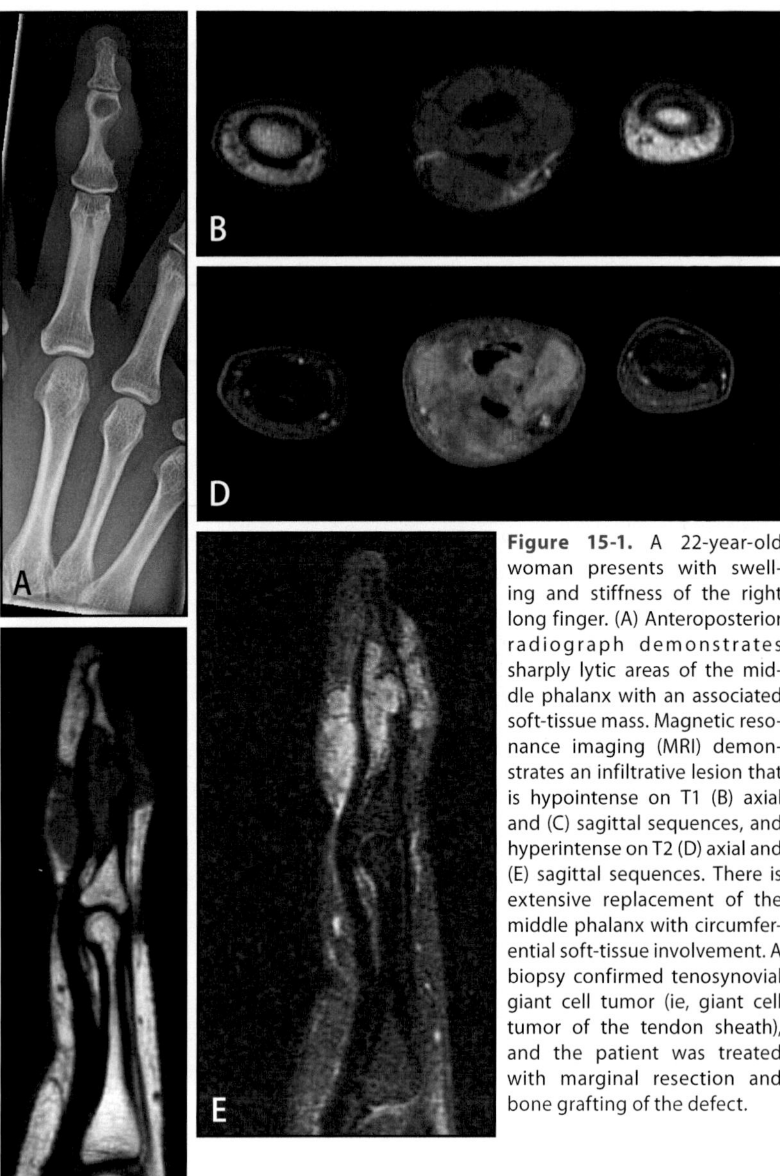

Figure 15-1. A 22-year-old woman presents with swelling and stiffness of the right long finger. (A) Anteroposterior radiograph demonstrates sharply lytic areas of the middle phalanx with an associated soft-tissue mass. Magnetic resonance imaging (MRI) demonstrates an infiltrative lesion that is hypointense on T1 (B) axial and (C) sagittal sequences, and hyperintense on T2 (D) axial and (E) sagittal sequences. There is extensive replacement of the middle phalanx with circumferential soft-tissue involvement. A biopsy confirmed tenosynovial giant cell tumor (ie, giant cell tumor of the tendon sheath), and the patient was treated with marginal resection and bone grafting of the defect.

accounts for many errors in diagnosis and management when the index of suspicion for malignancy is low and established principles of work-up and biopsy are not followed.

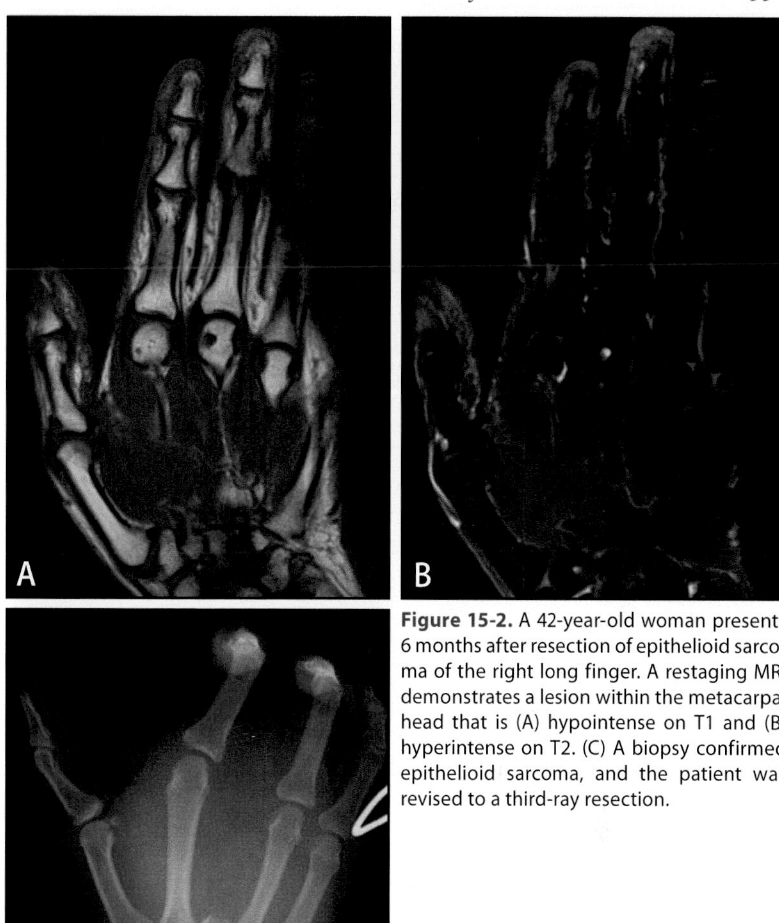

Figure 15-2. A 42-year-old woman presents 6 months after resection of epithelioid sarcoma of the right long finger. A restaging MRI demonstrates a lesion within the metacarpal head that is (A) hypointense on T1 and (B) hyperintense on T2. (C) A biopsy confirmed epithelioid sarcoma, and the patient was revised to a third-ray resection.

The complex structuring of hand and foot anatomy presents unique surgical challenges for resection and reconstruction. Well-defined lesions that respect anatomic boundaries are easily managed by conventional techniques such as marginal resection and intralesional curettage and bone grafting. For locally aggressive tumors, the close proximity of bone, tendon, and neurovascular structures and the frequent lack of physical boundaries to tumor growth often require sacrifice or ablation of significant portions of the distal extremity for malignant growths (Figure 15-2). Reconstructions after resection are likewise challenging. Sacrifice of critical soft-tissue structures

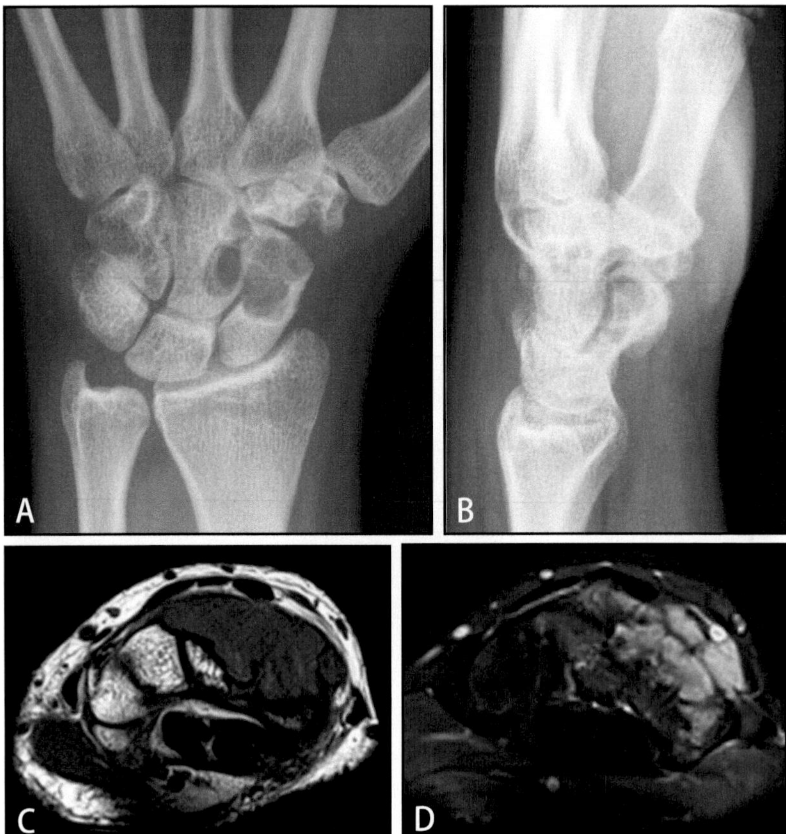

Figure 15-3. A 22-year-old man presents with left wrist pain. (A) Posteroanterior and (B) lateral radiographs demonstrate a lytic process involving the scaphoid, capitate, and trapezium of the left wrist. Axial (C) T1 and (D) T2 MRI demonstrate an associated soft-tissue mass spanning multiple carpal bones. A biopsy demonstrated giant cell tumor of bone. The patient was managed with extended curettage with high-speed burring, cryotherapy, and autograft filling across the defect.

such as nerves, muscles, and tendons can lead to significant functional impairment without predictably successful reconstructive options. Bony resections that compromise the integrity or stability of a joint generally do not have reconstructive options that preserve joint function, and arthrodesis is frequently required (Figure 15-3).

Skin Cancers

The hands are a common location for skin cancers, which develop secondary to ultraviolet ray exposure. Squamous cell carcinomas account for the majority of skin malignancies in the hand, which present as ulcerative or pebbly growths in sun-exposed areas. Basal cell carcinomas are the second most common skin malignancy, and present as raised nodules with telangiectasias and ulcerations. Malignant melanomas are the most lethal skin malignancies, 2% of which occur in the hands.[1] Of the subtypes of malignant melanoma, lentigo maligna, which commonly occurs on the dorsum of the hand, and acral lentiginous melanoma of the palmar and subungual surfaces are the most common. Ulcerated, nodular, and pigmented skin lesions should be investigated with a punch biopsy for diagnostic confirmation. Staging workup for squamous cell tumors and melanoma should include regional lymph node evaluation.

Management of skin cancers consists primarily of wide surgical resection. Basal cell carcinomas can be resected with a margin of 2 mm, squamous cell carcinomas 1 cm or more, and melanomas 2 cm to 3 cm, which often requires amputation of the affected digit or ray (Figure 15-4).

Glomus Tumor

Glomus bodies consist of smooth muscle tissue around a network of blood vessels that regulate blood flow of the skin. Tumors of glomus bodies are classically located in the subungual regions, the sides of the digits, and palmar surfaces. They are often bluish in coloration, and are exquisitely painful to pressure and cold temperatures. When identified, a marginal excision is typically curative, which may require removal of the nail and exposure through the nail bed for subungual lesions.

Epidermal Inclusion Cyst

After ganglions and tenosynovial giant cell tumors, epidermal inclusion cysts are the third most common lesion of the hand. Penetrating trauma, usually over the palmar and plantar surfaces, embeds squamous epithelial tissue into subcutaneous areas, which then continue to produce keratin that cannot be shed as normal. These cysts will continue to grow, and may erode bone and surrounding structures. Excision is curative (Figure 15-5).

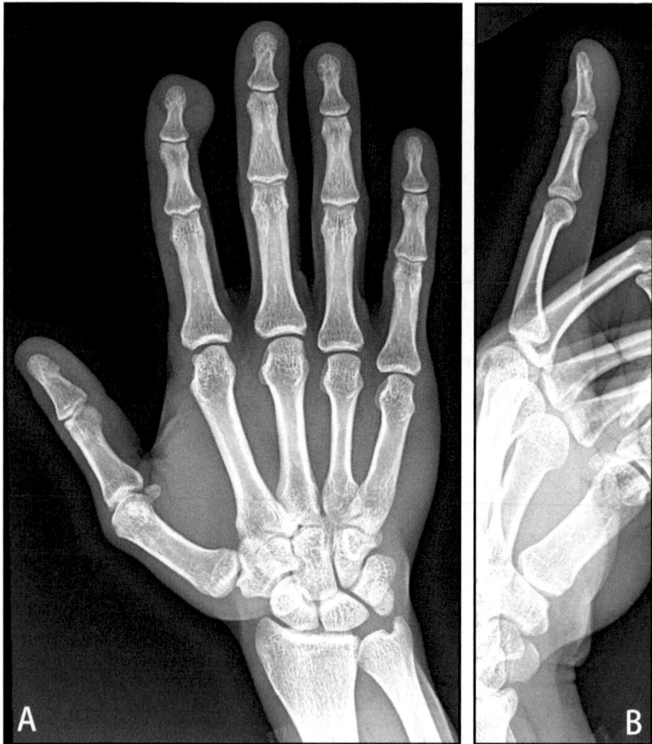

Figure 15-4. A 45-year-old man presents with a painless, nodular mass of the right index finger. (A) Posteroanterior radiograph of the hand and (B) lateral radiograph of the index finger demonstrate soft-tissue swelling over the ulnar aspect of the distal phalanx. A punch biopsy confirmed invasive squamous cell carcinoma, and the patient was managed with amputation through the distal interphalangeal joint.

Giant Cell Reparative Granuloma

Giant cell reparative granulomas are expansile lesions of the tubular bones of the hands and feet. Giant cell reparative granuloma is a reactive process that mimics many benign active bone tumors such as aneurysmal bone cyst and giant cell tumor of bone, and a biopsy is required for diagnosis. Intralesional resection is appropriate, but recurrences are common.[2]

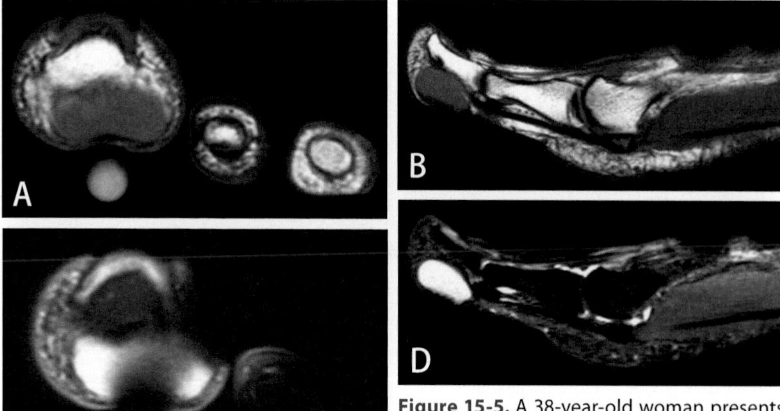

Figure 15-5. A 38-year-old woman presents with a firm nodule of the plantar surface of the right great toe. MRI demonstrates a well-defined soft-tissue mass plantar to the distal phalanx of the hallux, intimately associated with the dermis. The mass is hypointense on (A) axial and (B) sagittal T1 and hyperintense on (C) axial and (D) sagittal T2 sequences. Biopsy confirmed epidermal inclusion cyst, and the patient underwent resection of the lesion.

Reactive Periosteal Lesions

The small tubular bones of the hands and feet are common locations for a unique group of surface-based reactive lesions. It is proposed that an initial traumatic event results in subperiosteal hemorrhage over the affected bone.[3] This progresses to a stage of ill-defined mineralized density known as florid reactive periostitis (Figure 15-6). This resembles early callus formation, which may then mature into a well-defined cap of mixed cartilage and mature bone known as bizarre parosteal osteochondromatous proliferation, also known as Nora's lesion (Figure 15-7). As the lesion matures and fuses to the underlying cortex, it becomes a stable turret exostosis, also known as an acquired osteochondroma. These frequently occur in the subungual region, where overlying nail bed deformity is common. Treatment by marginal excision is appropriate, but given the post-traumatic, reactive nature of these lesions, there is a notable risk of recurrence.

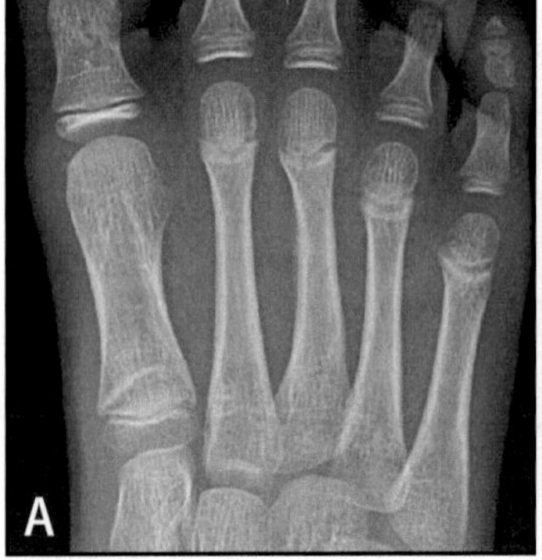

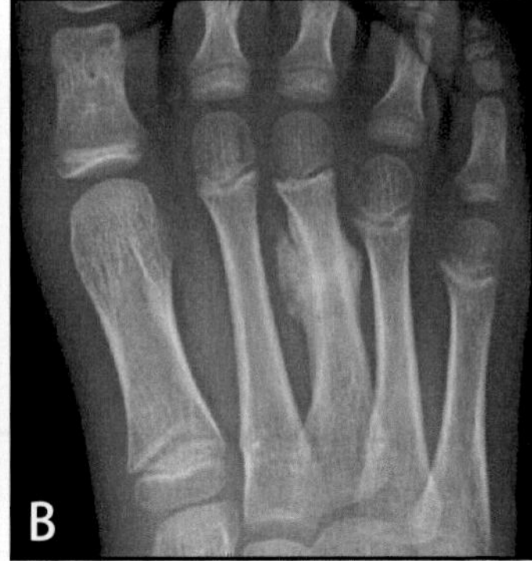

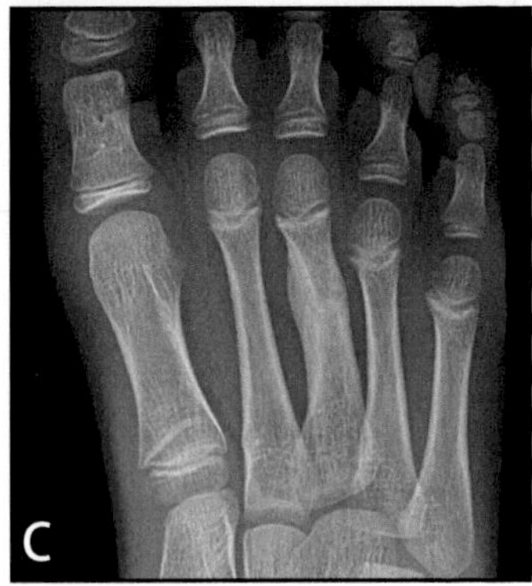

Figure 15-6. An 8-year-old boy presents with pain and swelling 3 weeks after an object fell onto his right foot. (A) Anteroposterior radiograph at the time of presentation demonstrates subtle periostitis of the shaft of the third metatarsal without discernable fracture. (B) This then progresses to florid reactive periostitis 2 months after injury, (C) which then stabilizes to normal bone at 6 months.

Take-Aways

1. Benign, malignant, and reactive lesions in the hands and feet can affect multiple adjacent bony and soft-tissue compartments, with similar radiologic appearances. Cautious adherence to standard principles of work-up and biopsy are essential.
2. Owing to regular sun exposure, the hands are frequent locations for common skin cancers. Wide resection is the mainstay of treatment, which may require complex reconstruction or amputation of the affected area.
3. Reactive periosteal lesions mature in stages similar to fracture callus, and can be very cellular and misleading histologically. These lesions must be recognized clinically and radiographically to avoid misdiagnosis and amputation of a perceived malignancy.

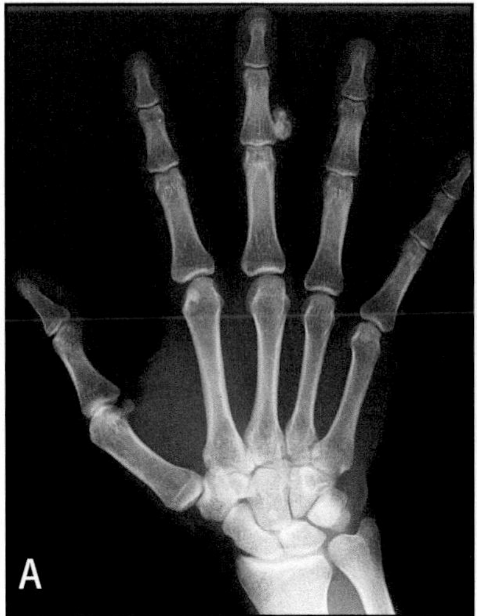
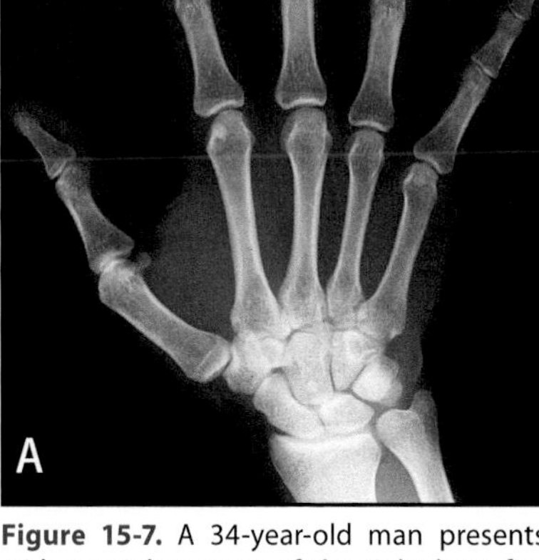

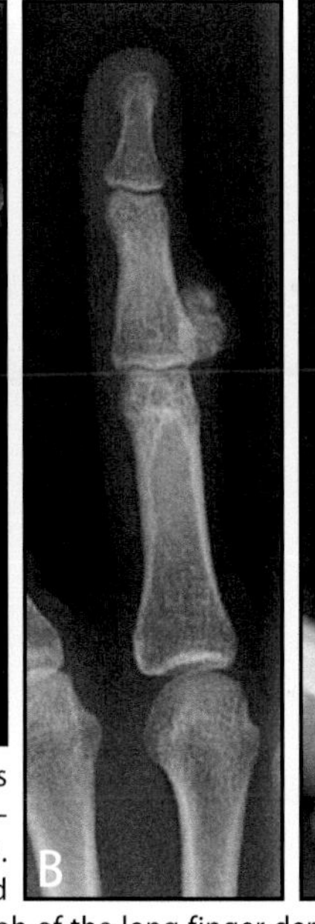

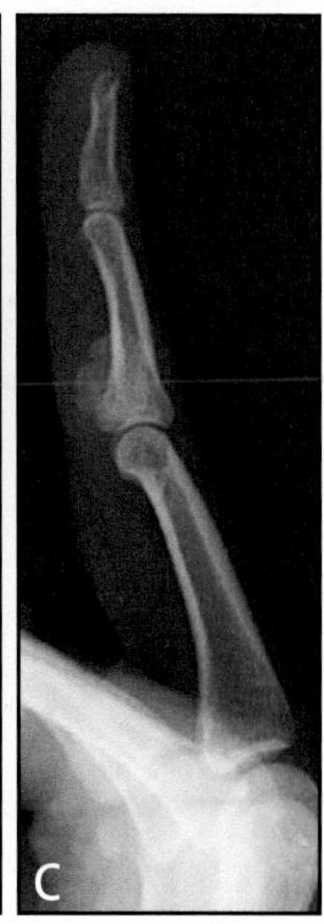

Figure 15-7. A 34-year-old man presents with a painless mass of the right long finger that interferes with writing and typing. Posteroanterior radiographs of (A) the hand and (B) long finger, and (C) lateral radiograph of the long finger demonstrate a lobulated, mineralized lesion abutting the ulnar cortex of the middle phalanx of the long finger. Excision of the lesion demonstrated bizarre parosteal osteochondromatous proliferation, also known as Nora's lesion.

Commonly Tested Topics for Trainees

- Malignant finger tumors distal to the insertion of the flexor digitorum superficialis at the level of the middle phalanx can be managed with partial digital amputation with good functional results. Tumors more proximal to this level are best managed with ray resection to avoid a defect in the middle of the hand.
- Glomus tumors are often subungual, bluish in coloration, and sensitive to pressure and cold temperature. This clinical presentation is diagnostic and resection is curative.

References

1. Warso M, Gray T, Gonzalez M. Melanoma of the hand. *J Hand Surg Am.* 1997;22(2):354-360. doi:10.1016/S0363-5023(97)80178-5.
2. Ratner V, Dorfman HD. Giant-cell reparative granuloma of the hand and foot bones. *Clin Orthop Relat Res.* 1990;260:251-258. doi:10.1097/00003086-199011000-00041.
3. Reactive lesion of the bone surface. In: Dorfman HD, Czerniak B. *Bone Tumors.* St Louis, MO: Mosby; 1998:1139-1152.

Conclusion

Team-Based Approach to Care

Musculoskeletal tumors encompass a broad category of lesions that range in presentation from common to exceedingly rare, from benign to malignant, from childhood to elderly adulthood, and from extremity to axial locations. Safe diagnosis and effective management are best accomplished with the input of an experienced team across multiple disciplines, and the benefit of open and frequent communication between members of the care team cannot be overstated. Discussion of patients at regularly scheduled multidisciplinary conferences and simultaneous evaluation of the patient by multiple practitioners in combined-specialty clinics are excellent practices to optimize patient care, facilitate expedient treatments, and improve patient convenience and engagement with the care team.

The diagnosis and management of musculoskeletal tumors can be compared to a relay race, with different disciplines involved within each phase of care. Throughout the process, focus must always remain on the patient, and it is important for cross-communication between disciplines for any new developments or changes. No single practitioner should feel compelled to provide comprehensive care for complex diseases that may strain the boundaries of his or her knowledge or technical comfort.

Phase 1

Diagnosis and Staging

Encountering Practitioners

Primary care providers, emergency medicine providers, musculoskeletal specialists, and surgeons: the discovery of the tumor and recognition of appropriate work-up is the most important initial step in managing musculoskeletal lesions. A delay in diagnosis is much more common and preventable than other medical errors.

Wallace, MT
Handbook of Musculoskeletal Tumors (pp 241-244).

Radiological Specialists

Radiologists and interventional colleagues are necessary to provide timely and accurate interpretations of imaging studies and to assist in obtaining diagnostic tissue by percutaneous sampling techniques when appropriate.

Surgeons

The surgeon who is expected to provide definitive surgical management of the patient must be the one to perform or guide the biopsy so that tissue for diagnosis can be obtained in a safe manner that does not compromise the surgical site and the ability to perform salvage of critical structures. The surgeon should also be familiar with the appropriate staging studies to obtain after the diagnosis is made.

Pathologists

Tissue diagnosis of many musculoskeletal diseases is a complex undertaking of histopathological, cytopathological, and genetic analyses that must be performed by or in consultation with experts in musculoskeletal pathology. The role of genomic and proteomic profiling of tumors is likely to expand in the future.

Phase 2

Treatment

Surgeons

The treating surgeon should take the most ownership of the patient's initial care. The surgeon must determine what surgical management, if any, is necessary, and be able to provide definitive surgical management for the lesion as required. The surgeon must discuss and determine the plan of treatment with the rest of the musculoskeletal care team, relay this information effectively to the patient, and coordinate the timing of surgery with other treatments as necessary.

Interventional Practitioners

Interventional radiologists are consulted for percutaneous interventions including thermal ablations, cement injection, and embolization.

Medical Specialists: Oncologists, Endocrinologists, Primary Care Providers

Systemic treatments such as chemotherapy, immunotherapy, stem cell transplantation, hormonal, and antiresorptive therapies are coordinated with medical practitioners.

Radiation Oncologists

Radiotherapy has applications for a wide range of musculoskeletal lesions, and these treatments are coordinated with radiation oncology specialists.

Pain Management

Patients should receive diligent symptom management so that treatments remain well tolerated. Pain management specialists assist in coordinating regimens of narcotic, non-narcotic, and percutaneous needle modalities to improve patient comfort and daily living.

Patient Coordinators and Social Workers

Patients frequently need assistance coordinating visits between multiple practitioners, arranging transportation, and navigating the significant financial burdens that tumor care can impose.

Rehabilitation Specialists

Physical and occupational therapists and rehabilitation practitioners should be involved as early in the treatment phase as feasible to ensure maintenance of functional mobility and quality of life.

Phase 3

Surveillance/Aftercare

Oncologists

The surgical and medical oncologic practitioners should be involved in the regular evaluation of the patient and restaging of the disease. Recurrence of disease may then be detected and managed swiftly.

Support Groups

Patient support groups provide a resource of support for patients and their families, and can assist in the emotional and social adjustments that patients undergo during and after treatment.

Geneticists

Tumorigenesis is largely a genetically driven process, and genetic counselors can guide patients and their families as to the future risk to the patient and genetic relatives, which can guide further screenings.

Palliative Care Specialists

For some patients, disease progression in spite of treatments will lead to worsening pain, function, and life expectancy. The goals of treatment for these patients may shift away from survival and disease remission, but should be no less aggressive in symptom management and optimizing function and quality of life. Palliative care specialists should be involved earlier rather than later in this process to provide a plan of care and a frame of reference to guide symptom management.

Take-Away

1. Safe and effective management of musculoskeletal tumors requires an accurate recognition and work-up of the lesion, followed by an appropriate biopsy and staging. Treatment is frequently multidisciplinary, and it is incumbent on one practitioner, typically the treating surgeon, to direct and coordinate this process.

Appendix

Pathology, Genetics, and Histology of Selected Cases

Wallace, MT
Handbook of Musculoskeletal Tumors (pp 245-293).

Table A-1

Common Immunohistochemical Stains

DIFFERENTIATION	STAIN	DIAGNOSES
Epithelial	Cytokeratins (CK7, CK20)	Carcinomas Synovial sarcoma Epithelioid sarcoma Adamantinoma Chordoma
	Prostate-specific antigen	Prostate carcinoma
	Estrogen/progesterone receptors	Breast carcinoma
	Epithelial membrane antigen (EMA)	Carcinoma Synovial sarcoma Epithelioid sarcoma
Hematopoietic	CD45	Lymphoid
B Lymphocytes	CD20, PAX-5	B-Cell lymphoma
T Lymphocytes	CD3, CD4, CD8	T-Cell lymphoma
Neural crest and melanocytic	S100	Schwanoma Neurofibroma Malignant peripheral nerve sheath Tumor Chordoma Melanoma Clear cell sarcoma Langerhans' cell histiocytosis Chondroblastoma
Mesenchymal	Vimentin	Sarcoma Melanoma +/- Renal, endometrial, thyroid Carcinoma

continued

Table A-1 continued

Common Immunohistochemical Stains

DIFFERENTIATION	STAIN	DIAGNOSES
Myogenic	Desmin	Smooth and skeletal muscle tumors
Smooth muscle	Smooth muscle actin	Leiomyoma Leiomyosarcoma Glomus tumor
Skeletal muscle	Myogenin, myoglobin, MyoD1	Rhabdomyosarcoma
Fibroblastic and vascular	CD34	Neurofibroma Solitary fibrous tumor Dermatofibrosarcoma protuberans Angiosarcoma Hemangioendothelioma
Neuroendocrine	CD99	Ewing sarcoma/PNET Alveolar soft part sarcoma Synovial sarcoma Mesenchymal chondrosarcoma
Polysaccharides	Periodic acid-Schiff (PAS)	Ewing sarcoma Alveolar soft part sarcoma
Immunoglobulin	Lambda/kappa light chains	Multiple myeloma Plasmacytoma
Elastic fiber	Elastin	Elastofibroma

Abbreviation: PNET, peripheral neuroectodermal tumor.

Table A-2

Genetics of Musculoskeletal Tumors

MUTATION/ TRANSLOCATION	RESULT	ASSOCIATED CONDITION
t (11;22) t (21;22)	EWS-FLI1 EWS-ERG	Ewing sarcoma, PNET
t (12;16)	TLS-CHOP	Myxoid liposarcoma
t (X;18)	SYT-SSX 1, 2, or 4	Synovial sarcoma
t (2;13) t (1;13)	PAX3-FHKR PAX7-FHKR	Alveolar rhabdomyosarcoma
t (9;22)	CHN-EWS TEC-EWS	Extracellular myxoid chondrosarcoma
t (12;22)	ATF1-EWS	Clear cell sarcoma
t (17;22)	CollA1-PDGF β-1	Dermatofibrosarcoma protuberans
p53	Li-Fraumeni syndrome	Osteosarcoma Soft-tissue sarcoma Numerous other malignancies
RB1	Retinoblastoma	Osteosarcoma Retinoblastoma Numerous other malignancies
EXT 1, 2, 3	Multiple hereditary exostosis	Osteochondromatosis Secondary chondrosarcoma
MDM2 amplification	Deregulation of p53	Soft-tissue sarcomas Atypical lipomatous tumor/well-differentiated liposarcoma
Ring chromosome 12	Oncogene amplification	Atypical lipomatous tumor/well-differentiated liposarcoma
NF-1	Neurofibromatosis-1	Neurofibroma Malignant peripheral nerve sheath tumor (MPNST)

continued

Table A-2 continued

Genetics of Musculoskeletal Tumors

MUTATION/ TRANSLOCATION	RESULT	ASSOCIATED CONDITION
Chromosome 5 APC	Familial adenomatous polyposis	Colon cancer Extra-abdominal desmoid Numerous other malignancies
GNAS	G-protein alpha subunit Gs-α	Fibrous dysplasia McCune-Albright syndrome Mauzabraud's syndrome

Abbreviations: APC, adenomatous polyposis coli; MDM2, murine double minute 2; PNET, peripheral neuroectodermal tumor.

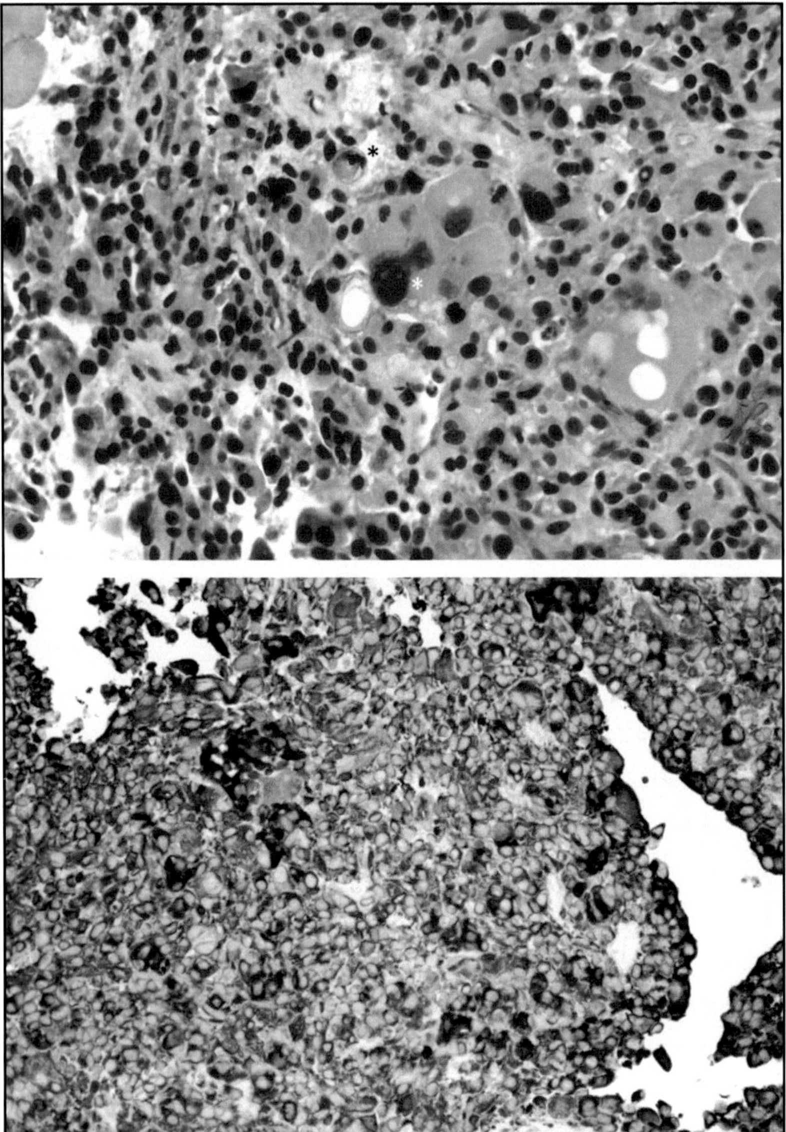

Figure 2-2. Pleomorphic rhabdomyosarcoma. Hematoxylin and eosin stain (above) demonstrates pleomorphic and atypical cells, with mitotic figures (black asterisk) and enlarged anaplastic cells (white asterisk). A desmin stain (below) confirms myogenic differentiation.

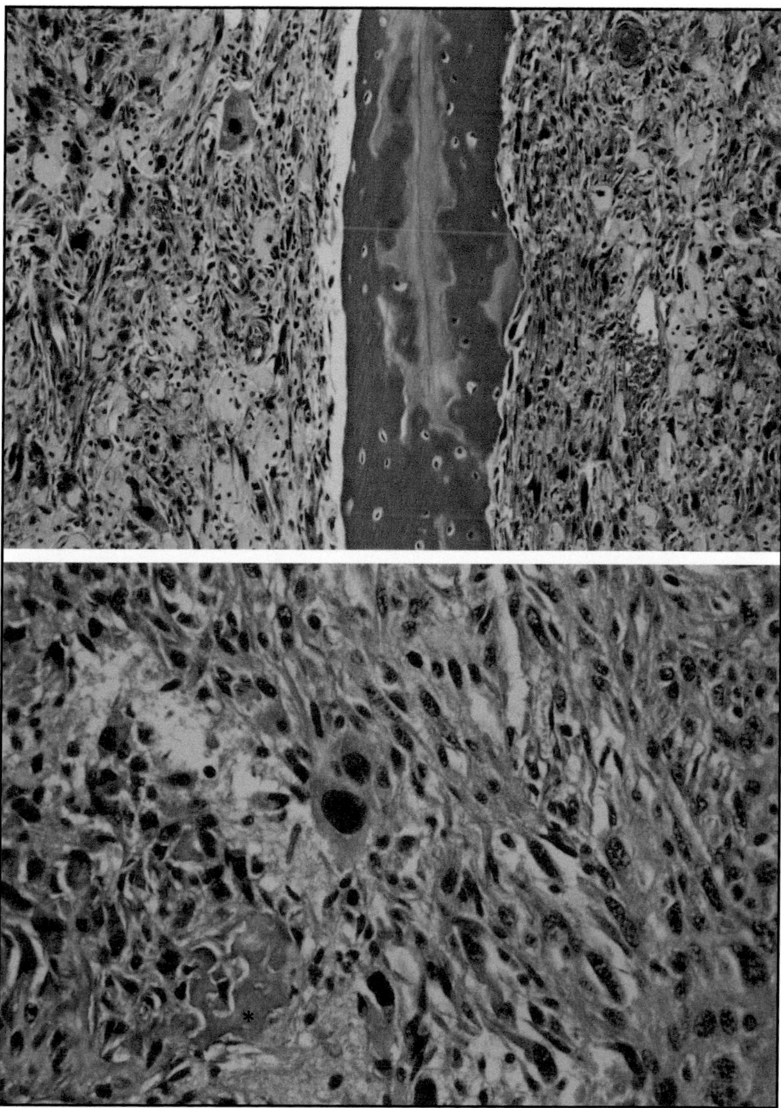

Figure 3-1. Conventional osteosarcoma. Hematoxylin and eosin stain demonstrates pleomorphic and hyperchromatic spindle cells with marked atypia and extracellular osteoid production (black asterisk).

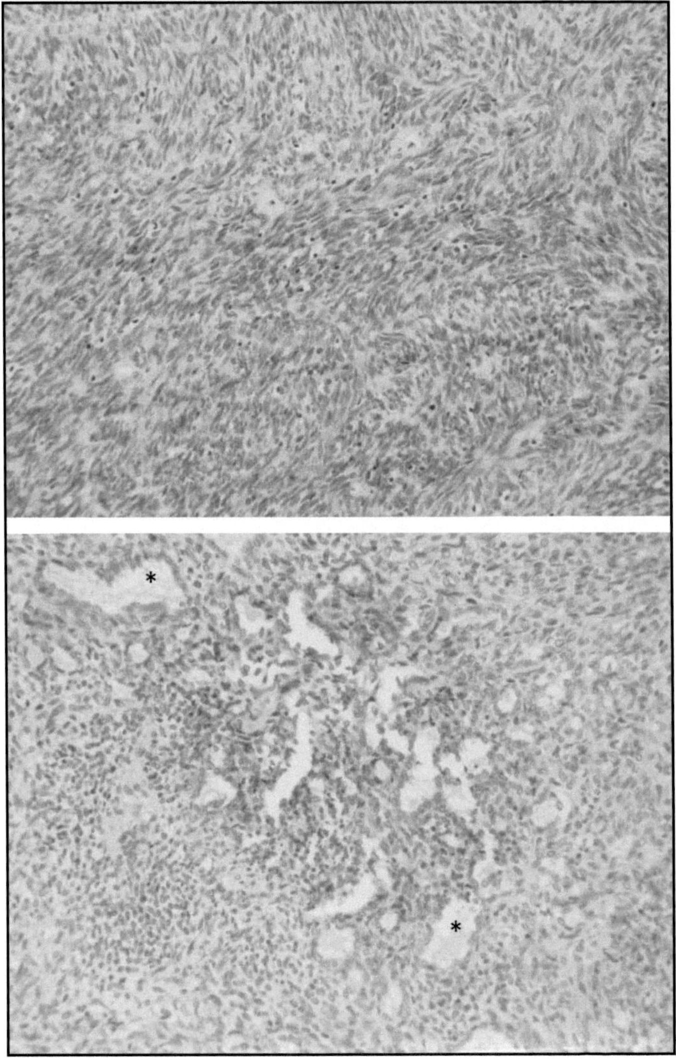

Figure 3-3. Synovial sarcoma. Hematoxylin and eosin stain demonstrates biphasic histology consisting of sheets of elongated, moderately pleomorphic spindle cells with areas of cuboid cells forming glandular structures (black asterisk).

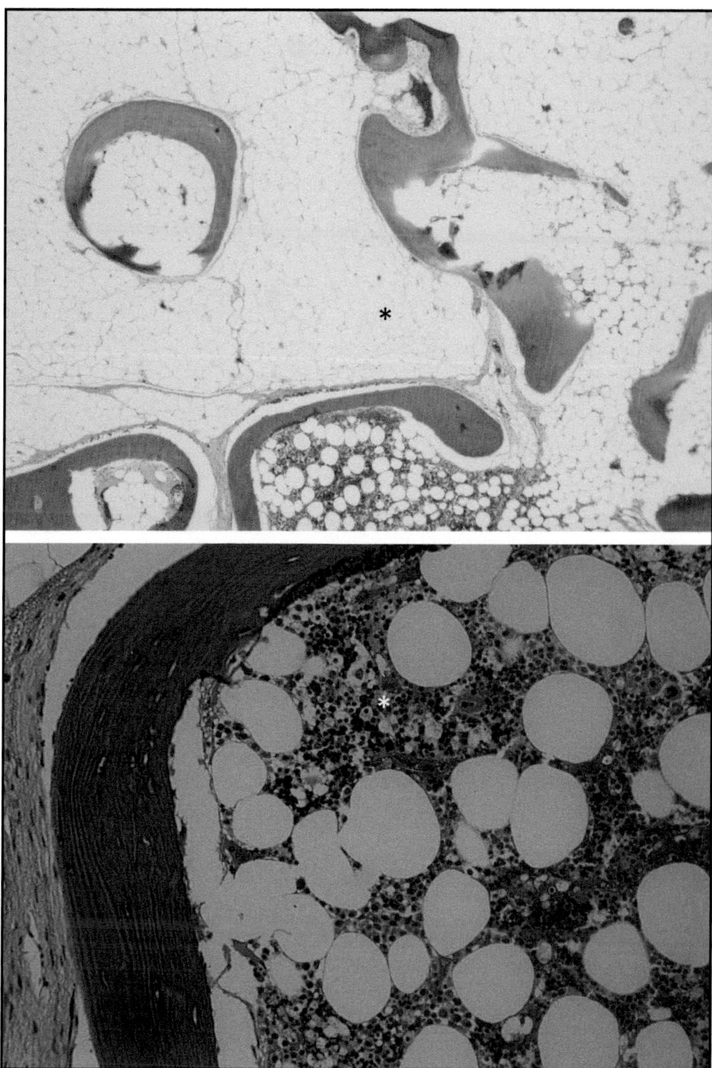

Figure 3-8. Myositis ossificans. Hematoxylin and eosin stain demonstrates mature lamellar bone with intralesional fat (black asterisk) and normal marrow elements (white asterisk).

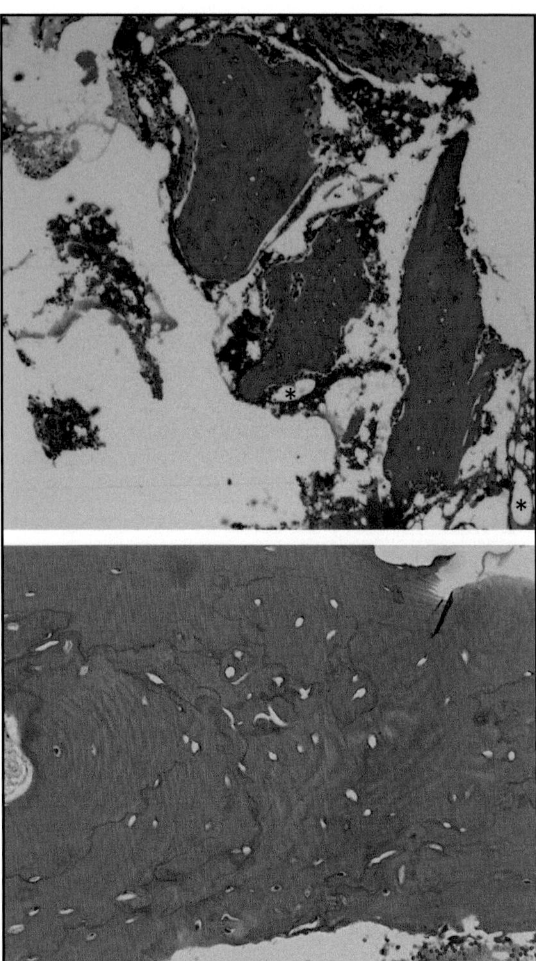

Figure 5-6. Paget's disease of bone. Hematoxylin and eosin stain demonstrates enlarged trabeculae of mature bone with a mosaic pattern of visible cement lines and prominent vascularity (black asterisk).

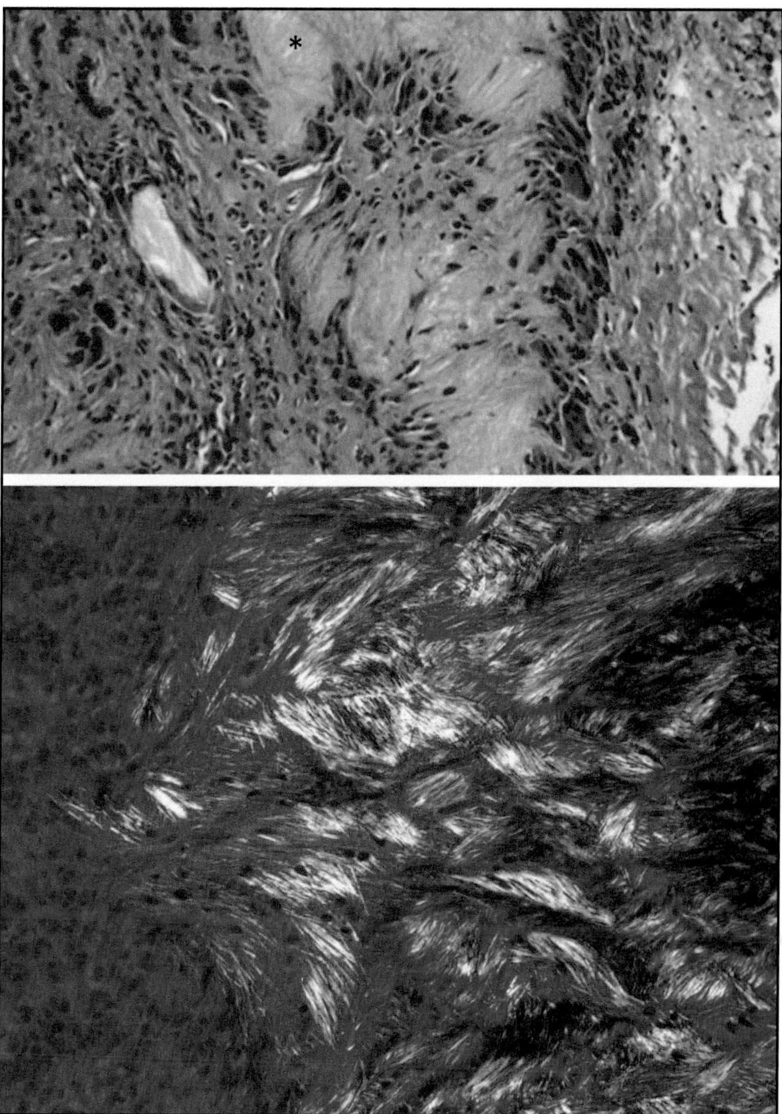

Figure 5-7. Gout. Hematoxylin and eosin stain (above) demonstrates fibroinflammatory tissue surrounding deposits of tophaceous material (black asterisk) with (below) negatively birefringent needle-shaped crystals on polarized microscopy.

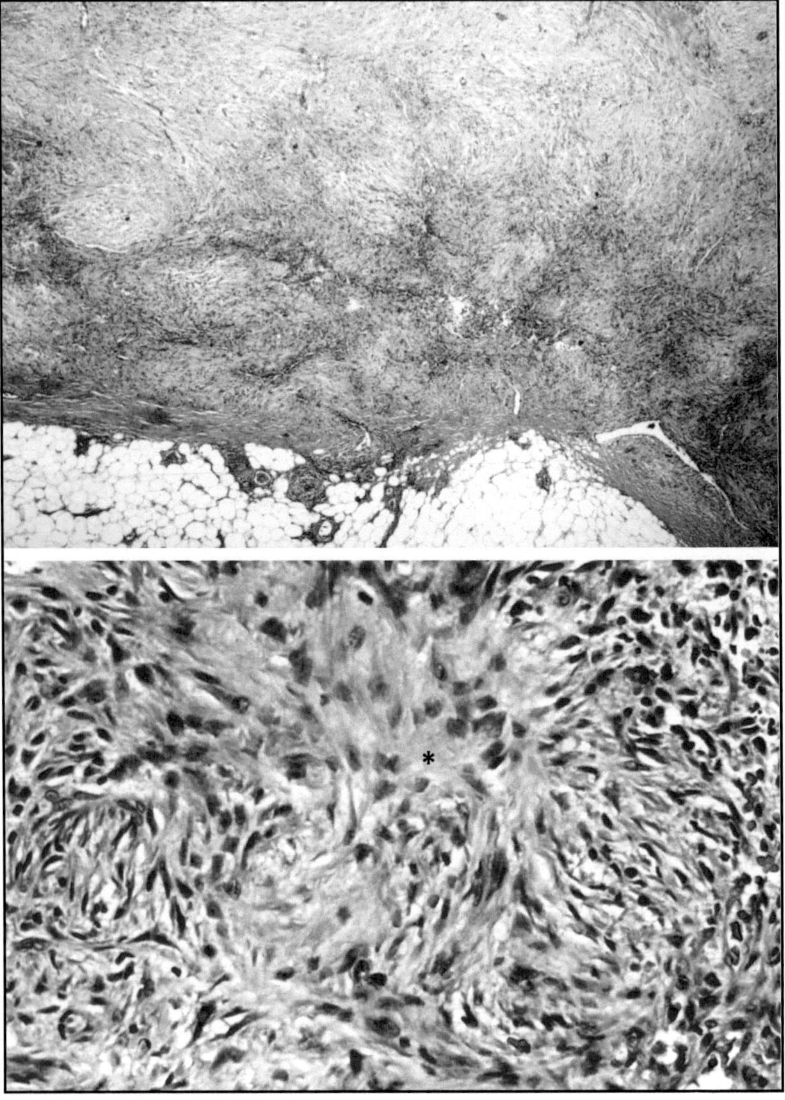

Figure 5-8. Nodular fasciitis. Hematoxylin and eosin stain demonstrates a nodular lesion that is hypocellular at toward the center and hypercellular at the periphery. The cellular zones are composed of elongated myofibroblasts without atypia in a storiform or "feathered" pattern (black asterisk).

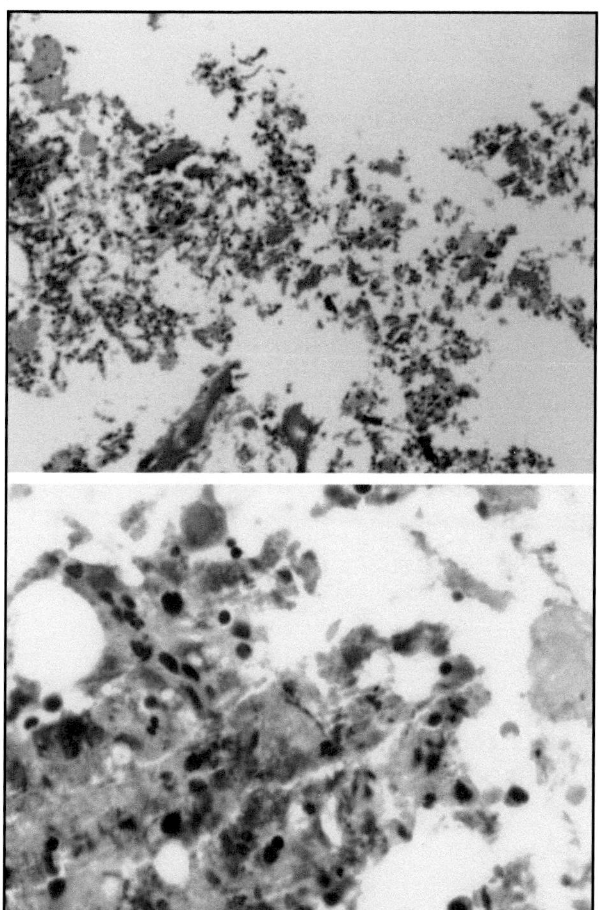

Osteomyelitis. Hematoxylin and eosin stain demonstrates fragments of devitalized bone in a loose collection of mixed inflammatory cells including lymphocytes, segmented neutrophils, and macrophages.

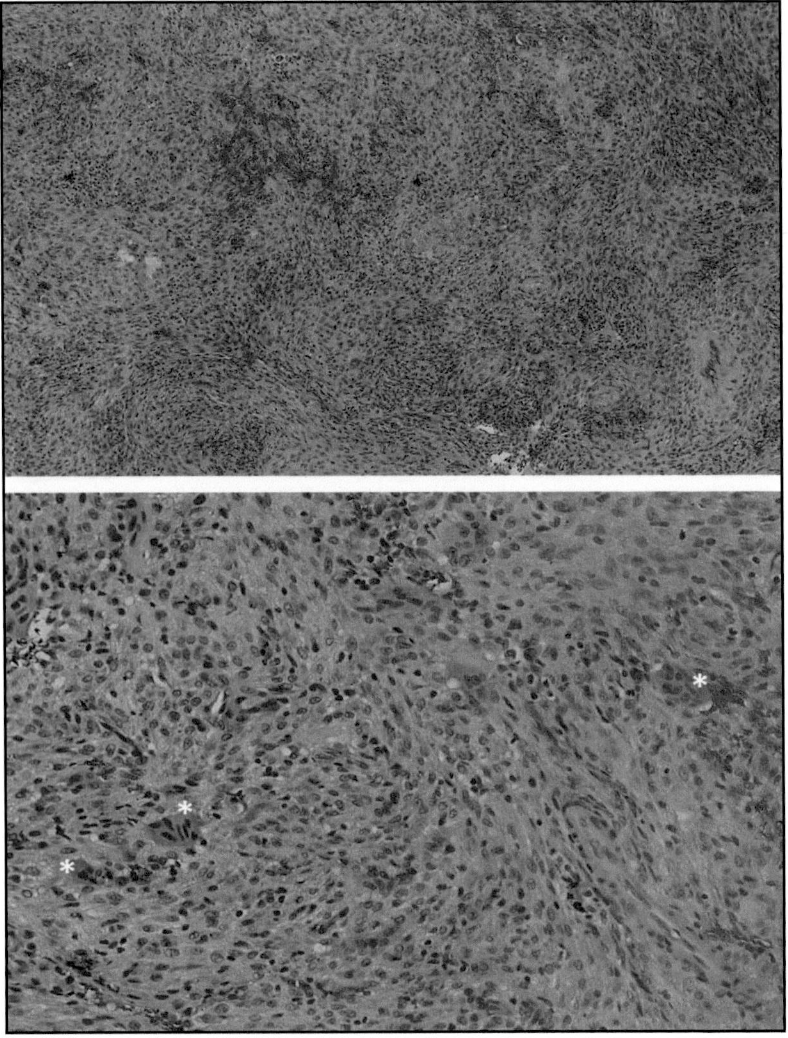

Figure 6-3. Nonossifying fibroma. Hematoxylin and eosin stain demonstrates spindle cells with areas of whorled "storiform" patterning and scatter giant cells (white asterisk). The nuclei within the background spindle cells are regular without atypia.

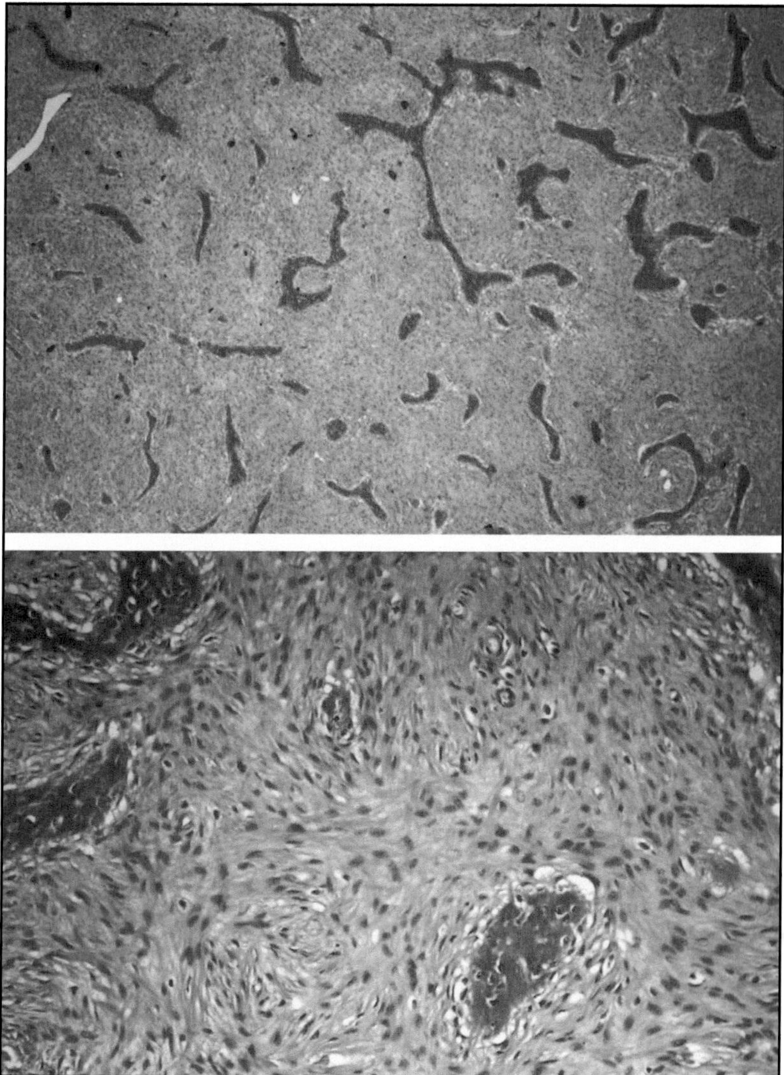

Figure 6-4. Fibrous dysplasia of bone. Hematoxylin and eosin stain demonstrates haphazard osteoid trabeculae in a background of fibroblasts without atypia. There are areas of relative clearing around the trabeculae, noting an absence of surrounding osteoblasts.

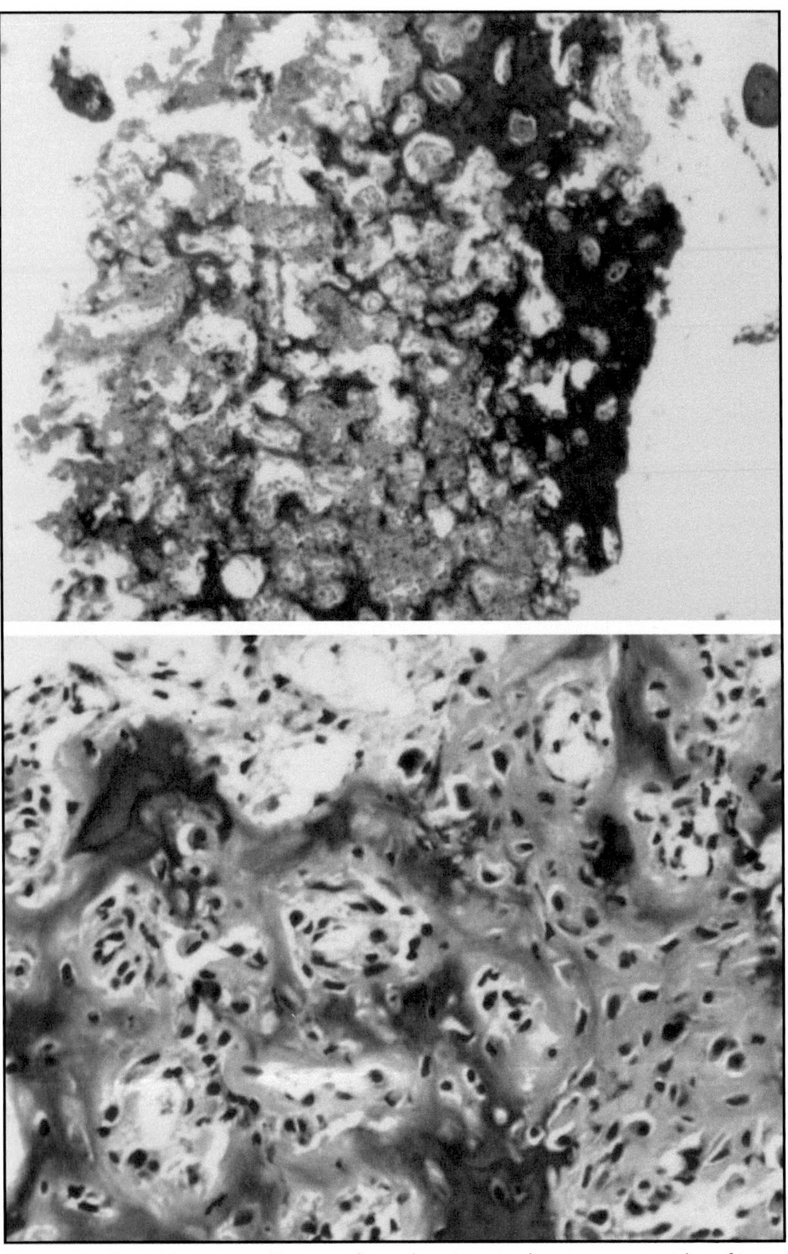

Figure 7-1. Osteoid osteoma. Hematoxylin and eosin stain demonstrates a nidus of interlacing osteoid trabeculae with a margin of dense sclerosis and uniform lining osteoblasts in a fibrovascular background.

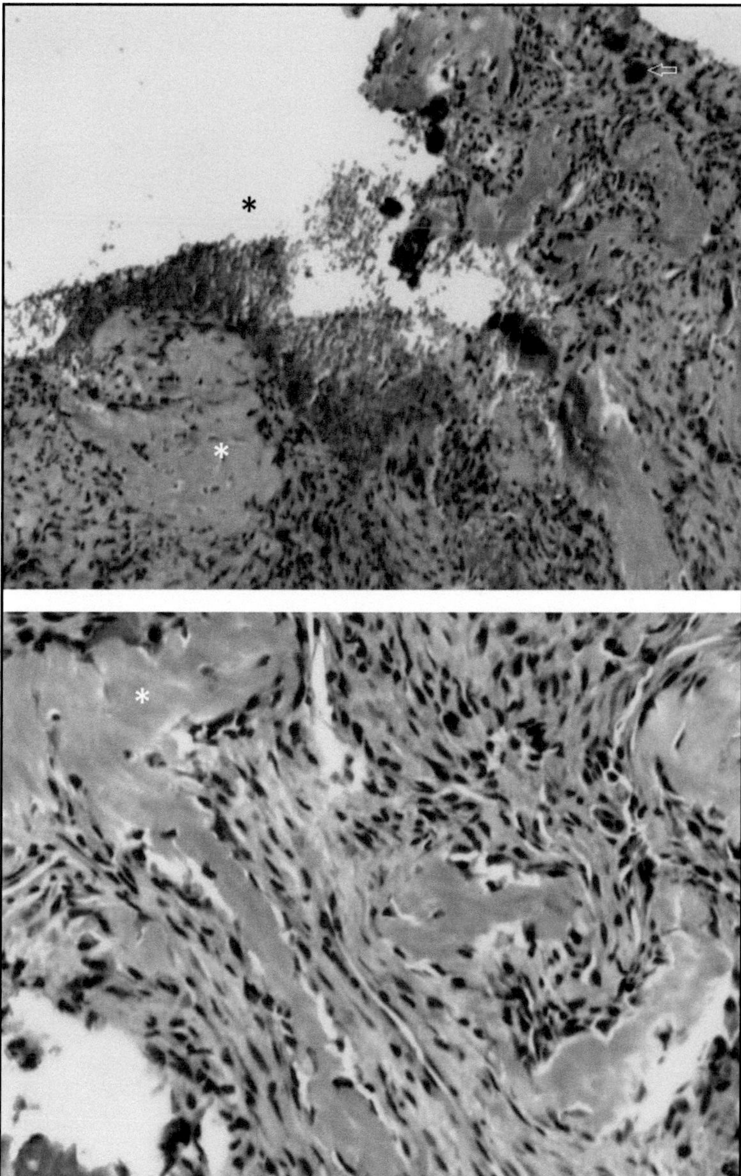

Figure 7-2. Aneurysmal bone cyst. Hematoxylin and eosin stain demonstrates blood-filled spaces (black asterisk) separated by a thickened lining of solid spindle cell proliferation with bone production (white asterisk) and occasional giant cells (white arrow). The spindle cell population is relatively regular, and lacks atypia and pleomorphism, differentiating this tumor from telangiectatic osteosarcoma.

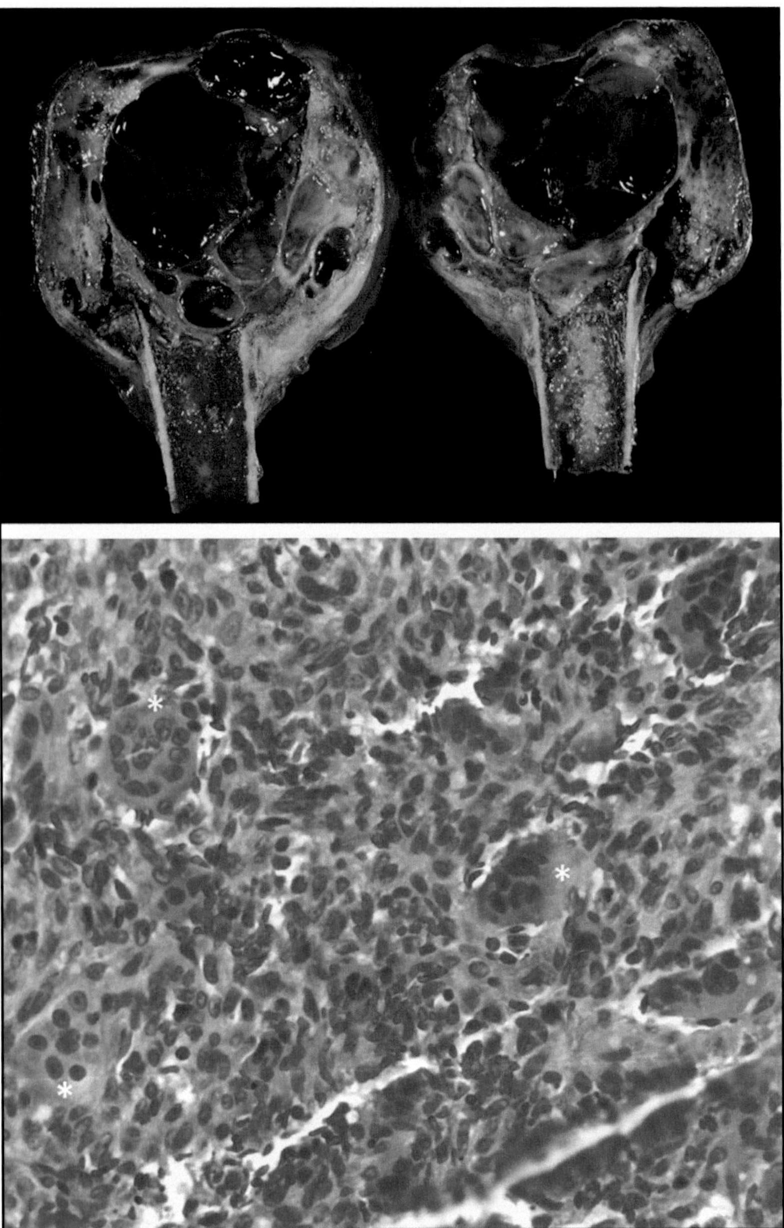

Figure 7-3. Giant cell tumor of bone. (Above) Gross examination demonstrates expansion of the bone with areas of tan-brown solid tumor mixed with areas of aneurismal cyst formation. (Below) Hematoxylin and eosin stain demonstrates uniformly scattered giant cells in a background of monocytoid stromal cells without atypia. Note that the nuclei within the stromal cells is identical to those within the giant cells.

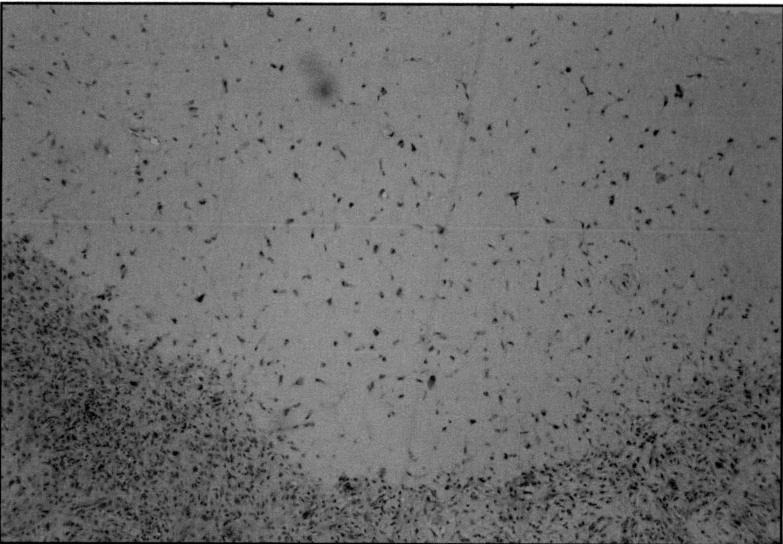

Figure 7-7. Chondromyxoid fibroma. Hematoxylin and eosin stain demonstrates a lobular pattern with hypocellular myxoid tissue with characteristic "stellate" cells centrally and peripheral hypercellularity.

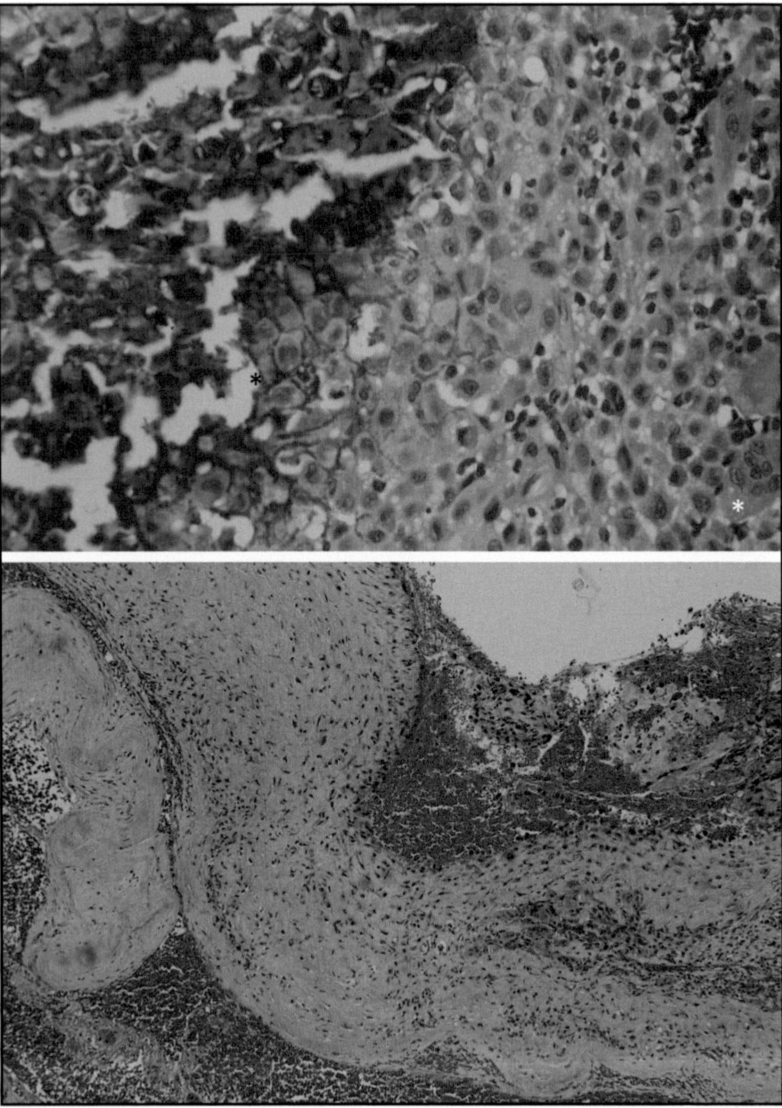

Figure 7-8. Chondroblastoma. (Above) Hematoxylin and eosin stain of the primary lesion demonstrates a population of pale, blue chondroblastic cells with abundant cytoplasm, occasional giant cells (white asterisk) and areas of mineralization that may form a "chicken-wire" pattern of intercellular calcification. (Below) Hematoxylin and eosin stain of adjacent tissue demonstrates large blood-filled areas adjacent to a thickened fibroblastic lining consistent with secondary aneurysmal bone cyst formation.

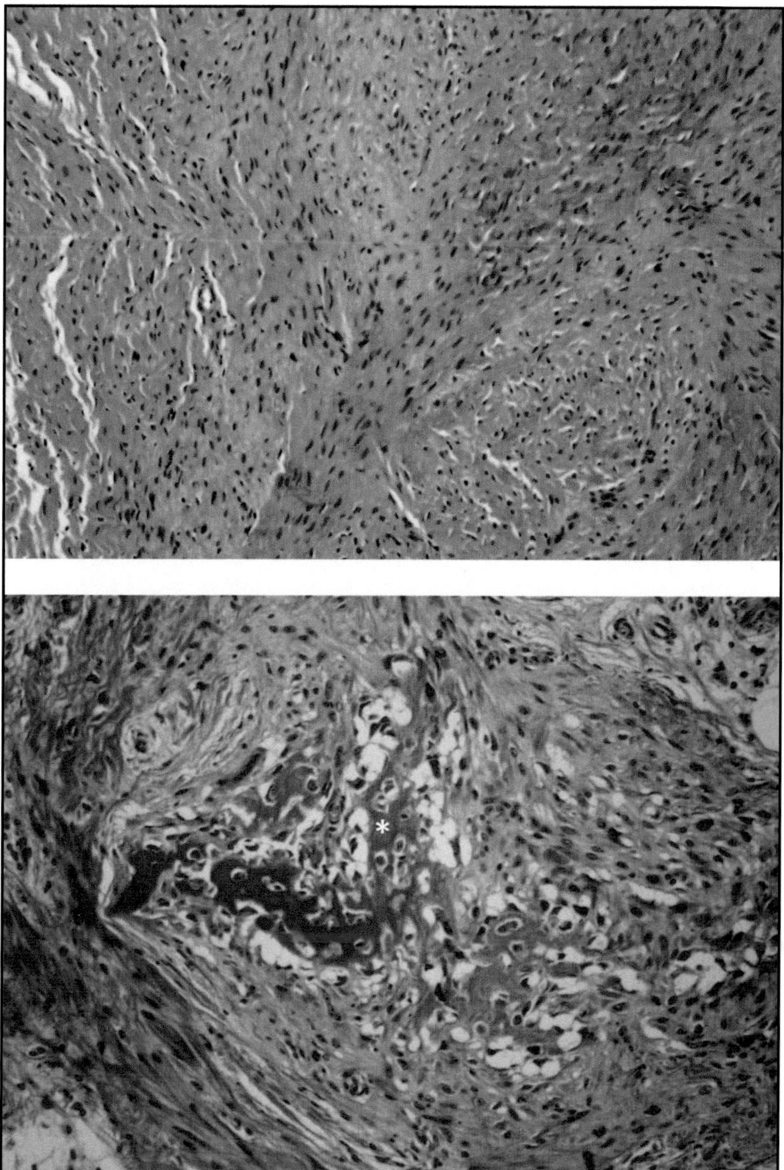

Figure 8-1. Low-grade osteosarcoma. Hematoxylin and eosin stain demonstrates a proliferation of bland spindle cells in a densely fibrous background and areas of mild atypia with malignant osteoid production (white asterisk).

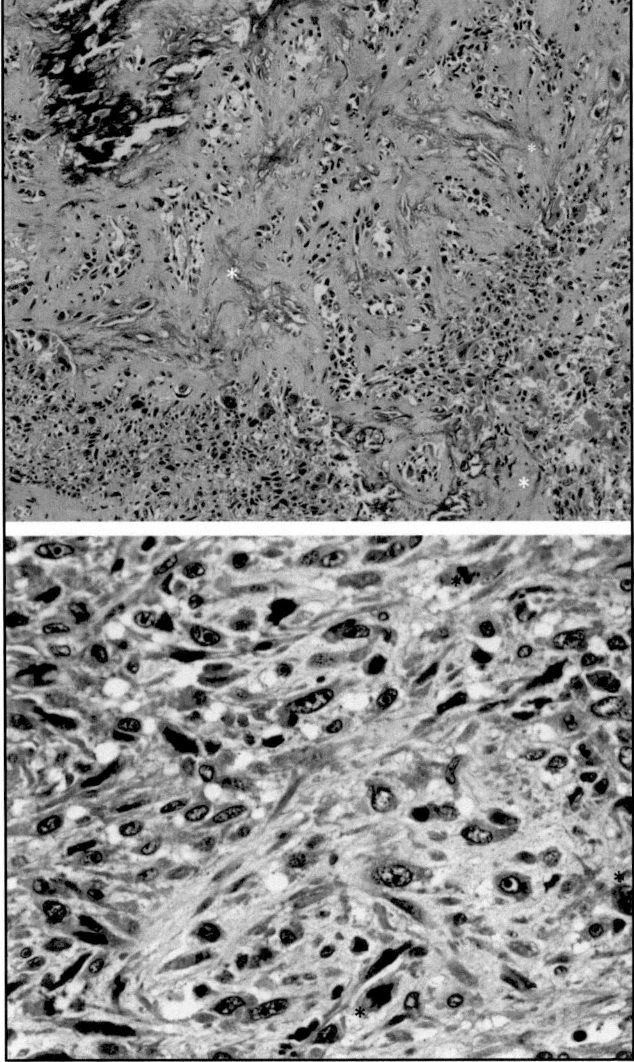

Figure 8-2. Osteosarcoma. Hematoxylin and eosin stain demonstrates a high-grade spindle cell malignancy with marked pleomorphism, atypia, and abundant malignant osteoid production (white asterisk) and numerous mitotic figures (black asterisk).

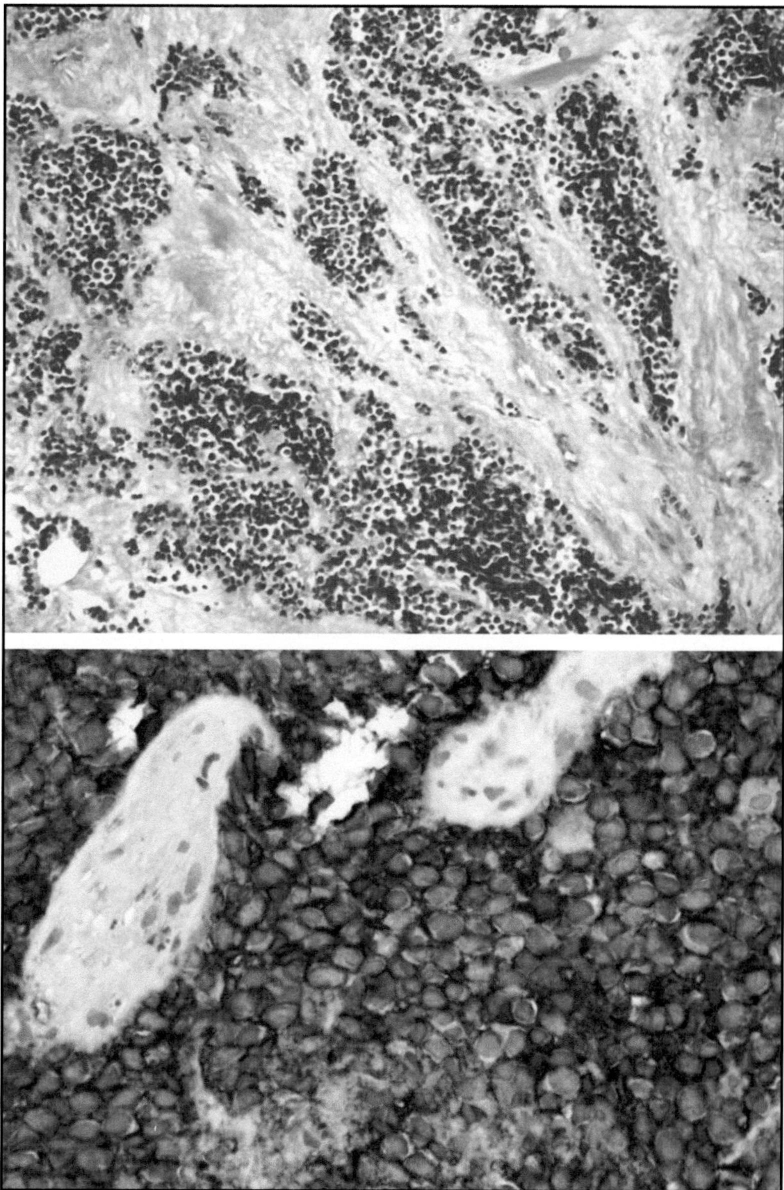

Figure 8-3. Ewing sarcoma. (Above) Hematoxylin and eosin stain demonstrates populations of hyperchromatic small round blue cells with scant cytoplasm. (Below) CD99 stain confirms the diagnosis of Ewing sarcoma.

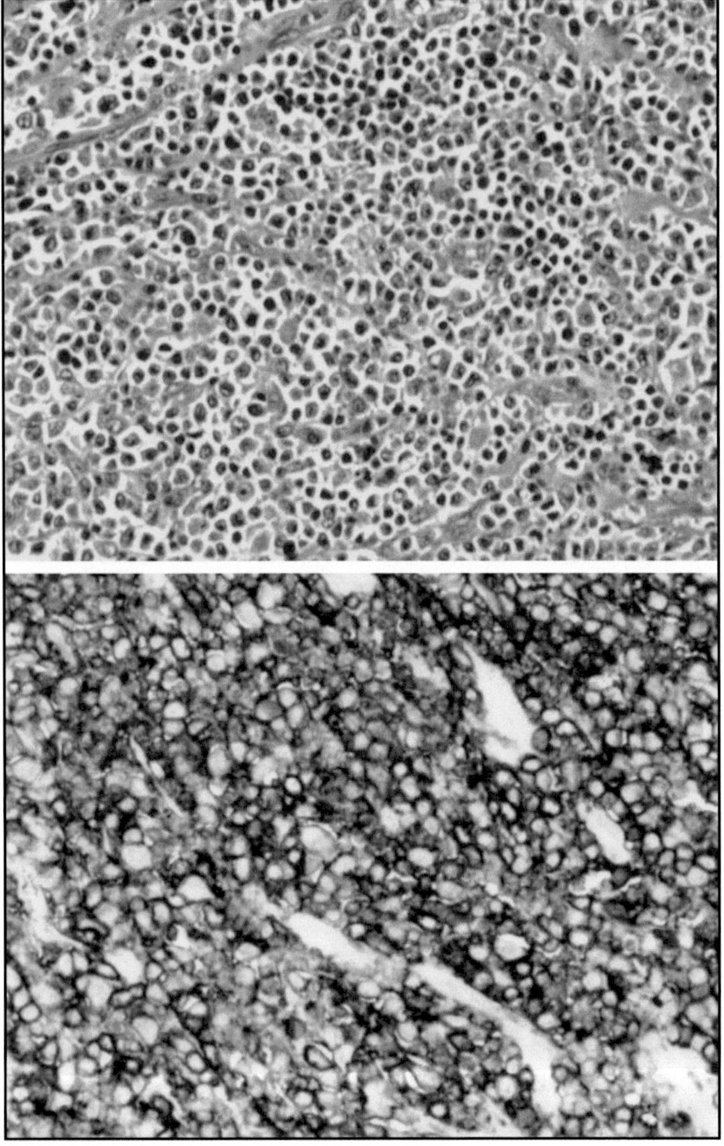

Figure 8-5. B-cell lymphoma of bone. (Above) Hematoxylin and eosin stain demonstrates sheets of monotonous small round blue cells. (Below) CD20 stain confirms a B-cell lymphoid cell population consistent with lymphoma.

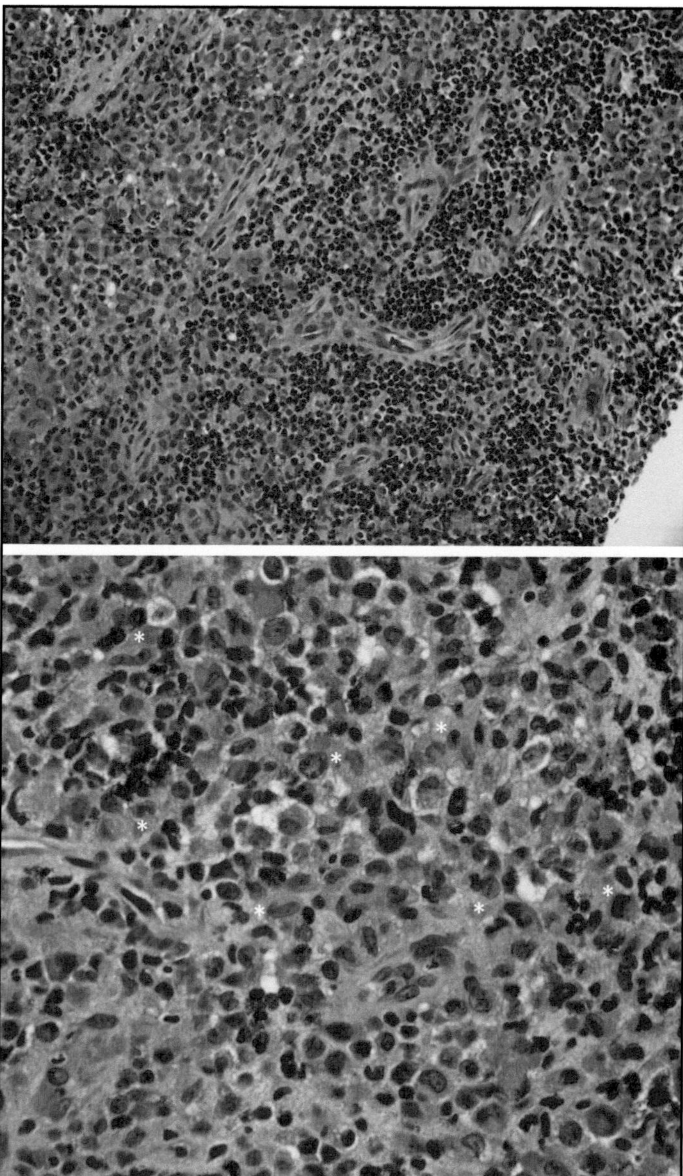

Figure 8-6. Eosinophilic granuloma. Hematoxylin and eosin stain demonstrates a polymorphous collection of inflammatory cells, including abundant eosinophils, histiocytes, and lymphocytes. The key cells of note are the Langerhan cells (white asterisk), which can be identified by a folded or indented nucleus with stippled chromatin and abundant cytoplasm.

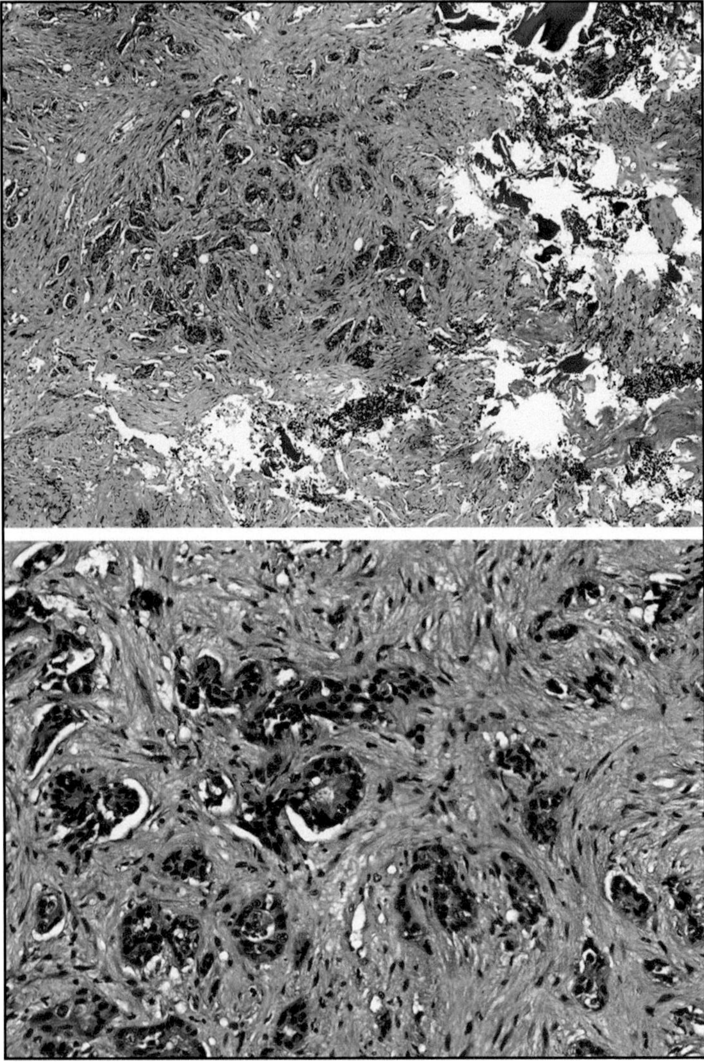

Figure 9-2. Metastatic carcinoma of the breast. Hematoxylin and eosin stain demonstrates infiltrative destruction of bone by a hyperchromatic lesion with glandular differentiation consistent with metastatic carcinoma.

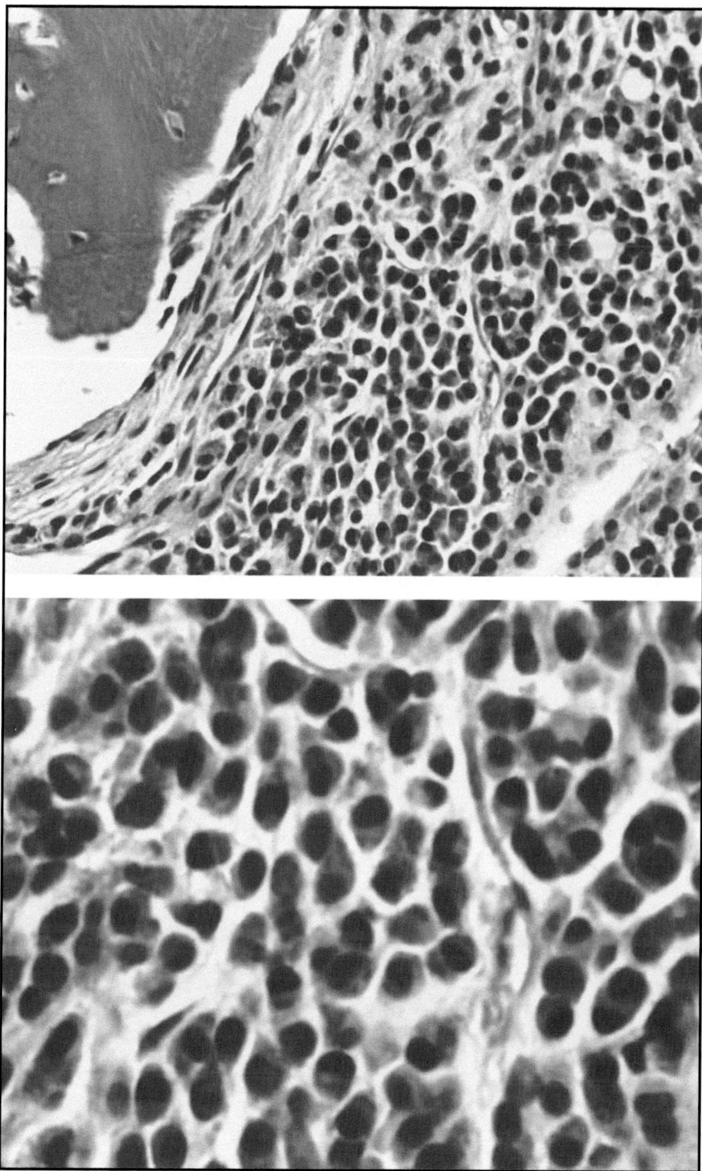

Figure 9-11. Plasmacytoma. Hematoxylin and eosin stain demonstrates bony destruction and sheets of uniform plasma cells, with abundant pink cytoplasm.

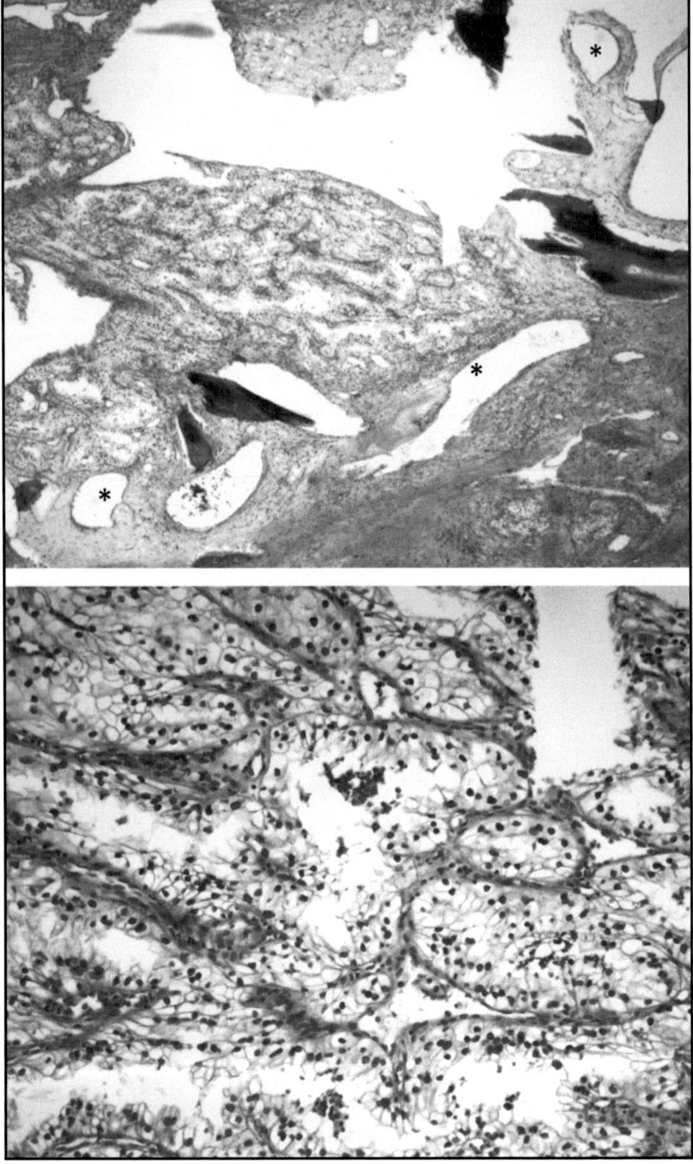

Figure 9-14. Metastatic renal cell carcinoma. Hematoxylin and eosin stain demonstrates bony destruction with a hypervascular proliferation with large vascular spaces (black asterisk) and areas of glandular differentiation with large, pale cells consistent with clear cell carcinoma.

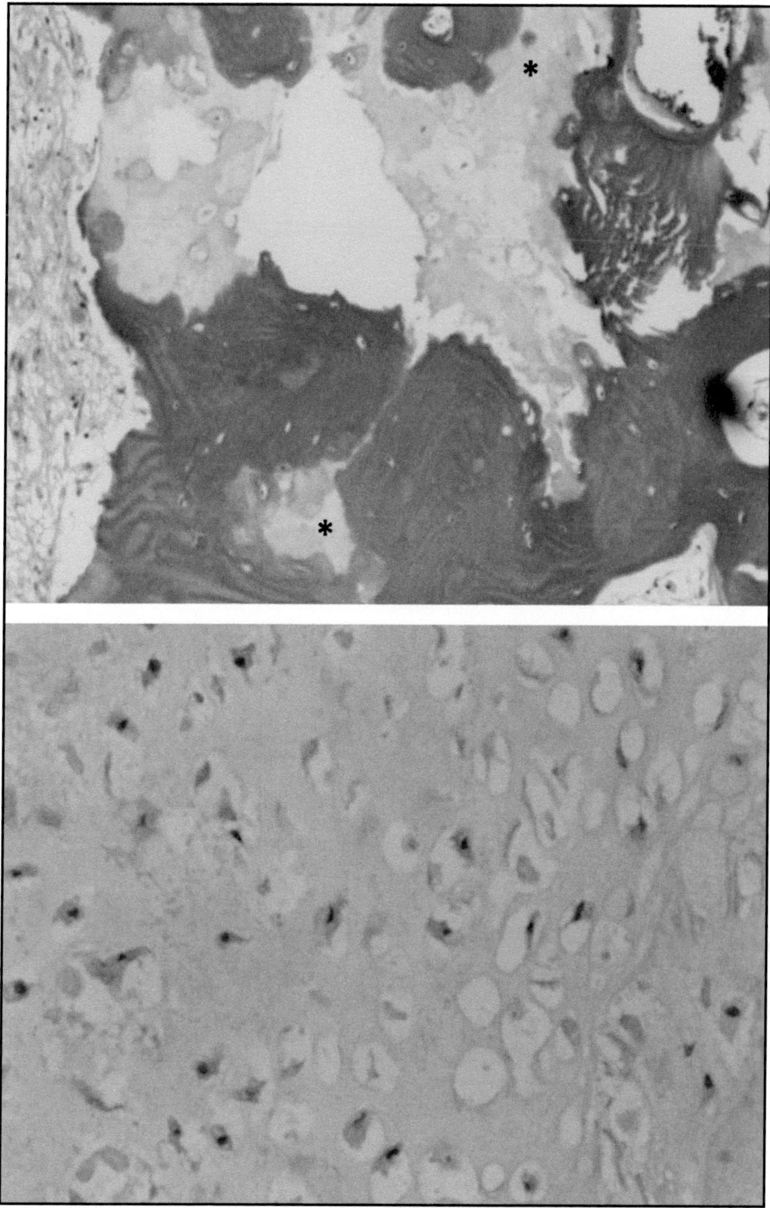

Figure 10-1. Chondrosarcoma. Hematoxylin and eosin stain demonstrates proliferation of bland-appearing cartilage with areas of permeation through lamellar bone (black asterisk). The cartilage is mildly hypercellular, without enlarged or pleomorphic cells.

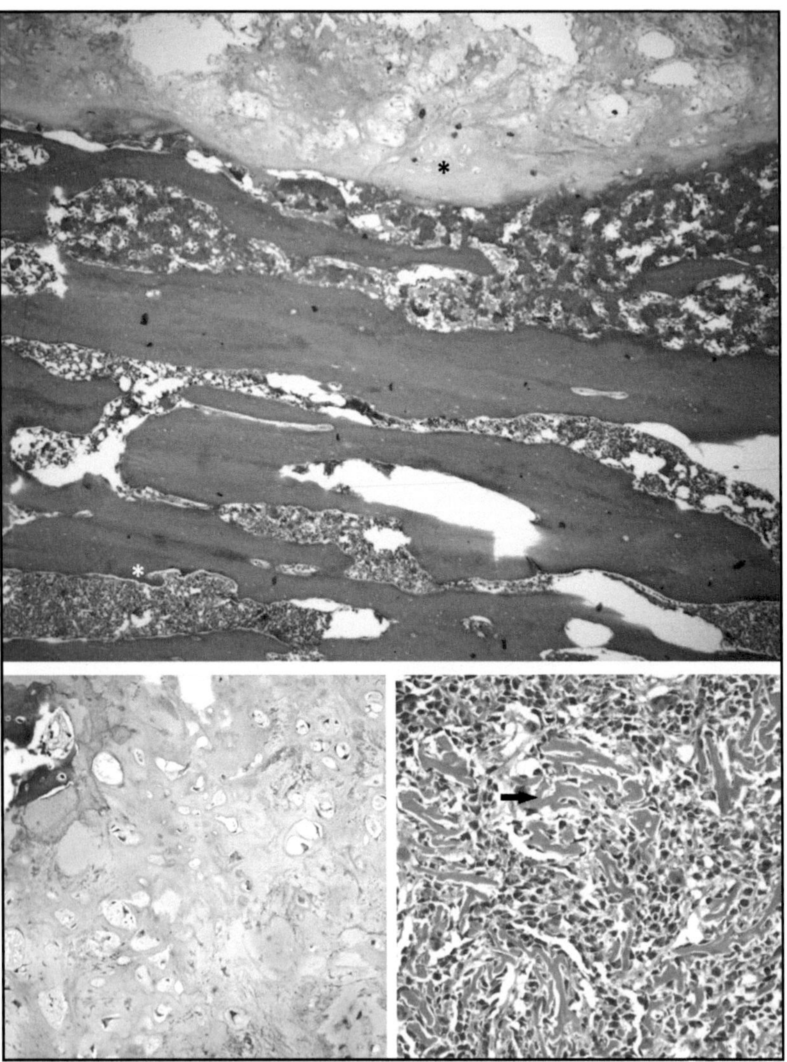

Figure 10-2. Dedifferentiated chondrosarcoma. Hematoxylin and eosin stain demonstrates an area of atypical but well-differentiated cartilage (black asterisk and bottom left) adjacent to an area of permeation of normal lamellar bone (white asterisk) by hypercellular, pleomorphic, and high-grade spindle cell sarcoma (bottom right). Malignant osteoid production (black arrow) confirms osteosarcomatous dedifferentiation.

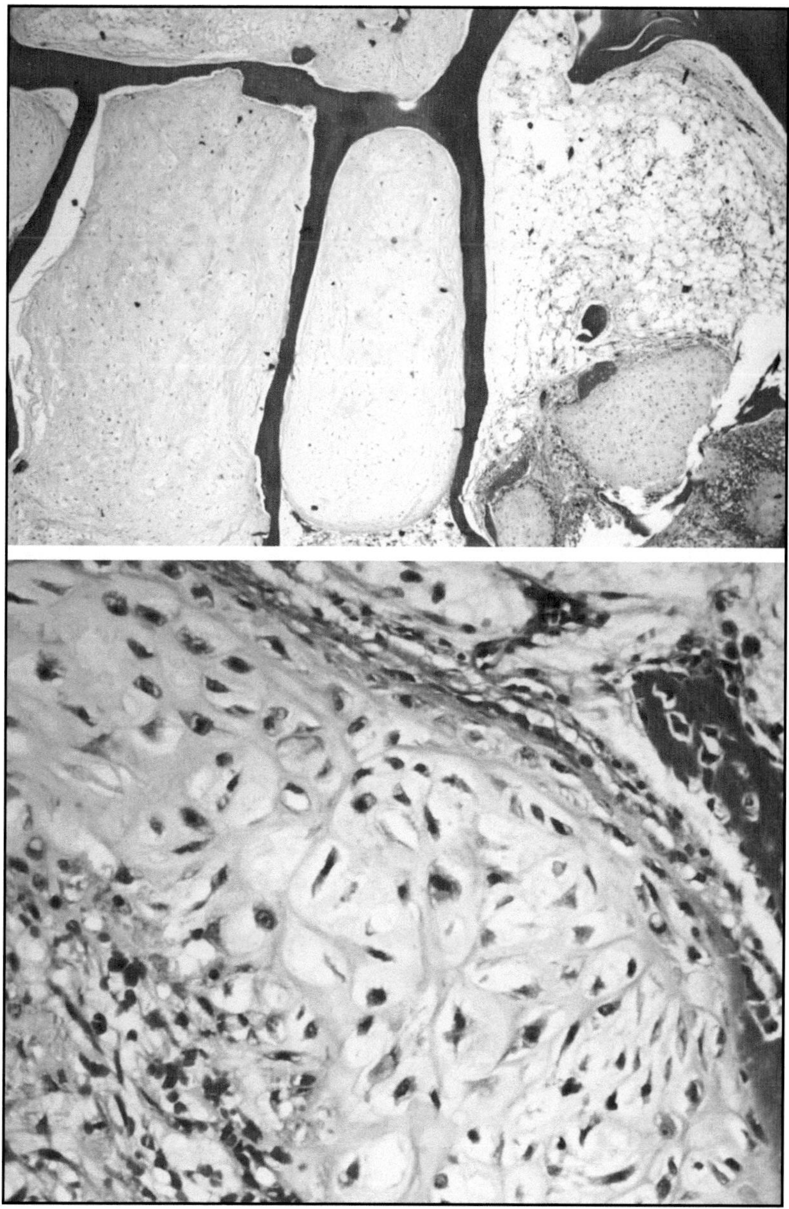

Figure 10-3. Chondrosarcoma. Hematoxylin and eosin stain demonstrates permeation and entrapment of trabecular bone with mildly hypercellular cartilage.

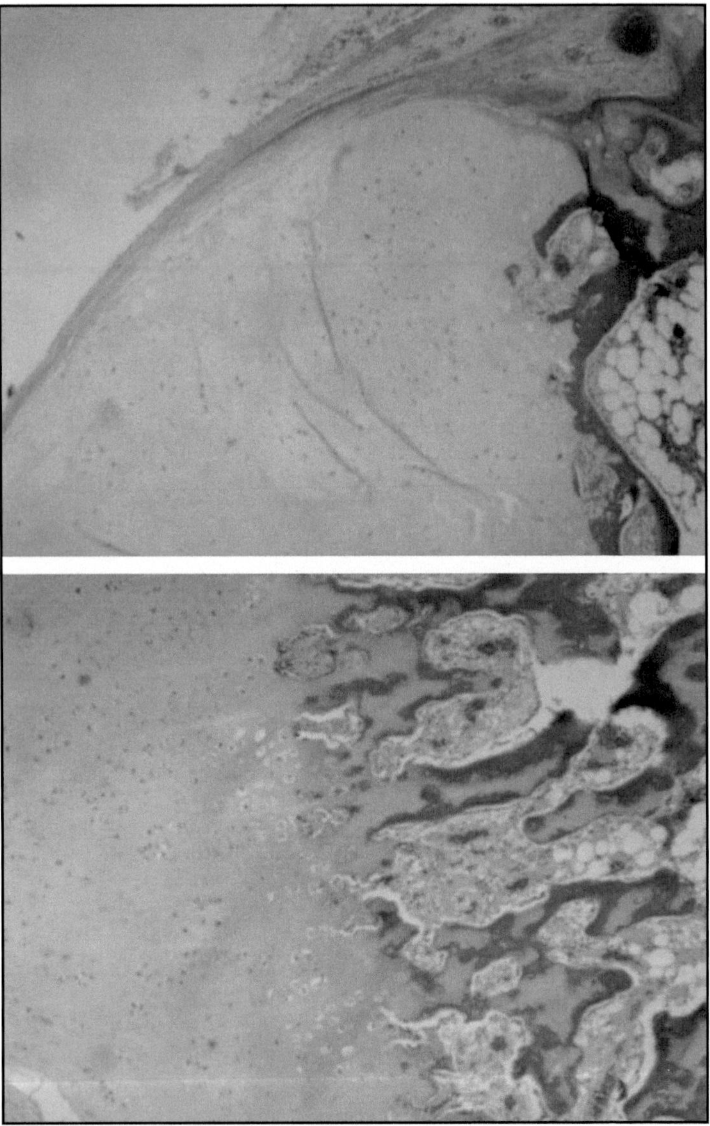

Figure 10-5. Osteochondroma. Hematoxylin and eosin stain demonstrates a bland hyaline cartilage cap confluent with normal trabecular bone with normal marrow elements.

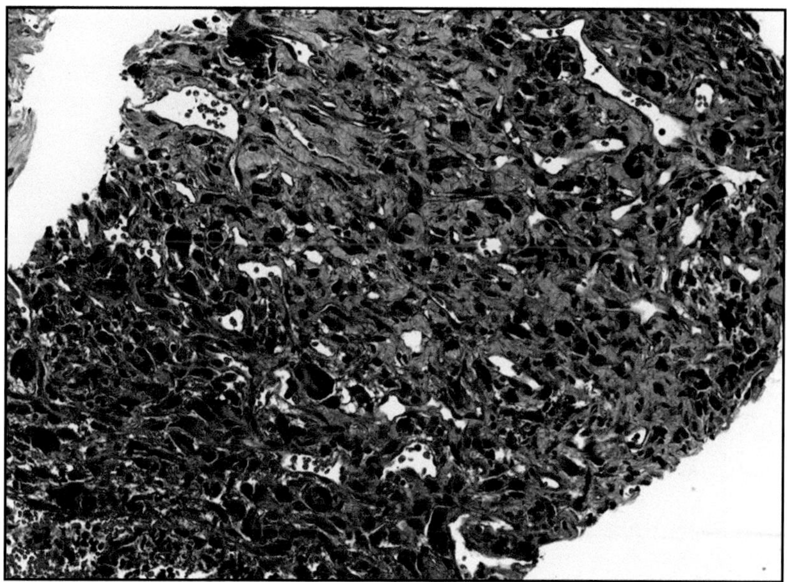

Figure 10-8. Malignant fibrous histiocytoma/undifferentiated pleomorphic sarcoma of bone. Hematoxylin and eosin stain demonstrates a hyperchromatic, pleomorphic, and highly atypical spindle cell population without clear differentiation.

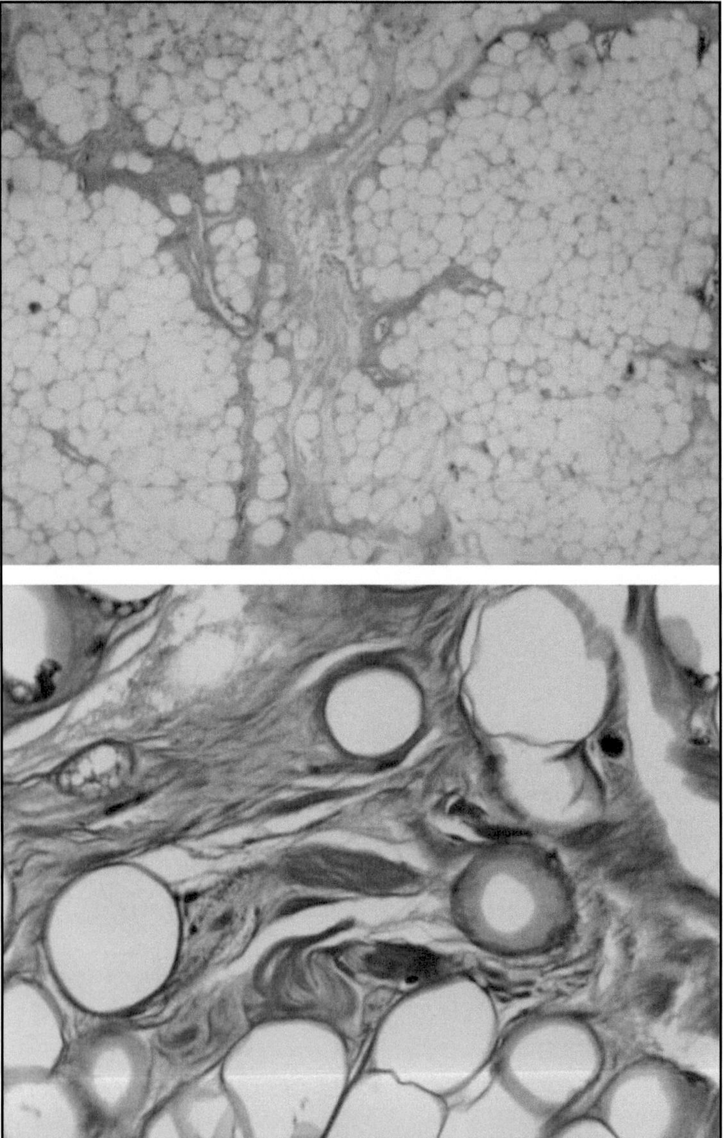

Figure 11-2. Atypical lipomatous tumor. Hematoxylin and eosin stain demonstrates well-differentiated fat separated by bands of fibrovascular tissue. No cellular atypia is present.

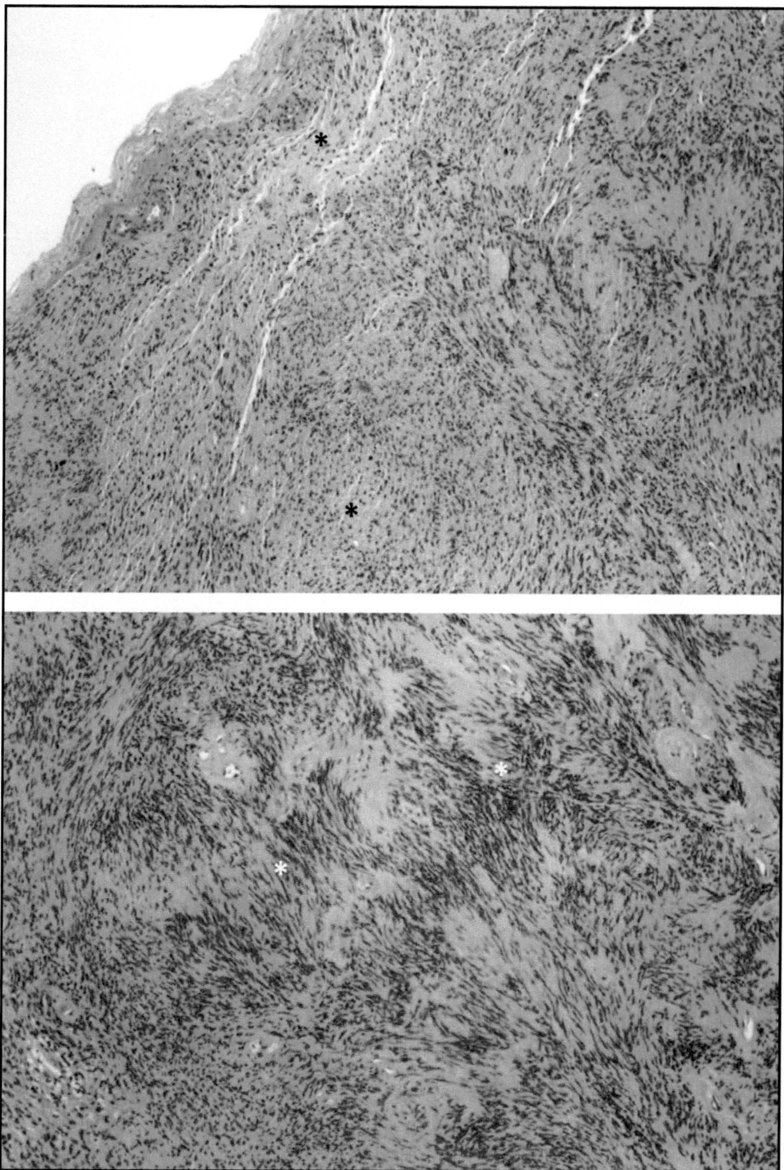

Figure 11-3. Schwannoma. Hematoxylin and eosin stain demonstrates a bland spindle cell lesion with Antoni A areas of palisading elongated nuclei (white asterisk) and loose, pale blue myxoid-containing Antoni B areas (black asterisk).

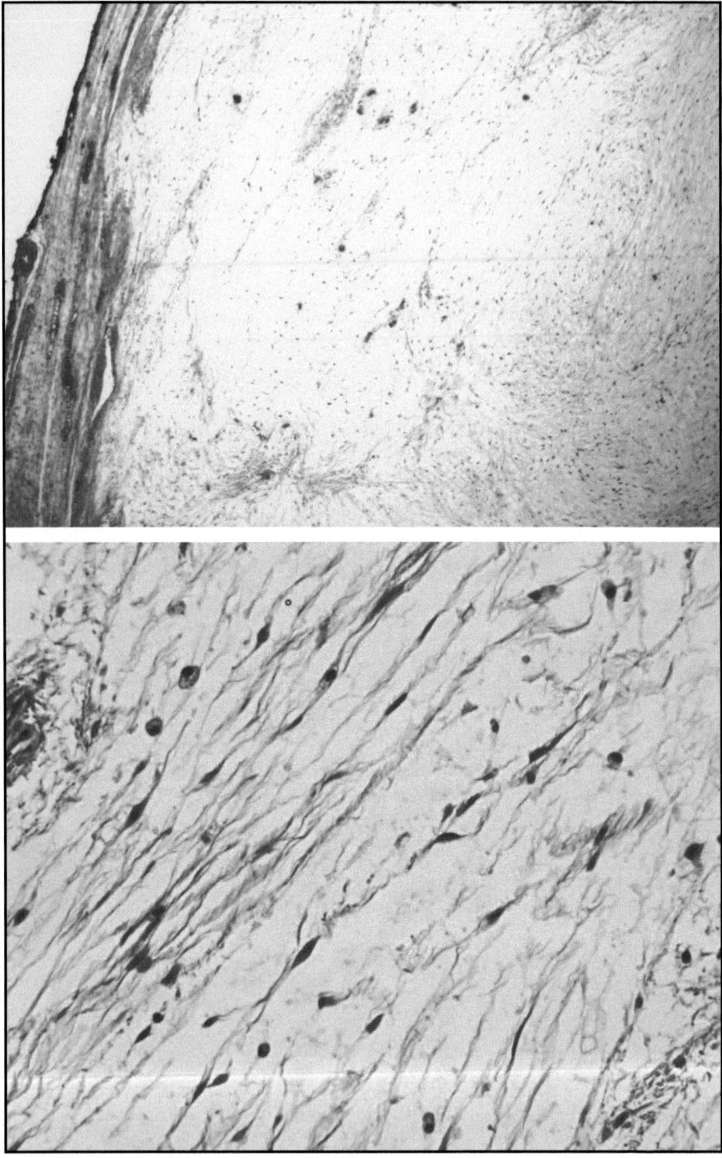

Figure 11-4. Intramuscular myxoma. Hematoxylin and eosin stain demonstrates a well-encapsulated lesion of loose, pale blue myxoid stroma with a sparse arrangement of bland spindle cells without atypia or mitotic activity.

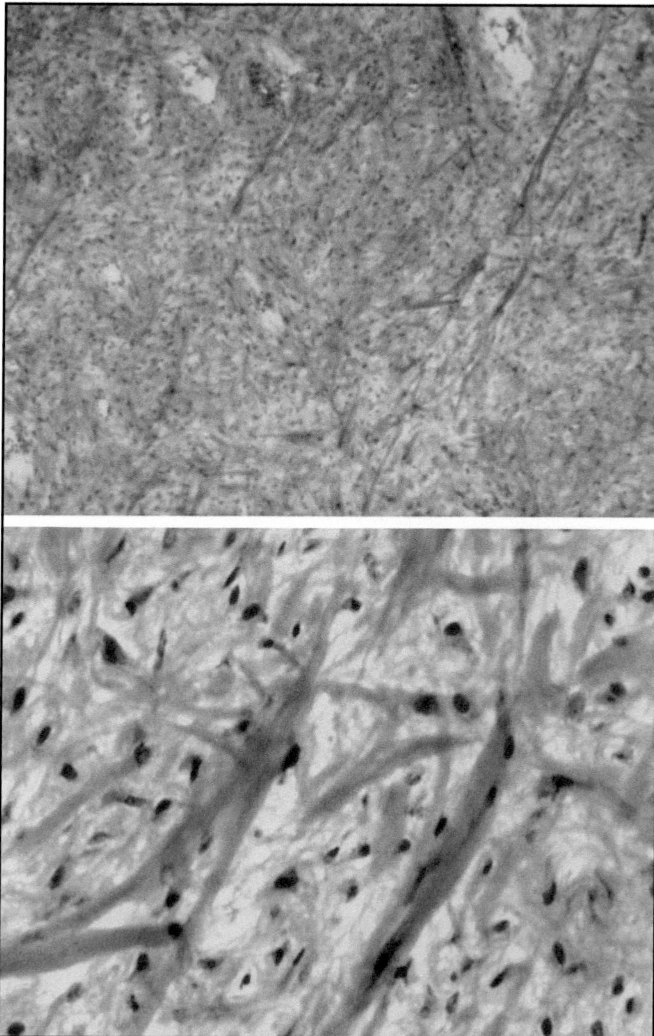

Figure 11-5. Fibromatosis/extra-abdominal demoid. Hematoxylin and eosin stain demonstrates a low-grade spindle cell population in a background of ropey collagen bundles.

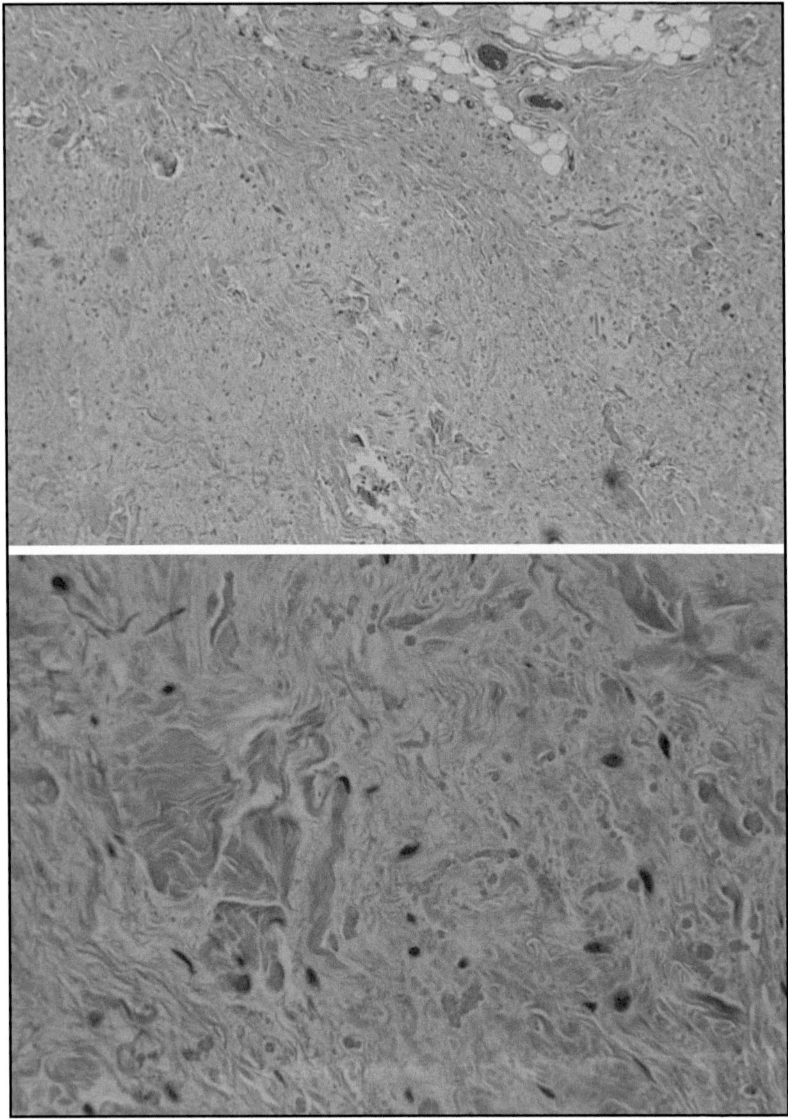

Figure 11-6. Elastofibroma. Hematoxylin and eosin stain demonstrates a sparse population of spindled fibroblastic cells in a background of wavy elastin fibers.

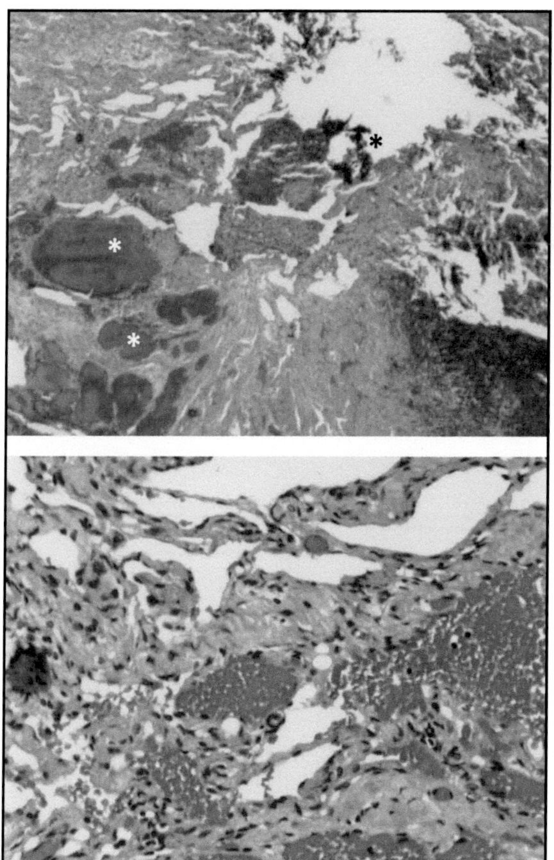

Figure 11-7. Hemangioma. Hematoxylin and eosin stain demonstrates multiple vascular spaces (white asterisk) separated by fibrous septae lined with endothelial cells. Calcified areas (black asterisk) are consistent with thrombus or phlebolith formation.

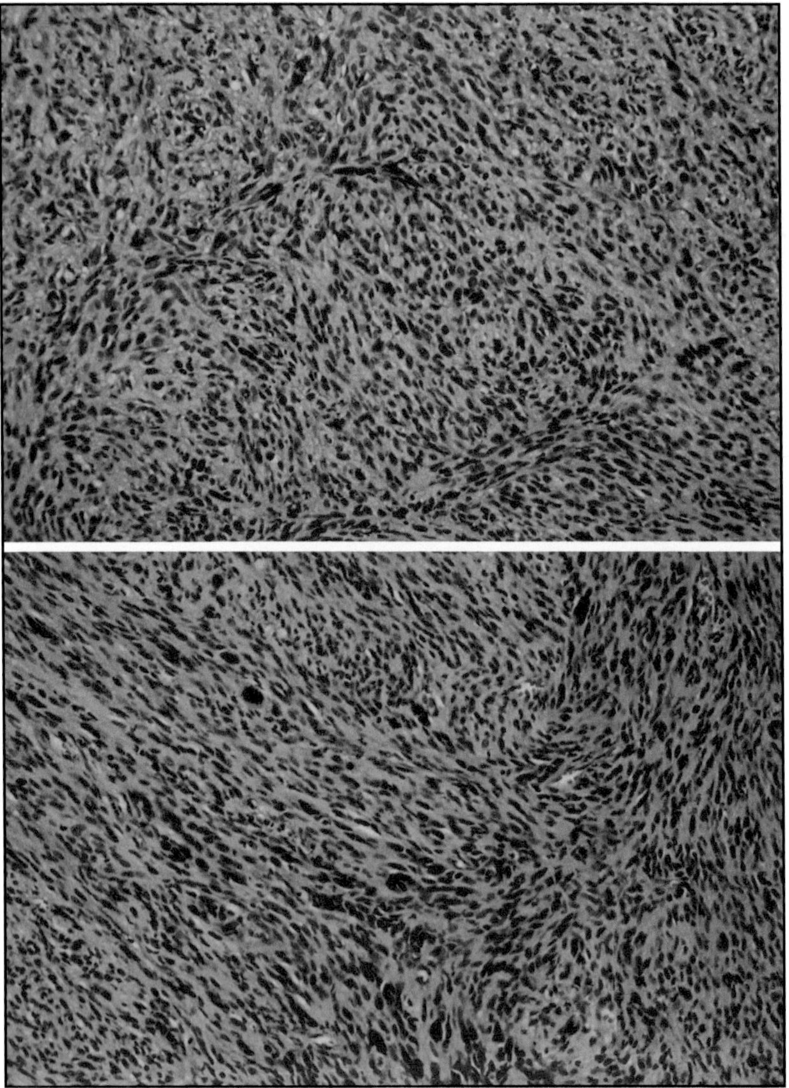

Figure 12-3. Undifferentiated pleomorphic sarcoma. Hematoxylin and eosin stain demonstrates a pleomorphic spindle cell population with nuclear atypia arranged in a whorled "storiform" pattern without other features of differentiation.

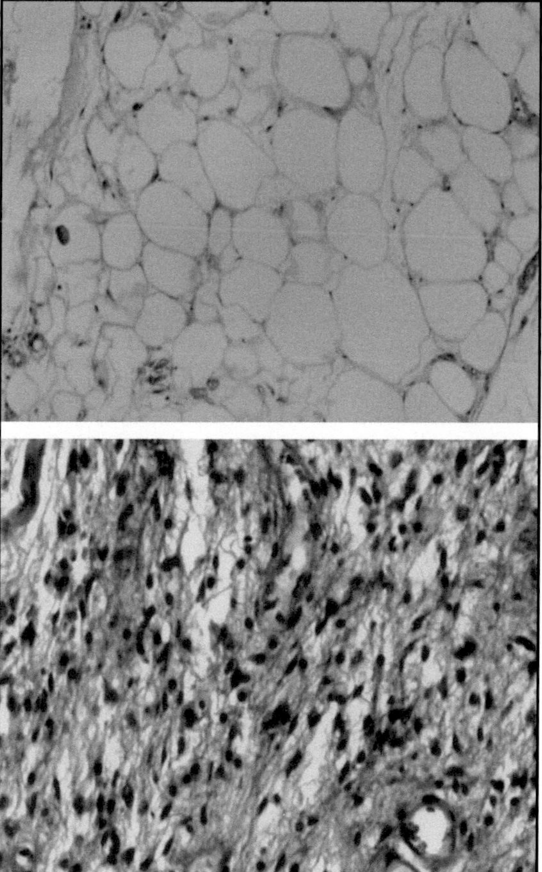

Figure 12-4.
Dedifferentiated liposarcoma. Hematoxylin and eosin stain demonstrates (above) an area of well-differentiated fat indistinguishable from normal fat and (below) an area of pleomorphic spindle cell proliferation without differentiating features.

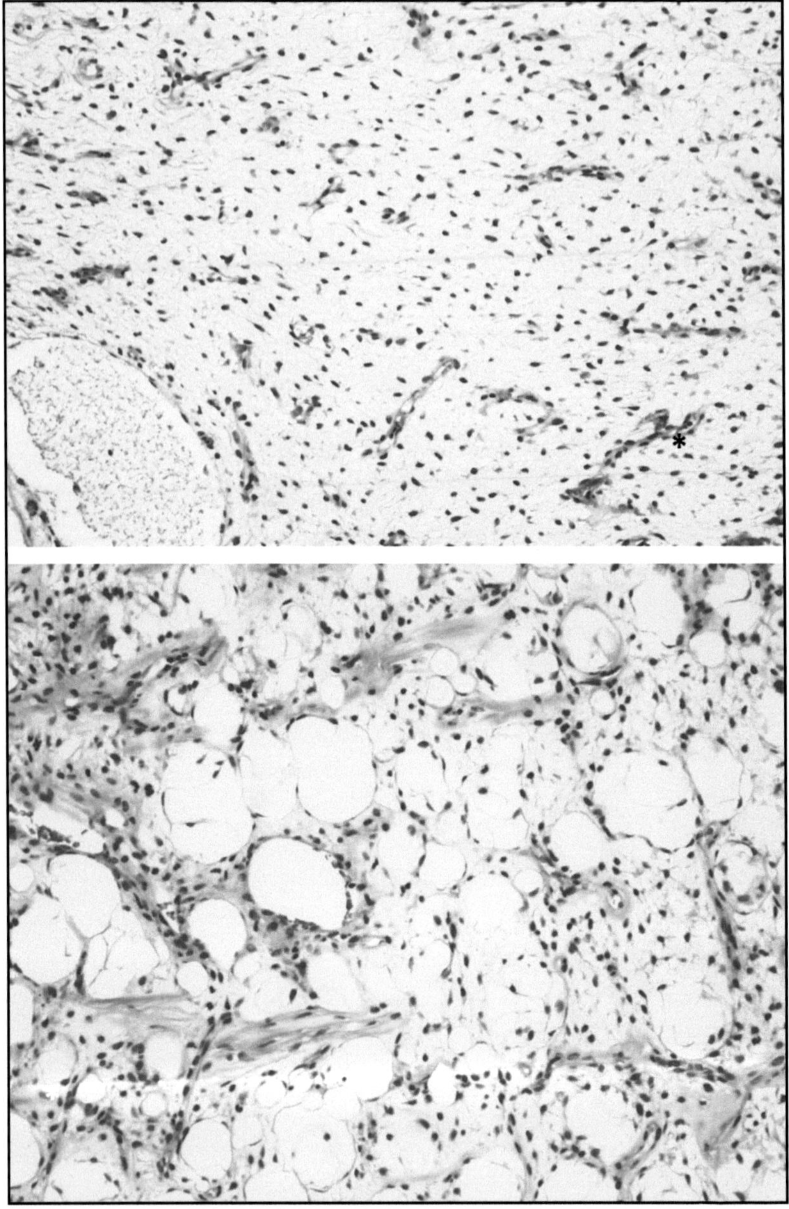

Figure 12-7. Myxoid liposarcoma. Hematoxylin and eosin stain demonstrates a spindle cell population in a pale blue myxoid background with arborizing blood vessels (black asterisk) and lipogenic areas including signet ring lipoblasts (white asterisk).

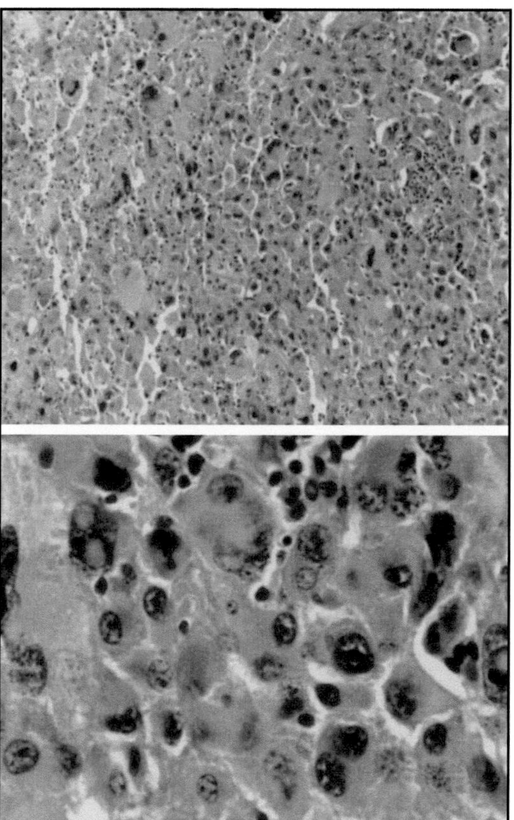

Figure 12-8. Undifferentiated pleomorphic sarcoma. Hematoxylin and eosin stain demonstrates a pleomorphic spindle cell population with marked atypia, enlarged nuclei, and mitotic figures without areas of obvious differentiation.

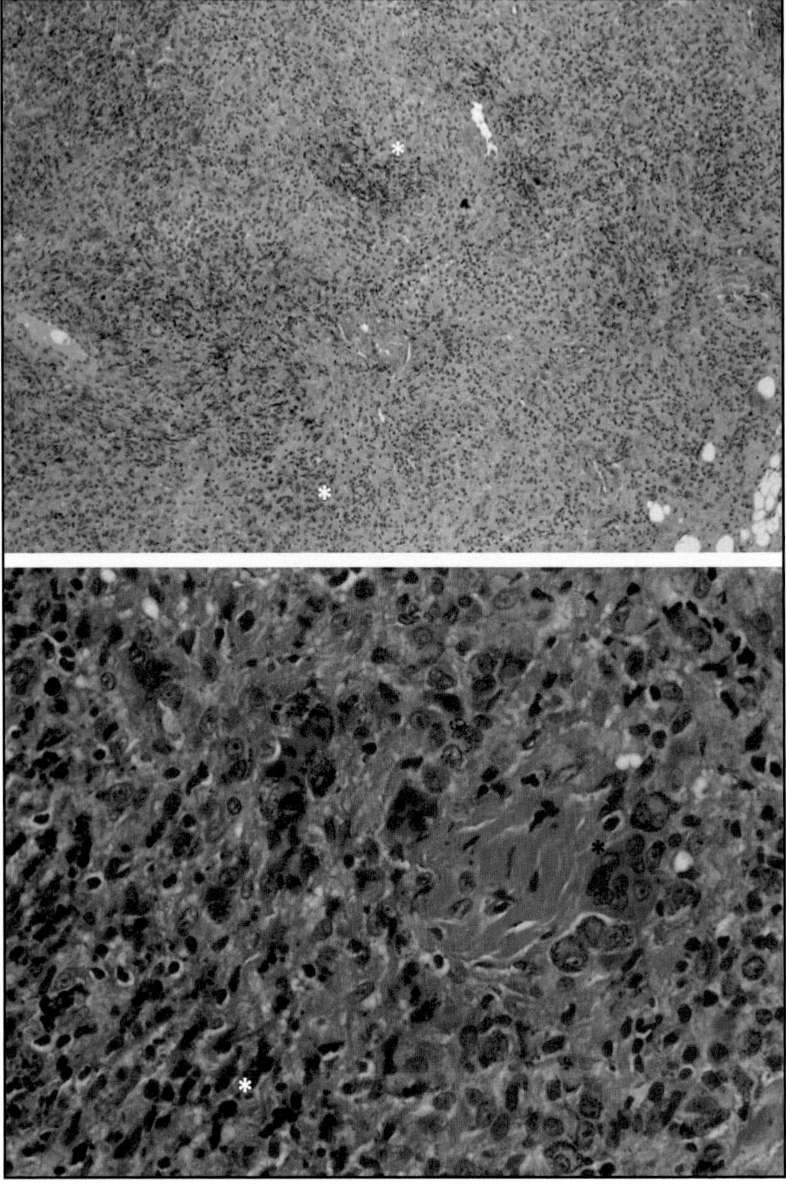

Figure 13-1. Pigmented villonodular synovitis. Hematoxylin and eosin stain demonstrates a nodule of histiocytic proliferation with collagen bundles (black asterisk) and macrophages laden with brown hemosiderin pigment (white asterisk).

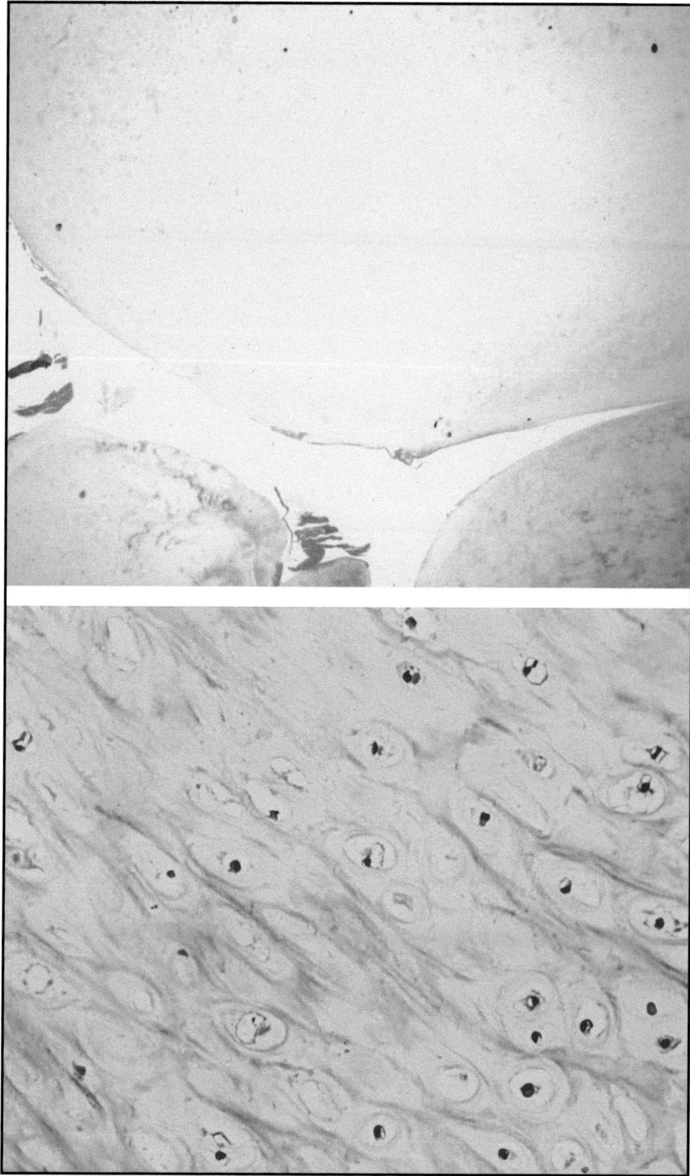

Figure 13-2. Synovial chondromatosis. Hematoxylin and eosin stain demonstrates lobules of bland hyaline cartilage without hypercellularity, atypia, or pleomorphism.

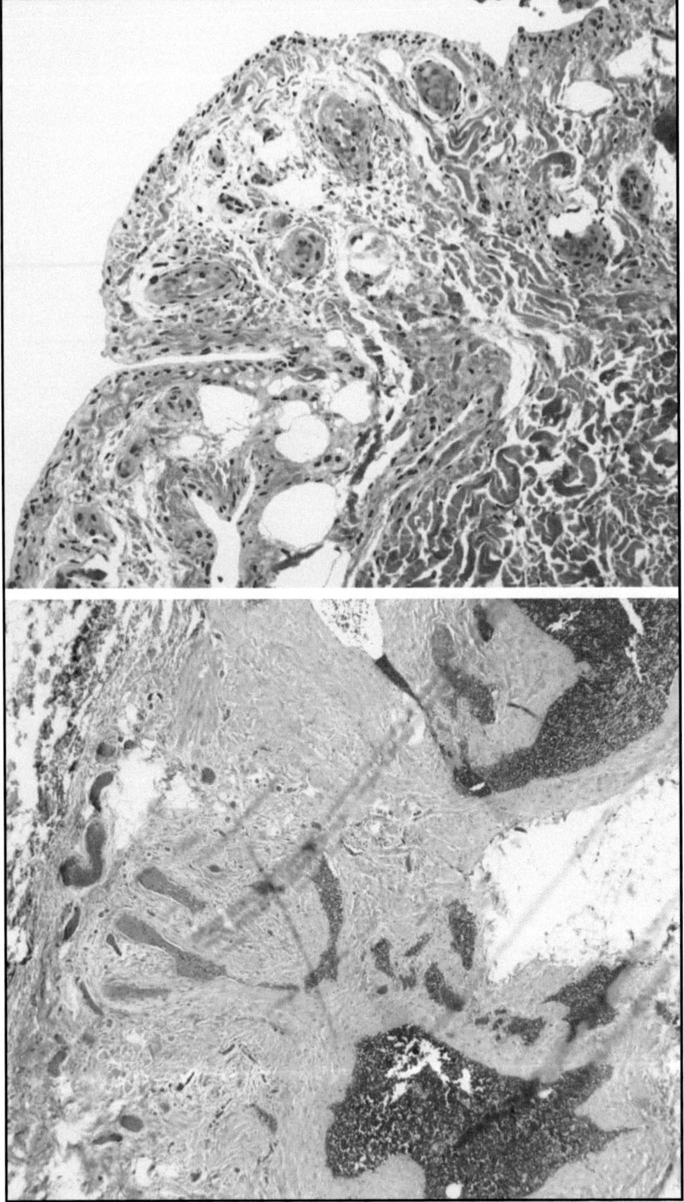

Figure 13-3. Synovial hemangioma. Hematoxylin and eosin stain demonstrates a synovial lining with multiple blood-filled spaces and smaller vascular channels separated by fibrous septae.

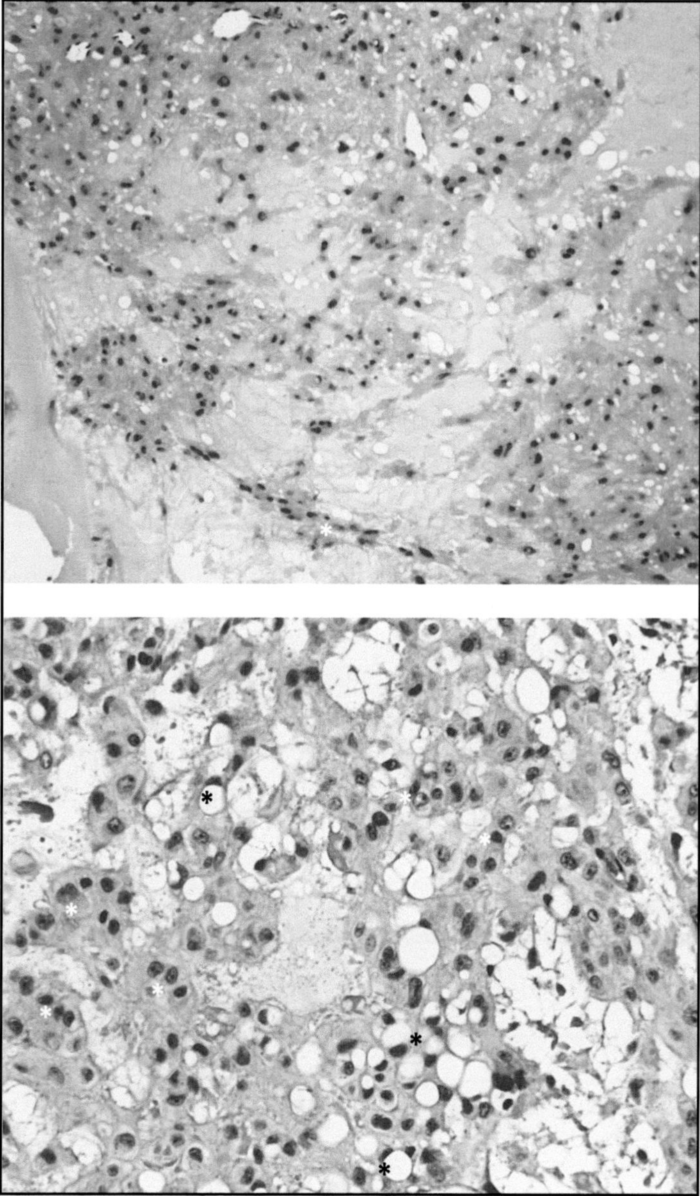

Figure 14-2. Sacral chordoma. Hematoxylin and eosin stain demonstrates a lobule of pleomorphic cells within a pale mucinous background, with areas of occasional linear filing known as "chording" (white asterisk) and cells with vacuolated cytoplasm known as physaliferous cells (black asterisk).

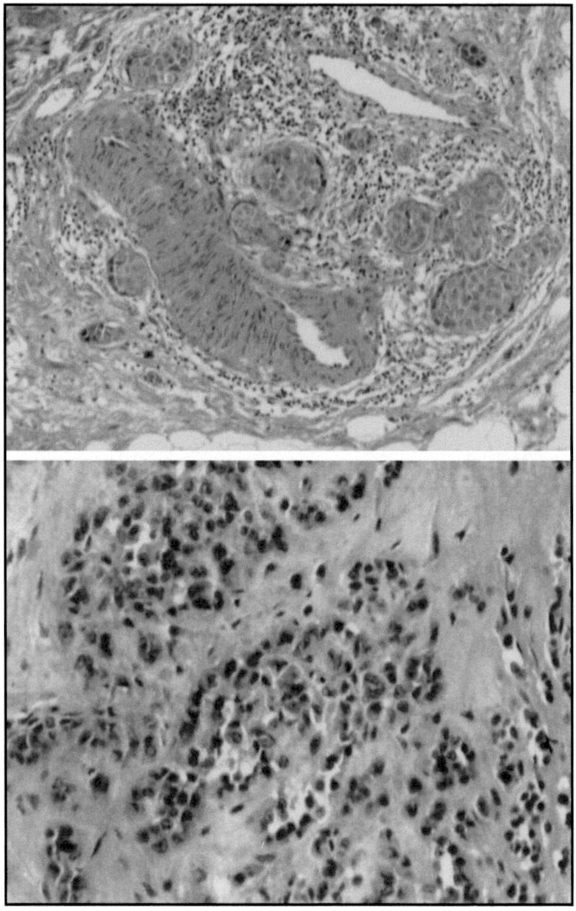

Figure 15-2. Epithelioid sarcoma. Hematoxylin and eosin stain demonstrates a nodular collection of epithelioid cell clusters within a pleomorphic spindle cell background.

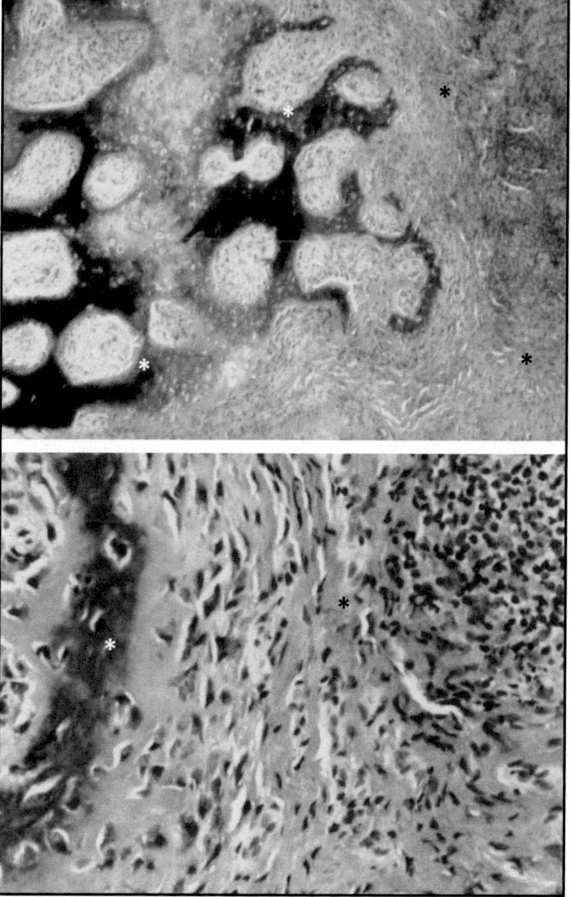

Figure 15-7. Bizarre parosteal osteochondromatous proliferation/known as Nora's lesion. Hematoxylin and eosin stain demonstrates disorganized areas of endochondral ossification of cartilage (white asterisk) separated from a uniform spindle cell proliferation by fibrovascular zones (black asterisk).

Index

Wallace, M. T.
Handbook of Musculoskeletal Tumors (pp 295-306).

Printed in the United States
by Baker & Taylor Publisher Services